Praise for Leslie Beck

"Canada's nutrition guru has mapped out a plan that guarantees a new you. If you follow her 12-week plan, you will lose weight. Period."

—*Calgary Herald*

"Packed with information on foods to avoid, those to eat more often, proper serving sizes, recipes and easy-to-implement suggestions for minimizing risk."

—*Best Health Magazine*

"One of the most sensible 'diet books' out there."

—*The Georgia Straight*

"Adolescence is a critical period for developing healthy eating and exercise habits, and the guidance provided in this book is invaluable."

—Chris Carmichael, personal coach to eight-time Tour de France champion Lance Armstrong and author of *Chris Carmichael's Food for Fitness*

"Covers the subject extensively ... Beck's tools are based on a common sense approach to eating ."

—*Daily Press* (Timmins, Ontario)

"Teenagers are constantly confronted with fast food, poor cafeteria choices and eating on the go. *Healthy Eating for Teens and Preteens* provides them with straightforward, useable tools for making the right food choices."

—Dr. Marla Shapiro, medical consultant, CTV

"Leslie Beck offers indispensable advice for healthy living."

—James F. Balch, MD, co-author of *The Prescription for Nutritional Healing*

"If you'd like to eat more healthfully, Leslie Beck is a must-read."

—*Homemakers* magazine

"Leslie Beck, one of Canada's leading authorities on nutrition, has written another well researched, fabulously written and perfectly executed book, this time on boosting heart health. It's chock full of useful information and tips as well as scrumptious heart healthy recipes."

—Pauline Anderson, family health editor, *Canadian Living*

"[Beck's] book offers plenty of sound nutrition information and evidence-based diet strategies that can help protect you from coronary heart disease. It's all about implementing a sustainable, heart healthy lifestyle. The tools in this book will help you achieve this."

—Dr. Rob Myers, director of cardiology, Medcan Clinic

"A comprehensive nutrition book aimed at teens that also includes terrific information for the whole family. It includes the most up-to-date information that will help your teen form a great foundation for a healthy lifestyle."

—Sally Brown, CEO, Heart and Stroke Foundation of Canada

"Parents and teens need all the help they can get, including nutrition advice. This book is so practical and thorough that I plan to share it with my daughter and son."

—Linda Lewis, editor-in-chief, *Today's Parent*

"It is a relief to have Leslie Beck's well-researched, approachable and up-to-date guide to lifelong healthful eating."

—Elizabeth Baird, *Canadian Living*

"A very sensible approach to eating, diet and nutrition."

—*The London Free Press*

"Practical, easy to follow strategies to help transform your relationship with food."

—*The Hamilton Spectator*

"Trying to eat healthfully can be a daunting task. Advice is plentiful, but often conflicting or scientifically suspect. Enter Leslie Beck and *Leslie Beck's 10 Steps to Healthy Eating*, a valuable home reference with a wealth of practical 'how-to' strategies."

—*The Vancouver Sun*

"Leslie Beck has done a superb job of rounding up all the latest nutritional information to guide women healthfully through their menopausal years. Not only does she review the current scientific literature and make sense of it—no mean feat—but she also provides you with her expert dietician's opinion on everything ... a must-have for 40-plus women who want to make informed choices."

—June Rogers, health editor, *Chatelaine*

"Finally, a map that women can use to chart their voyage through menopause the natural way."

—Marilyn Linton, health editor, *Toronto Sun*, and author of *Taking Charge by Taking Care: A Canadian Guide to Women's Health*

"Leslie Beck has written the first book that specifically outlines the relationship between nutrition and certain symptoms associated with the peri- and post-menopausal years. This book can help alleviate stressful side effects of menopause and lower the risk of disease through diet and nutrition."

—Rose Reisman, bestselling author of *The Balance of Living Well*

"A guide for women of all ages seeking to manage their health and well-being."

—Dr. Jean Marmoreo, *National Post* columnist, "Dr. Jean Marmoreo on Middle-Aged Women"

"If you believe that we are what we eat—and I do—*Leslie Beck's Nutrition Guide for Women* serves up food for thought and more to help you take charge of your own good health."

—Charlotte Empey, editor-in-chief, *Canadian Living*

"*Leslie Beck's 10 Steps to Healthy Eating* contains everything you need to know to get healthy and stay healthy by eating right. The 'Getting Ready' section is especially impressive and helpful!"

—Christiane Northrup, MD, author of *Women's Wisdom* and *The Wisdom of Menopause*

"If you are looking for a comprehensive resource *Leslie Beck's Nutrition Guide to a Healthy Pregnancy* is a must-read."

—*Toronto Sun*

PENGUIN CANADA

Foods That Fight Disease

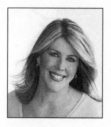

LESLIE BECK, a registered dietitian, is a leading Canadian nutritionist and the bestselling author of seven nutrition books. Leslie writes a weekly nutrition column in *The Globe and Mail,* is a regular contributor to CTV's *Canada AM,* and can be heard one morning a week on CJAD Radio's *The Andrew Carter Show.*

Leslie has worked with many of Canada's leading businesses and international food companies and runs a thriving private practice at the Medcan Clinic in Toronto. She also regularly delivers nutrition workshops to corporate groups across North America.

Visit Leslie Beck's website at www.lesliebeck.com.

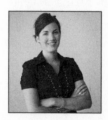

MICHELLE GELOK, BASc, is a Toronto-based nutritionist who completed her degree in Food and Nutrition at Ryerson University and is currently pursuing her dietetic internship at University Health Network in Toronto. Michelle has worked extensively with Leslie Beck since 2004. In that time, she developed recipes for two of Leslie's books, *The No-Fail Diet* and *Foods That Fight Disease.* In addition to her passion for creating recipes, Michelle writes on nutrition and food for Leslie's website, www.lesliebeck.com, and is a regular contributor to the health section of CBC online.

Also by Leslie Beck

Leslie Beck's Nutrition Encyclopedia

Leslie Beck's Nutrition Guide for Women

Leslie Beck's Nutrition Guide to a Healthy Pregnancy

Healthy Eating for Preteens and Teens

10 Steps to Healthy Eating

Leslie Beck's Nutrition Guide to Menopause

The No-Fail Diet

Heart Healthy Foods for Life

The Complete A–Z Nutrition Encyclopedia

The Complete Nutrition Guide for Women

FOODS THAT FIGHT DISEASE

A NUTRITION GUIDE TO STAYING HEALTHY FOR LIFE

Leslie Beck, RD

Michelle Gelok, BASc, nutritionist
Recipe development and nutritional analysis

PENGUIN
CANADA

PENGUIN CANADA

Published by the Penguin Group

Penguin Group (Canada), 90 Eglinton Avenue East, Suite 700, Toronto, Ontario, Canada M4P 2Y3
(a division of Pearson Canada Inc.)

Penguin Group (USA) Inc., 375 Hudson Street, New York, New York 10014, U.S.A.
Penguin Books Ltd, 80 Strand, London WC2R 0RL, England
Penguin Ireland, 25 St Stephen's Green, Dublin 2, Ireland (a division of Penguin Books Ltd)
Penguin Group (Australia), 250 Camberwell Road, Camberwell, Victoria 3124, Australia
(a division of Pearson Australia Group Pty Ltd)
Penguin Books India Pvt Ltd, 11 Community Centre, Panchsheel Park, New Delhi – 110 017, India
Penguin Group (NZ), 67 Apollo Drive, Rosedale, North Shore 0632, New Zealand
(a division of Pearson New Zealand Ltd)
Penguin Books (South Africa) (Pty) Ltd, 24 Sturdee Avenue, Rosebank, Johannesburg 2196,
South Africa

Penguin Books Ltd, Registered Offices: 80 Strand, London WC2R 0RL, England

First published in a Penguin Canada paperback by Penguin Group (Canada),
a division of Pearson Canada Inc., 2008
Published in this edition, 2010

1 2 3 4 5 6 7 8 9 10 (WEB)

Recipe development and nutritional analysis: Michelle Gelok, BASc, nutritionist

This publication contains the opinions and ideas of its author and is designed to provide useful
information in regard to the subject matter covered. The author and publisher are not engaged
in health or other professional services in this publication. This publication is not intended to provide
a basis for action in particular circumstances without consideration by a competent professional.
The author and publisher expressly disclaim any responsibility for any liability, loss, or risk,
personal or otherwise, which is incurred as a consequence, directly or indirectly, of the use
and application of any of the contents of this book.

Manufactured in Canada.

LIBRARY AND ARCHIVES CANADA CATALOGUING IN PUBLICATION

Beck, Leslie
Foods that fight disease : a nutrition guide to staying healthy for life / Leslie Beck.

Includes bibliographical references and index.
ISBN 978-0-14-305658-4

1. Diet therapy. 2. Diet in disease. 3. Medicine, Preventive. 4. Cookery. I. Title.

RA784.B424 2010   613.2   C2009-906281-X

Visit the Penguin Group (Canada) website at **www.penguin.ca**

Special and corporate bulk purchase rates available; please see
www.penguin.ca/corporatesales or call 1-800-810-3104, ext. 477 or 474

Contents

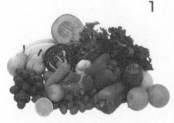
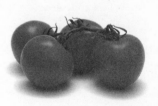
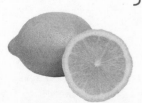

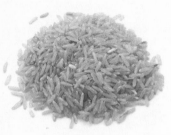
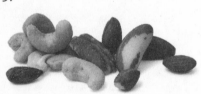
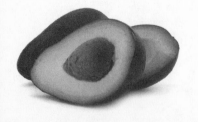

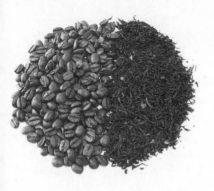

Acknowledgments

If it were not for the commitment of my dedicated team, my clients, my husband, and my family and friends, this book would not have been completed. The following people deserve a special thanks for their contributions, support, and encouragement.

Michelle Gelok, whose creativity and passion for cooking allowed her to develop each and every recipe for this book. I am grateful for the dedication, thoroughness, and enthusiasm she brought to this project.

Gia Gelok, Michelle's mother, who once again so generously lent us her spacious kitchen and her time to help test more than a hundred recipes!

Dawn Bone and Rosemary Chubb, my amazingly efficient, professional, and considerate assistants, who help me manage a busy private practice as I research and write my books. Thank you for your unwavering support; every day you help build the success of my business.

My private practice clients, whose questions allow me to continue to learn and grow professionally.

Andrea Magyar and the entire team at Penguin Group (Canada), who continue to support my vision and bring my work to the public.

Darrell, my husband and my closest friend, whose constant support, love, and praise make me believe I can accomplish anything.

Introduction

The notion that foods can fight disease is certainly not new. Food as medicine began 3500 years ago, when ancient Egyptians discovered that night blindness—caused by a lack of vitamin A—could be treated with certain foods. Much later, in the mid-1700s, a Scottish surgeon named James Lind learned that some unknown substance in limes prevented scurvy in British sailors.

Despite that we've used foods to heal for thousands of years, nutrition is a relatively new science. Only less than a century ago did scientists discover vitamins and minerals and determine that very small amounts could cure diseases such as rickets, goiter, beri beri, and pellagra.

Fast forward to the twenty-first century. No longer are North Americans plagued by diseases caused by a lack of vitamin and minerals. We have easy access to an abundance of foods, many of them fortified with nutrients and with vitamin supplements.

Instead, the diseases that are killing us are caused by over-nutrition—eating too much food, rather than too little. Today, cardiovascular disease (heart disease and stroke), cancer, chronic obstructive lung disease (emphysema and bronchitis), and diabetes are the leading causes of death and disability around the world. In Canada, nearly two-thirds of all deaths are due to these chronic diseases. As our national waistline continues to expand, the number of cases of type 2 diabetes—a major cause of heart disease—is expected to continue to rise.

Our lifestyle choices are clearly linked to the diseases that plague us in modern times. A poor diet high in overly processed foods—many high in saturated and trans fats, sodium, and refined sugars—with too few fruits, vegetables, and whole grains contributes to weight gain, high blood pressure, high blood cholesterol, and elevated blood sugar, which are all risk factors for future disease. And a lack of regular physical activity also shares some of the blame.

But there is good news. The majority of today's chronic diseases are preventable. During the past few decades, scientists have learned how phytochemicals like beta carotene (in carrots), anthocyanins (in blueberries), lutein (in spinach), and catechins (in tea) can help guard against cancer, heart disease, cataract, even Alzheimer's disease. Almost every day study findings are reported that link certain diets, foods, and food components to disease prevention.

It seems that Canadians are also aware of the link between nutrition and health. According to the most recent national survey conducted by the Canadian Council of Food and Nutrition, the majority of Canadians strongly believe that fibre, omega-3 fats, and trans fat play a role in their health. What's more, 75% of Canadians consult nutrition labels when deciding what foods to buy. Among label readers, nearly two-thirds use them to check how much of a particular nutrient is in a food product. Many of us are seeking foods with more omega-3 fats, fibre, whole grains, and vitamins and little or no trans fat, sugar, and sodium.

Indeed, an increasing number of people are turning to the foods they eat as a way to reduce the risk of disease and stay healthy, active, and energetic as they age. The desire to eat the right foods to ward off disease is evident in my private practice. Every day I meet clients who want to know what foods they should be eating more of, and which ones they need to eat less of in order to prevent heart disease, type 2 diabetes, cancer, osteoporosis, and obesity. Often I am consulted for advice on what to eat to lower blood pressure, blood cholesterol, or blood sugar levels. Clients at increased risk for developing a health problem are highly motivated to improve the quality of their diet to ward off disease and, if possible, avoid taking a prescription drug.

Eating to reduce your risk of chronic disease is more than just limiting high-fat animal foods, refined grains, sugary desserts, heavily processed foods, and fast foods. Don't get me wrong, that is important. But when it comes to fighting disease, the foods you *include* in your diet are just as important as the ones you exclude.

Foods That Fight Disease is a comprehensive guide to disease-fighting foods. It's a manual of which foods to eat—how often, in what amounts, and how to add them to your family's diet in unique and delicious ways. *Foods That Fight Disease* will help you discover power foods—nutrient-packed whole foods that have been shown in scientific studies to lower the risk of many chronic diseases.

Although this book focuses on the foods you should be including in your diet, I'd be remiss not to mention foods that you should limit in an effort to stay healthy. You'll find tips throughout the book on how to cut sodium, saturated fat, and added sugars from your diet. You'll also read about the pros and cons of red wine and other alcoholic beverages. Most of all, however, *Foods That Fight Disease* is about the enjoyment of tasty and healthful foods.

How to use *Foods That Fight Disease*

The information and practical tips in this book will help you boost the nutritional quality of your diet. Each chapter provides everything you need to know about a category of power foods—vegetables, fruits, whole grains, protein foods, dairy foods, vegetables oils, and beverages that are nutritional standouts when it comes to fighting disease.

There is no right or wrong place to start. Choose a group of foods that you want to learn more about or you want to increase your intake of. While some people might start with vegetables, others might prefer to begin eating more whole grains. For each power food, I share with you the study findings that support its disease-fighting powers, how it works in the body, and notable nutrients and phytochemicals it contains.

While it's nice to know the science behind how foods keep you healthy, you need to know how to incorporate them into your diet. Many of my clients say they know that legumes are healthy, but they don't know what to do with them. *Foods That Fight Disease* arms you with the information you'll need to put my recommended intakes into action: tips for buying, storing, and preparing, and plenty of ideas for creative ways to incorporate each food into meals and snacks.

To help you gradually increase your intake of power foods, I recommend you make copies of my Power Foods Checklist, which you'll find at the back of the book. Here, you'll also find suggestions for adding phytochemical-rich herbs and spices to meals, as well as a label-reading tips.

Over a hundred recipes that fight disease

Every recipe in this book was developed, tested, and analyzed by Michelle Gelok, a nutritionist who has worked with me as a research assistant for the past three years. (At the time of writing, Michelle was completing her dietetic internship in Toronto.) Along with my tips to add power foods to breakfasts, lunches, dinners, and snacks, you'll find delicious and easy-to-prepare recipes created by Michelle—recipes that will add leafy greens, berries, legumes, fish, even green tea to your meals. Each recipe is accompanied by a nutrient analysis: a breakdown of its calories, fat, protein, fibre, and so on.

We've come a long way in our understanding of how foods fight disease since the days of the ancient Egyptians. Yet, we still have more to learn as nutrition and food scientists seek answers to questions that remain unanswered. In the meantime, I hope you will use this book as a resource—one that's based on our current scientific knowledge—to help you and your family eat the healthiest diet possible.

Leslie Beck, RD
Toronto, 2008

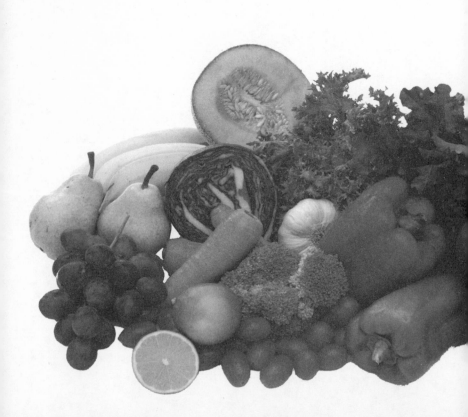

1

What your body needs

- ★ carbohydrates
- ★ fat
- ★ minerals
- ★ phytochemicals
- ★ protein
- ★ vitamins
- ★ water

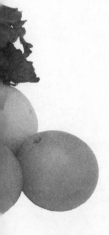

Nutrition is a three-step process by which we use foods to nourish our body. First we consume the food. Then our body breaks down that food into individual nutrients. Finally, those nutrients travel in the bloodstream to different parts of the body where they're used for energy, cell growth, and tissue maintenance, and to fight disease. Simply put, nutrition is all the good we get from the foods we eat that keeps our bodies healthy. As you'll learn in later chapters, some foods and beverages—called "power foods"—do an exceptional job of maintaining good health.

Foods that promote health contain thousands of natural compounds that work together to exert their beneficial effects. Some of these compounds, such as protein, fatty acids, vitamins, and minerals, cannot be made by your body, so they must be obtained from the foods you eat. Others, such as phytochemicals, are not essential but have been linked in many studies with disease prevention. As you read about each power food, you'll learn how its unique nutrients and phytochemicals help guard against many diseases and promote healthy aging.

This chapter is intended to help you become familiar with the many nutrients and phytochemicals you will read about in later chapters. Consider the information that follows a crash course in nutrition. You'll learn how each nutrient keeps you healthy, how much you need, and the best food sources.

What are power foods?

I make repeated reference to "power foods" in this book. And if you scan the table of contents of this book, you will see a list of many power foods, including green leafy vegetables, citrus fruit, fish, legumes (dried beans, peas, and lentils), and unsaturated fats. What exactly are power foods? Well, they're not foods that will miraculously treat disease or give you instant energy to run a marathon. Simply put, *power foods are whole foods rich in nutrients and phytochemicals that contain no synthetic or artificial additives.* What's more, to qualify as a power food each food must have been shown by scientific research to reduce the risk of chronic disease and/or have demonstrated properties that help fight disease. To sum up, the power foods described in this book are:

- *Whole foods.* Power foods have not been highly processed and so retain their naturally occurring nutrients and phytochemicals. Power foods also retain the flavour, colour, and texture that nature intended.
- *Nutrient dense.* Power foods provide the most nutrients per serving for the fewest number of calories. Consider, as an example, a slice each of white bread and whole-wheat bread. Each contains roughly the same number of calories, but the whole-wheat bread offers more fibre, B vitamins, vitamin E, magnesium, and numerous phytochemicals than does its white counterpart.
- *Free of synthetic additives.* Since power foods are processed little, if at all, they don't contain artificial chemicals. Unlike highly processed foods that require synthetic additives to add texture, flavour, colour, or preservatives, whole foods have not been adulterated.
- *Linked to disease prevention.* The foods you will learn about have been shown in scientific studies—animal and human—to lower the risk of many chronic diseases. These foods contain ingredients that can help combat free radicals, lower blood fats, boost your immune system, and/or enhance body processes that prevent or halt cancer growth.

To help you create the healthiest diet possible, I provide details about more than 40 power foods. The best way to make these foods work for you is to include as many as possible in your daily diet, rather than focusing on just one or two. I challenge you to add as many as possible to your family's meals each day. To help you track your progress, you'll find a Power Foods Checklist in Appendix 1. Make copies of this checklist and post one on your refrigerator each week.

Carbohydrates, fibre, and the glycemic index

Fruit, vegetables, grains, legumes, and nuts are all sources of carbohydrates. Dairy products are as well, since they contain lactose, a type of carbohydrate. Carbohydrates in foods are essential for health. They provide about half of all the energy used by your muscles, nerves, and other body tissues. In fact, carbohydrates are your brain's preferred fuel source—it relies on a steady supply of carbohydrate to function properly.

The term *carbohydrate* encompasses sugars, starches, and fibres.

SUGARS

Often called simple sugars, these carbohydrates are single sugar molecules (glucose, fructose, galactose) or pairs of two sugar molecules linked together (sucrose, lactose, maltose). Sugars can be naturally occurring (e.g., fructose in fruit, lactose in milk) or added to foods during processing. Added sugars are refined sugars; these you'll see listed as sucrose, glucose, dextrose, liquid sugar, honey, fructose, and high fructose corn syrup. Although there's no evidence that sugar causes diabetes, heart disease, cancer, or hyperactivity, too much can add a surplus of calories to your diet and promote weight gain.

The most controversial added sugar is high fructose corn syrup, an inexpensive sweetener that's added to soft drinks, fruit drinks, baked goods, and canned fruit. Researchers have linked our increased use of corn syrup sweeteners over the past 20 years with rising obesity rates. This correlation doesn't prove that high fructose corn syrup causes weight gain. But some experts contend that fructose in high fructose corn syrup is processed differently from glucose in cane or beet sugar. Fructose doesn't trigger hormone responses that regulate appetite and satiety, which could trick you into overeating.

The following tips will help you reduce your intake of added sugars:

- Limit sugary drinks. Replace soft drinks and fruit drinks with water, low-fat milk, vegetable juice, or tea.
- Satisfy your sweet tooth with natural sugars. Choose fresh fruit, yogurt, and homemade smoothies over candy, cakes, cookies, and pastries.
- Order smaller portions. Avoid the temptation to order king-sized desserts, pastries, and candy bars when eating away from home.

- Choose breakfast cereals that have no more than 8 grams of sugar per serving. Exceptions include cereals with dried fruit and 100% bran cereals.
- Sweeten foods with spices instead of sugar. Add cinnamon and nutmeg to hot cereals, a dash of vanilla to coffee and lattes, and grated ginger-root to fruit and vegetables.
- Reduce sugar in recipes. As a rule, you can cut the sugar in most recipes for baked goods by one-third.

STARCHES

Unlike sugars, starches are complex chains of hundreds or thousands of sugar units linked together. You'll find plenty of starch in foods such as breads, cereals, rice, pasta, corn, and potatoes. Starchy foods have very little fat, saturated fat, or cholesterol. In their unprocessed forms, starchy foods are good sources of fibre, vitamins, and minerals. As you'll learn in Chapter 4, some starchy foods definitely deserve a place in your diet.

DIETARY FIBRE

Dietary fibre is the material in plant foods such as fruits, vegetables, whole grains, and legumes that your body's digestive enzymes can't break down. As a result, fibre passes though the small intestine—where most nutrients are digested and absorbed—and ends up in the large intestine. Here, bacteria in the colon break down the fibre and, in the process, produce substances that help keep colon cells healthy.

To many people, fibre is synonymous with certain types of breakfast cereal. But if you rely on one single food to get your fibre, you're short-changing yourself. That's because foods provide two types of fibre, soluble and insoluble. Although both types are present in varying proportions in foods, some foods may be rich in one or the other.

Soluble fibre

Soluble fibre dissolves in water. Dried peas, beans, lentils, oats, barley, psyllium husks, apples, and citrus fruits are good sources of soluble fibre. When you consume these foods, their soluble fibre forms a gel in your stomach and slows the rate of digestion and absorption. A diet rich in soluble fibre can help keep you feeling full after eating, stabilize blood sugar, and reduce elevated blood cholesterol levels.

Foods such as wheat bran, whole grains, nuts, and vegetables contain mainly *insoluble fibre*. This fibre doesn't dissolve in water, but it does have a significant capacity for retaining water. In this way, insoluble fibre increases stool bulk and promotes regularity. By preventing constipation, a high-fibre diet can ease symptoms of irritable bowel syndrome and prevent diverticulosis and possibly colon cancer.

High-fibre diets are usually fairly low in fat and calories, thus helping you maintain a healthy weight—yet another reason to boost your fibre intake. The tables below show how much fibre you need to consume each day and good food sources of fibre.

Recommended daily fibre intake (grams)

Age	
1–3 years	19
4–8 years	25
Females, 9–18 years	26
Females, 19–50 years	25
Females, 51+ years	21
Males, 9–13 years	31
Males, 14–50 years	38
Males, 51+ years	30

Fibre content of selected foods (grams)

Cereals and grains	
100% bran cereal, 1/2 cup (125 ml)	12.0
Bran flakes, 3/4 cup (175 ml)	6.3
Kellogg's All Bran Buds, 1/3 cup (75 ml)	12.0
Oat bran, cooked, 1 cup (250 ml)	4.5
Oatmeal, cooked, 1 cup (250 ml)	3.6
Quaker Corn Bran, 1 cup (250 ml)	6.3
Bread, 100% whole-wheat, 2 slices	4.0

Fibre content of selected foods (grams), cont'd.

Flaxseed, ground, 2 tbsp (25 ml)	4.0
Pita pocket, whole-wheat, 1 pocket	4.8
Rice, brown, cooked, 1 cup (250 ml)	3.1
Spaghetti, whole-wheat, cooked, 1 cup (250 ml)	4.8
Wheat bran, 2 tbsp (25 ml)	3.0
Legumes and nuts	
Almonds, 1/4 cup (50 ml)	4.0
Beans and tomato sauce, 1/2 cup (125 ml)	10.0
Black beans, cooked, 1/2 cup (125 ml)	6.0
Lentils, cooked, 1/2 cup (125 ml)	4.5
Peanuts, 1/4 cup (50 ml)	3.5
Fruit	
Apple, 1 medium with skin	2.6
Apricots, dried, 1/4 cup (50 ml)	2.6
Blueberries, 1/2 cup (125 ml)	2.0
Figs, dried, 5	8.5
Orange, 1 medium	2.4
Pear, 1 medium with skin	5.1
Prunes, dried	33.0
Raisins, seedless, 1/2 cup (125 ml)	2.8
Strawberries, 1 cup (250 ml)	3.8
Vegetables	
Broccoli, 1/2 cup (125 ml)	2.0
Brussels sprouts, 1/2 cup (125 ml)	2.6
Carrots, 1/2 cup (125 ml)	2.2
Corn niblets, 1/2 cup (125 ml)	2.3
Green peas, 1/2 cup (125 ml)	3.7

Fibre content of selected foods (grams), cont'd.

Potato, 1 medium, baked, with skin	5.0
Sweet potato, mashed, 1/2 cup (125 ml)	3.9

Source: Canadian Nutrient File, 2007.

CARBOHYDRATES AND THE GLYCEMIC INDEX

All carbohydrate-containing foods—starch, sweets, fruit, even milk—ultimately end up in the bloodstream as glucose, the major fuel source for the body's metabolism. How quickly that glucose enters your bloodstream can affect your hunger, your weight, and your long-term health. Nutritionists use a scale called the glycemic index (GI) to rank carbohydrate-rich foods by how fast they raise blood sugar levels compared with pure glucose, which is ranked 100.

Foods with a high GI value are digested quickly and cause a rapid rise in blood sugar and, therefore, an outpouring of insulin (a hormone that removes sugar from the blood and stores it in cells). This surge of insulin can trigger hunger and overeating. What's more, a steady intake of high GI carbohydrates can lead to chronically elevated blood glucose and insulin levels and eventually insulin resistance, a precursor for type 2 diabetes.

Foods that are ranked high on the GI scale (70 or higher) include white bread, whole-wheat bread, baked potatoes, refined breakfast cereals, instant oatmeal, cereal bars, Pop-Tarts, raisins, dates, ripe bananas, carrots, honey, and sugar.

Foods with a low GI (less than 55) release sugar more slowly into the bloodstream and don't produce a rush of insulin. These include grainy breads with seeds, steel-cut oats, 100% bran cereals, brown rice, sweet potatoes, pasta, apples, citrus fruit, grapes, pears, legumes, nuts, cow's milk, yogurt, and soy milk.

Studies suggest that diets based on low GI foods guard against obesity, type 2 diabetes, and colon cancer.

Adopting a low glycemic diet might sound easy, but it's not always as straightforward as it seems. You shouldn't rely on the glycemic index as the only basis for choosing foods. If you limit your diet to include only foods with a low GI value, you'll miss out on important nutrients found in some higher GI foods. Take whole-wheat bread, for example. It's definitely a more nutritious choice than fluffy white bread, but because both are finely milled, they both have a high GI. Carrots have a high GI but are loaded with the disease-fighting antioxidant beta carotene. Bananas are also high on the GI scale but are an excellent source of potassium, a mineral that helps keep blood pressure in check.

On the flip side, not all low GI foods are good for you. The glycemic index of ice cream is 38, but its high saturated fat and sugar content makes it a relatively unhealthy food.

Glycemic index values are based on eating single foods on an empty stomach. The size of a meal, its fat content, and the variety of foods eaten together can skew the glycemic index. For instance, eating a banana (high GI) with a bowl of bran cereal (low GI) and milk (low GI) results in a meal that has a low to medium glycemic index.

Keep these tips in mind when choosing foods:

- Use common sense. Unprocessed fresh foods such as whole grains, legumes, fruits, and vegetables have a low GI value. High glycemic foods are usually highly processed and may have a concentrated amount of sugar.
- Include at least one low GI food per meal, or base two of your meals on low GI choices.
- Pay attention to breads and breakfast cereals, since these foods contribute the most to the high glycemic load of our North American diet.
- Avoid eating high GI snacks such as pretzels, corn chips, cereal bars, and rice cakes, as these can trigger hunger and overeating. Opt for fresh fruit, low-fat dairy products, nuts, or plain popcorn.
- Choose fruits that are acidic (e.g., oranges, grapefruit, cherries), as these have a low GI and will lower the glycemic load of a meal.
- Use salad dressings made with vinegar or lemon juice—the acidity will result in a further reduction in the GI of your meal.

Protein and amino acids

Protein is used by the body to make many critical body compounds. Proteins that are the structural components in the body—muscle tissue, connective tissue, and the support tissue inside bones—are all derived from the protein we eat. Many of these body proteins are in a continual state of breakdown, repair, and maintenance. Proteins are also used to make hormones, enzymes, and immune compounds that attack foreign invaders and prevent infection. Other proteins in your blood help maintain your body's fluid balance.

All these proteins in your body are made up of *amino acids,* the building blocks of protein. Protein in food supplies 20 amino acids, all of which are needed for good health. Eleven of these can be made by your body and are called *non-essential* amino acids. The remaining nine, however, are *essential* amino acids and must be supplied by food because your body cannot synthesize them on its own.

Protein-rich foods include meat, poultry, fish, eggs, dairy products, legumes, nuts, tofu, and soy products. Animal-source protein contains all nine essential amino acids in sufficient quantities to support growth, repair, and maintenance of body tissues. With the exception of soybeans, vegetarian protein foods are low or lacking in one or more essential amino acids.

Our daily protein requirements are really requirements for essential amino acids. Without an adequate intake of essential amino acids, the body's rate of protein building slows down. Eventually, your body will break down its own protein tissues to get these amino acids. Sedentary individuals require 0.8 grams of protein per kilogram of body weight per day. For a 130-pound (59 kg) woman, this translates into roughly 50 grams of protein per day. During the second and third trimesters of pregnancy, as well as when exclusively breastfeeding, protein requirements increase by 25 grams per day.

Exercise also increases the body's need for protein. Extra protein is needed to repair muscle damage that occurs during exercise and to support muscle building.

Endurance athletes, for example, marathon runners, need to consume 1.2 grams of protein per kilogram of body weight per day. Resistance exercise such as weight lifting increases protein needs even more. It's recommended that strength athletes consume 1.6 to 1.7 grams of protein per kilogram body weight per day.

Most people, including athletes, get enough protein by eating a mixed diet. Even vegetarians can meet their protein requirements without resorting to protein powders and protein bars, so long as they eat a variety of plant protein foods throughout the day. The table on page 17 illustrates why it's easy to meet your daily protein needs by diet alone.

Protein content of selected foods (grams)

Meat, poultry, and fish	
Meat, 3 oz (90 g)	21–25
Chicken, 3 oz (90 g)	21
Salmon, canned and drained, 3 oz (90 g)	25
Tuna, canned and drained, 1/2 cup (125 ml)	30
Eggs	
Egg, 1 whole, large	6
Egg, 1 white, large	3
Dairy products	
Cheddar cheese, 1 oz (30 g)	10
Milk, 1 cup (250 ml)	8
Yogurt, 3/4 cup (175 g)	8
Soy products	
Soybeans, cooked, 1 cup (250 ml)	30
Soy beverage, 1 cup (250 ml)	8
Tofu, firm, 3/4 cup (175 ml)	21
Veggie burger, soy-based, 1 patty 2.5 oz (75 g)	11–17
Legumes and nuts	
Kidney beans, cooked, 1 cup (250 ml)	6.3
Lentils, cooked, 1 cup (250 ml)	19
Almonds, 1/2 cup (125 ml)	12
Peanut butter, 2 tbsp (25 ml)	9

Source: Canadian Nutrient File, 2007.

Although meeting your daily protein requirements is important for overall health, consuming more is not better. Contrary to popular belief, increasing your protein intake beyond the daily recommended intake won't help build bigger muscles, since there's a limit to the rate at which protein can be synthesized into muscle. Unlike carbohydrate and fat, protein can't be stored in the body. That means excess protein will either be burned for energy or, if you're already getting the calories you need from your diet, tucked away as body fat.

MEAT AND CANCER RISK

A high intake of protein-rich foods can have other health consequences, too. Studies have linked high intakes of red meat with a higher risk of breast cancer. A University of Minnesota study of 41,836 women revealed that those who enjoyed their hamburger, steak, and bacon well done were almost five times as likely to develop breast cancer as were their peers who ate their meat rare or medium done.[1]

The harmful effect of meat may be because of its saturated fat content, or it may be because of the way it's prepared. Grilling, broiling, and frying meat at high temperatures creates chemicals called heterocyclic amines (HCAs) that are not present in uncooked meats. They're formed when amino acids and creatine (a natural compound found in muscle meats) react at high temperatures. Researchers have identified at least 20 different heterocyclic amines formed during cooking meat that may up cancer risk. Heterocyclic amines have been shown to cause breast tumours in animals.

A heavy intake of red meat, both fresh and processed, is also thought to increase the likelihood of colorectal cancer. A pooled analysis of 29 studies that examined the link between fresh meat (beef, pork) and processed meat (sausage, bacon, deli meats, hot dogs) concluded that a high intake of both increased the risk of colorectal cancer. Compared with people with low intakes of fresh and processed meat, those with high intakes are 20% to 30% more likely to develop colorectal cancer.[2]

In addition to the carcinogens formed during high-heat cooking, red meat contains heme iron, a compound that's been found to cause cancer tumours in laboratory studies. Some researchers also hypothesize that certain gut bacteria give off cancer-causing by-products when meat consumption is high. Until more is known about the effect of cooked meat, experts advise that we consume no more than 3 ounces (90 g) of red meat each day.

Poultry and fish have not been shown to increase cancer risk. In fact, some studies suggest that these so-called "white" meats may actually help prevent cancer. Poultry contains the nutrients selenium and calcium, which have been associated with lower risk of colon cancer. Fish is a good source of omega-3 fatty acids, shown in laboratory studies to inhibit the growth of cancer cells.

In Chapter 5, you'll learn which protein-rich foods you should be eating more often.

Dietary fats and cholesterol

Believe it or not, we do need some fat in our diet to maintain good health. Fat in foods and in the body is made up of building blocks called fatty acids. The body can make all but two fatty acids—linoleic acid and alpha-linolenic acid. Because these two fatty acids are vital to body function, they must be supplied from the diet. Certain types of fats in food supply these two essential fatty acids, which are used to maintain cell membranes and make hormone-like compounds called eicosanoids. Eicosanoids help regulate blood pressure, blood clot formation, blood fats, and the body's immune system.

In additional to supplying essential fatty acids, dietary fat provides fat-soluble vitamins—A, D, E, and K. Later in this chapter you'll learn how these fat-soluble vitamins support growth, development, and overall health. Fat in foods has another function: It adds flavour to meals, increasing the enjoyment and pleasure of eating. And because fat empties from the stomach slowly, it imparts satiety, or a feeling of fullness.

Once consumed, fat has many important roles in the body. Stores of body fat provide a significant source of energy for the body. In fact, about half of our daily energy requirements are supplied by stored fat. Stored body fat also acts as a layer of insulation protecting and cushioning our major organs. The layer of fat beneath our skin helps keeps the body warm. Our body's ability to store fat is pretty much unlimited, since fat cells increase in size if we consume more than we need. And we can always form new fat cells if our existing fat cells can't expand any more. Although stored body fat gives our cells the energy they need and helps insulate us, too much stored fat is clearly not healthy.

SATURATED VERSUS UNSATURATED FATS

Fatty acids in foods have various chemical structures that determine how they will behave in our body. A fatty acid that is completely full of hydrogen atoms is known as a *saturated* fatty acid. Meat, poultry, and high-fat dairy products contain mostly saturated fatty acids, as do coconut and palm oils. Fatty acids that are not saturated with hydrogen atoms are called *unsaturated* fats, which are divided into *monounsaturated* and *polyunsaturated* fats.

All dietary fats are a mixture of saturated, polyunsaturated, and monounsaturated fatty acids, but we call them by the name of the fatty acid they have the most of. Safflower oil, sunflower oil, corn oil, walnuts, Brazil nuts, and seeds contain high levels of polyunsaturated fats. Olive oil, canola oil, peanut oil, avocados, almonds, macadamia nuts, and hazelnuts contain a high proportion of monounsaturated fats.

Polyunsaturated vegetable oils help your body get rid of newly formed cholesterol and, as a result, keep blood cholesterol levels down. And both polyunsaturated and monounsaturated fats can help lower blood cholesterol when they're used in place of cholesterol-raising saturated fat. Olive oil's heart healthy reputation might also be due to oleocanthal, a naturally occurring anti-inflammatory chemical it contains.

OMEGA-3 FATS

Omega-3 fats belong to the family of polyunsaturated fats. Cold water fish such as salmon, lake trout, sardines, mackerel, and herring contain two omega-3 fats: DHA (docosahexaenoic acid) and EPA (eicosapentaenoic acid). Flaxseed, walnut, and canola oils contain another omega-3 fat, ALA (alpha-linolenic acid), an essential fatty acid.

Eating oily fish as little as once or twice per week is thought to decrease your risk of heart attack and stroke. Omega-3 fats in fish make your blood less likely to form clots, reduce blood fats called triglycerides, and protect against irregular heartbeats that cause sudden cardiac death. Although research suggests that a steady intake of ALA can protect from heart disease, the data are much less compelling compared with the evidence for DHA. Still, if you don't eat fish, getting ALA from your diet could lower the odds of developing heart disease. One study found that, among 76,763 healthy women who were followed for 18 years, those who consumed the most ALA (from oil-and-vinegar salad dressings) had a 40% lower risk of sudden cardiac death compared with women whose diets provided the least.[3]

DHA in oily fish may also reduce the risk of Alzheimer's disease. This omega-3 fatty acid is needed to keep the lining of brain cells flexible so memory messages can pass easily between cells. Research also suggests that fish oils can block the growth of certain types of cancer tumours.

TRANS FATS

Trans fats are formed through partial hydrogenation, a chemical process by which food manufacturers turn an unsaturated fat into a more solid fat, such as shortening or margarine. Roughly 90% of the trans fat in our food supply lurks in commercial baked goods (cookies, cakes, pastries, doughnuts), snack foods, fried fast foods, and some margarines. Trans fat occurs naturally in beef and dairy products, but in tiny amounts. It's also not known if trans fat in beef and dairy behaves the same way in the body as industry-produced trans fat.

Substantial evidence indicates that both saturated and trans fatty acids increase total and LDL (bad) cholesterol levels. But unlike saturated fat, consuming too much trans fat can lower your HDL (good) cholesterol. Compared with saturated fats, trans fats are linked to a 2.5- to 10-fold higher risk of heart disease. The harmful effects of trans fats aren't limited to heart disease: Research suggests that diets high in trans fat increase the risk of type 2 diabetes.

In June 2007, Health Canada called on Canada's food industry to virtually eliminate processed trans fats in Canadian-manufactured foods. The government mandated that the trans fat content of vegetable oils and soft, spreadable margarines be limited to 2% of the total fat content, and the trans fat content for all other foods to 5%, including ingredients sold to restaurants. These new regulations are expected to be implemented by 2010.

Sources of dietary fats

Fat	Food source
Saturated fatty acids	Fresh meat, bacon, sausage, poultry, butter, cheese, cream, whole cow's milk, whole-milk and Balkan-style yogurt, coconut oil, palm and palm kernel oils
Trans fatty acids	Baked products, commercial snack foods, fried fast food, margarine made with partially hydrogenated vegetable oil or shortening
Monounsaturated fatty acids	Olive, canola, and peanut oils; avocados, olives, non-hydrogenated margarines made from these oils
Polyunsaturated fatty acids	Corn, safflower, sesame, soy, and sunflower oils; non-hydrogenated margarines made from these oils; nuts and seeds

Fat	Food source
Omega-3 fatty acids	DHA, EPA: herring, mackerel, salmon, sardines, trout, some brands of fortified eggs, cheese, milk, fruit juice ALA: canola, flaxseed, and walnut oils; pecans, walnuts, soybeans, and some fortified foods such as eggs, yogurt, and juice

DIETARY CHOLESTEROL

Cholesterol in foods is a wax-like fatty substance found in meat, poultry, eggs, dairy products, fish, and other seafood. It's particularly plentiful in shrimp, liver, and egg yolks. The foods you eat account for only about 20% of the cholesterol in your body; the rest is produced mainly by your liver. Cholesterol in your body is used to make cell membranes, other components of cells, certain hormones, and vitamin D.

Many people worry that eating high-cholesterol foods—for example, eggs—will increase blood cholesterol levels. Although high-cholesterol diets cause high blood cholesterol in animals, this effect is not seen in humans. In fact, dietary cholesterol has little or no effect on most people's blood cholesterol. One reason is that our intestines absorb only half of the cholesterol we eat. The rest gets excreted in the stool. Our bodies are also efficient at turning cholesterol in the bloodstream into bile, a digestive aid that's stored in the gallbladder. That means there's less cholesterol available for transport in your blood. Even so, experts advise consuming no more than 300 milligrams of cholesterol per day, 200 milligrams if you have heart disease.

Cholesterol content of selected foods (milligrams)

Meat, poultry, and fish	
Beef sirloin, lean, 3 oz (90 g)	64
Calf's liver, fried, 3 oz (90 g)	416
Pork loin, lean, 3 oz (90 g)	71
Chicken breast, skinless, 3 oz (90 g)	73
Salmon, 3 oz (90 g)	54
Shrimp, 3 oz (90 g)	135

Cholesterol content of selected foods (milligrams), cont'd.

Eggs

1 egg, whole	190
1 egg, white	0

Dairy products

Milk, 2% milk fat (MF), 1 cup (250 ml)	19
Milk, skim, 1 cup (250 ml)	5
Cheese, cheddar, 31% MF, 1 oz (30 g)	31
Cheese, mozzarella, part-skim, 1 oz (30 g)	18
Cream, half and half, 12% MF, 2 tbsp (25 ml)	12
Yogurt, 1.5% MF, 3/4 cup (175 ml)	11
Butter, 2 tsp (10 ml)	10

Source: Canadian Nutrient File, 2007.

RECOMMENDATIONS FOR DIETARY FAT

Current guidelines emphasize the importance of minimizing our intake of the so-called bad fats—saturated and trans fats—while emphasizing healthy, unsaturated fats in our diet:

- *Consume no more than 35% of your daily calories from fat.* This means that there should be no more than 3.5 grams of fat for every 100 calories (the nutrition label will give you this information). But this does not mean that every food you eat must be low in fat. It's the big picture that counts. You can make up for eating one high-fat food by including plenty of low-fat foods in the rest of your meals that day.
- *Minimize your intake of saturated fat.* Choose lean cuts of meat, poultry breast, skim or 1% milk, yogurt with 1% milk fat or less, and part-skim cheese (20% milk fat or less). Use butter sparingly.
- *Minimize your intake of trans fat.* As often as possible when choosing packaged foods, avoid products that list *partially hydrogenated fat* as an ingredient. Read the Nutrition Facts box (see Appendix 3) and choose products with less than 0.5 grams of trans fat, or preferably none.
- *Eat fatty fish two times a week* to get heart-protective omega-3 fats. The oilier the fish, the better.

- *Include 2 to 3 tablespoons (25 to 50 ml) of unsaturated oils* in your daily diet to get essential fatty acids.
- *Limit your intake of dietary cholesterol to no more than 300 milligrams per day.* If you have heart disease, limit your intake to 200 milligrams.
- *Drizzle, don't pour.* Even the healthiest of oils can cause weight gain if you consume too much. A steady diet of fatty foods, high-fat spreads, and overly dressed salads can add unwanted pounds. Gram per gram, all types of fat—saturated and unsaturated—deliver almost double the calories that protein and carbohydrate do.

Water

It's easy to forget that water is an essential nutrient. Although a deficiency of other nutrients can take weeks, months, or even years to develop, we can survive only a few days without water. Water is the most abundant compound in the human body, making up roughly 60% of our body weight. Your body needs water to regulate its temperature, transport oxygen and nutrients to cells, keep skin hydrated, and cushion joints.

Normally, the average adult loses more than 10 cups (2.5 L) of water each day just by breathing, sweating, and excreting wastes. When it's hot outside, your body loses even more water through sweat, especially if you're active. For instance, an hour of singles tennis can drain 4 to 10 cups (1 to 2.5 L) of water from your body, and a round of golf as many as 16 cups (4 L).

Because your body is constantly losing water, you need to replace it by drinking fluids and, to a lesser degree, eating watery foods such as fruit and vegetables. If you don't consume enough fluid to replace losses, you'll start to feel dizzy, light-headed, and fatigued, and you may get a headache and develop muscle cramps. Other signs of mild to moderate dehydration include thirst, decreased urine output, flushed skin, dry mouth and eyes, nausea, and loss of appetite. A child's irritability on a hot day may also indicate he or she is dehydrated.

If dehydration progresses, extreme thirst, lack of sweating, low blood pressure, rapid heartbeat, muscle spasms, and heat injury can occur. Heat injury results from drinking too little fluid combined with heavy exercise and sweating. Symptoms range from mild heat cramps to potentially life-threatening heat stroke (when the body's sweating mechanism shuts down and the body is depleted of fluids).

Some people are at greater risk for suffering the effects of dehydration and need to pay close attention to their water intake. Young children, older adults, people working outdoors in hot weather, and people with poorly controlled diabetes and other chronic illnesses are more susceptible to becoming dehydrated.

How much water do you need to drink each day?

Age	Amount
1–3 years	4 cups (1 L)
4–8 years	5 cups (1.25 L)
9–13 years	8 cups (2 L)
Females, 14–18 years	8 cups (2 L)
Females, 19+ years	9 cups (2.2 L)
Males, 14–18 years	11 cups (2.7 L)
Males, 19+ years	13 cups (3 L)

Source: National Academy of Sciences, Institute of Medicine, Food and Nutrition Board. Dietary Reference Intakes for Water, Potassium, Sodium, Chloride, and Sulfate. The National Academy Press, Washington, DC, 2004.

WHEN YOU NEED MORE WATER

The above guidelines don't take into account factors that drive up your daily water requirements. Hot and humid weather cause your body to sweat more and increase your fluid needs. The low humidity on airplanes increases water losses through the skin and boosts your water requirements during air travel. Women who are pregnant or breastfeeding need to drink an additional 1 cup (250 ml) or 4 cups (1 L) per day respectively.

Although water is good for you, you can have too much of a good thing. If you drink too much water, the kidneys can't keep up and are unable to excrete the excess. Your blood becomes diluted, resulting in low blood sodium (hyponatremia), which can lead to swelling of the brain. But even if you drink a lot of water, you're unlikely to experience hyponatremia as long as you drink it over the course of the day, as opposed to drinking an enormous volume at one time. Endurance athletes, including marathon runners and triathletes, who drink large amounts of water in a short period are at greater risk.

During exercise, you do need to drink more water. That's because physical activity generates heat in your muscles, which your body releases through your skin as sweat. If you don't drink enough before, during, and after exercise, your body can't properly release this heat. As a result, your heart beats harder, your body temperature rises, and, ultimately, your performance suffers.

During exercise, it's important to drink 1/2 to 1 cup (125 to 250 ml) of water every 15 to 20 minutes. Sports drinks (e.g., Gatorade, Powerade) are recommended during exercise that lasts longer than an hour. The sodium added to sports drinks stimulates fluid absorption, maintains the desire to drink, and helps prevent hyponatremia in prolonged exercise. Plus, most beverages contain 6% to 9% carbohydrate in the form of liquid sugar and/or high fructose corn syrup to provide energy for working muscles. To determine how much fluid you lose during exercise, weigh yourself before and after your workout. For every pound you lose, it takes 2 cups (500 ml) of water to replenish what you've lost through sweat. Drinking water during exercise will help minimize your body's fluid loss.

WHAT COUNTS AS WATER?

The good news is that *all* beverages—with the exception of alcoholic beverages—count toward your daily water requirements. In addition to plain drinking water, fruit juice, milk, soy beverages, soft drinks, even coffee and tea help keep you hydrated. Although older studies demonstrated caffeine to have a weak, short-term diuretic effect, recent studies have not. We now know that the body adjusts to caffeine within 5 days of regular use, greatly reducing its mild effect of fluid loss.

Even so, some fluid choices are better than others, particularly if you're counting calories. Research suggests that we don't register the calories we drink as well as we do the calories we eat. Liquid calories add to, rather than displace, food calories, thereby increasing our total daily calorie intake. That liquid calories can easily lead to weight gain prompted a U.S. research panel to review the studies on beverages and health and propose a guide for choosing beverages. Published in 2006 in the *American Journal of Clinical Nutrition,* the Beverage Guidance System ranks beverages based on their calorie and nutrient content.

According to the report, plain water outranked all other beverages because it has no calories, no sugar, and no sodium, and may provide some calcium, magnesium, and fluoride. Water was followed by, in descending order, unsweetened coffee and tea, low-fat milk and soy beverages, diet drinks, calorie beverages with some nutrients (fruit juice, sports drinks), and, lastly, sugary beverages (soft drinks, fruit drinks).

To prevent consuming too many calories from beverages, experts recommend limiting beverage calories to no more than 10% of daily caloric intake. In other words, you shouldn't sip more than 200 calories, if you follow a 2000-calorie diet.

In Chapter 8, you'll learn which beverages have health benefits beyond keeping you hydrated.

Vitamins and minerals

Vitamins and minerals are essential nutrients the body can't make on its own, so your diet must supply them. They're needed in small amounts for normal growth and development, body function, and maintenance of healthy body tissues. Vitamins and minerals also participate in metabolic processes that generate energy for the body. Studies suggest that certain vitamins and minerals also keep us healthy by fending off chronic diseases, such as heart disease, stroke, arthritis, Alzheimer's, and certain cancers.

Use the guide below to choose nutrient-packed foods, to help you and your family eat a diet brimming with vitamins and minerals:

Key vitamin	Needed for	Best food sources
Vitamin A	Vision, growth, and development; healthy skin, hair, nails, bones, teeth Beta carotene–rich foods may protect from lung cancer and heart disease	Calf's liver, oily fish, milk, cheese, eggs; beta carotene: apricots, mango, peaches, broccoli, carrots, kale, spinach, sweet potato, winter squash
Vitamin B1 (thiamine)	Converting food into energy; healthy nerve, muscle, and heart function	Calf's liver, pork, fish, enriched breakfast cereals and breads, legumes, nuts, whole grains, wheat germ
Vitamin B2 (riboflavin)	Converting food into energy; vision; healthy skin and red blood cells	Red meat, eggs, cheese, milk, yogurt, fortified soy and rice milk, whole grains, legumes, nuts

Key vitamin	Needed for	Best food sources
Vitamin B3 (niacin)	Converting food into energy; healthy skin; digestion; nerve function	Calf's liver, red meat, poultry, fish, eggs, dairy products, peanuts, almonds, enriched breakfast cereals, wheat bran
Vitamin B6	Breaking down protein and fat; red blood cell formation May guard against heart disease, cognitive decline, and dementia	Calf's liver, red meat, poultry, fish, eggs, legumes, nuts, seeds, whole grains, avocados, bananas, green leafy vegetables, potatoes
Vitamin B12	Building and repairing DNA (genetic material of cells); making red blood cells; nerve function May help prevent heart disease, depression, cognitive decline, and Alzheimer's disease	Red meat, poultry, fish, eggs, dairy products, fortified soy or rice milk
Folate	Breaking down protein; red blood cell formation; prevents neural tube defects in newborns May guard against heart disease, colon cancer, breast cancer, cognitive decline, and Alzheimer's disease	Lentils, legumes, seeds, orange juice, artichokes, asparagus, spinach
Vitamin C	Forming connective tissue, bones, teeth, gums; absorbing iron; immune function; wound healing May reduce risk of heart attack, stroke, cataract, and lung cancer	Cantaloupe, citrus fruit and juices, kiwi, strawberries, bell peppers, broccoli, cabbage, cauliflower, tomato juice
Vitamin D	Strong bones and teeth; healthy blood pressure and immunity May guard against osteoporosis; hypertension; rheumatoid arthritis; type 1 diabetes; multiple sclerosis; and breast, colon, and prostate cancers	Milk, egg yolks, oily fish, fortified soy or rice milk

Key vitamin	Needed for	Best food sources
Vitamin E	Cell membranes, immune function, and red blood cell production High dietary intake may help prevent heart disease, cataract, and prostate cancer	Nuts, seeds, soybeans, whole grains, wheat germ, avocados, leafy green vegetables, vegetable oils
Vitamin K	Blood clotting and bone formation May reduce risk of osteoporosis and hip fractures	Calf's liver, broccoli, cabbage, green peas, leafy green vegetables
Calcium	Building bones and teeth; muscle and nerve function; blood clotting; maintaining healthy blood pressure May help prevent osteoporosis, colon cancer, kidney stones, and high blood pressure	Canned salmon (with bones), sardines, dairy products, fortified soy or rice milk, almonds, legumes, tofu, fortified fruit juice, broccoli, leafy green vegetables
Chromium	Blood sugar regulation; metabolism of carbohydrate, fat, and protein May reduce risk of type 2 diabetes	Red meat, turkey, whole grains, English muffins, apple with skin, grape juice, orange juice, broccoli, dried basil, dried garlic
Iron	Formation of hemoglobin, which transports oxygen to body tissues; making brain chemicals that aid in concentration	Red meat, poultry, eggs, salmon, tuna, lentils, baked beans, enriched breakfast cereals, whole grains, blackstrap molasses, raisins
Magnesium	Heart, muscle, and nerve function; protein building; bone growth May prevent hypertension and cardiovascular disease	Legumes, tofu, almonds, Brazil nuts, sunflower seeds, whole grains, dates, figs, prunes, leafy green vegetables
Potassium	Maintaining fluid balance in body; muscle and nerve function; maintaining healthy blood pressure May prevent stroke, osteoporosis, and kidney stones	Avocados, bananas, cantaloupe, oranges, orange juice, peaches, broccoli, Brussels sprouts, green peas, lima beans, spinach, tomato juice

Key vitamin	Needed for	Best food sources
Selenium	Thyroid function; immune function; synthesis of antioxidant enzymes May guard against skin, lung, and prostate cancers	Red meat, chicken, crab, halibut, salmon, shrimp, brown rice, Brazil nuts, whole-wheat bread
Zinc	Growth; sexual development; immune function wound healings May prevent advanced symptoms of macular degeneration	Beef, pork, lamb, crab, oysters, milk, yogurt, legumes, almonds, cashews, pumpkin seeds, wheat bran, wheat germ, whole grains, enriched breakfast cereals

SODIUM—AN OVERCONSUMED MINERAL

Although scientists agree that we need a minimal amount of salt (sodium chloride) to survive, the health implications of intaking too much salt are loudly heard by scientists, health professionals, and public watchdog groups. Sodium is needed to regulate fluid balance and blood pressure, and it keeps muscles and nerves working properly. As such, acceptable daily sodium intakes have been established to cover the needs of moderately active people.

People under the age of 50 need 1500 milligrams of sodium per day, people age 50 to 70 need 1300 milligrams, and older persons need 1200 milligrams. Endurance athletes, such as marathoners, need more sodium to cover sweat losses that occur during exercise. The daily upper limit of sodium for healthy adults is 2300 milligrams. People who are sodium sensitive—roughly 35% of Canadians—should limit their daily intake to fewer than 2300 milligrams. In salt-sensitive individuals, excess sodium can boost blood pressure. Older adults, African-Americans, and those who have a parent, sibling, or child with high blood pressure are particularly prone to a salt sensitivity.

The problem is that our daily sodium intake often greatly exceeds acceptable intakes and the upper limit. It's estimated that the average Canadian male consumes 4100 milligrams of sodium per day, and women, 2900 milligrams. The major risk of a high-salt diet is elevated blood pressure, a risk factor for heart attack, stroke, and kidney disease. Studies show that, on average, blood pressure rises progressively with increasing sodium intakes. Consuming too much sodium may also increase the risk of osteoporosis by causing the body to excrete calcium.

The vast majority (77%) of salt we consume each day is unseen, lurking in processed and restaurant foods. Only 11% of our daily sodium comes from salt that's added during cooking and while eating. The remainder occurs naturally in the foods we eat (e.g., in milk, shellfish, and tap water). To help reduce your daily sodium intake, practise the following:

* Read labels. Use nutrition labels to identify packaged foods that are low in sodium. The Nutrition Facts box lists the amount of sodium (in milligrams) per one serving of the food. To quickly determine if a food has a little or a lot of sodium, read the % Daily Value, which is set at 2400 milligrams. Foods low in sodium will have a % Daily Value of 5% or less; foods with a Daily Value of 25% or more are high in sodium. It's okay to include a high-sodium food in your diet as long as you balance that sodium intake by also choosing foods naturally low in sodium, such as fresh fruits and vegetables.

* Pay attention to portion size. Sodium numbers on a nutrition label will underestimate your intake if you consume more than the serving size indicated. So, if you eat more than the specified serving size, you'll need to adjust the sodium number.

* Limit your intake of processed meats, including bologna, ham, sausage, hot dogs, bacon, deli meats, and smoked salmon.

* Limit your use of bouillon cubes, Worcestershire sauce, soy sauce, and barbecue sauce.

* Rely less on convenience foods, including canned soups, frozen dinners, and packaged rice and pasta mixes.

* Choose premade entrees or frozen dinners that contain no more than 200 milligrams sodium per 100 calories.

* When possible, choose low-sodium products. Many sodium-reduced brands contain 25% less sodium than the original version, and some, such as V8 juice, contain 75% less. If your supermarket doesn't carry low-salt products, ask your grocer to stock them.

* Remove the salt shaker from the table to break the habit of salting food. Substitute herbs and spices for salt when cooking—try garlic, lemon juice, salsa, onion, vinegar, and herbs.

DO YOU NEED A DAILY MULTIVITAMIN?

If you follow Canada's Food Guide—and make a point of adding power foods to your daily diet—do you need a multivitamin supplement? Well, in fact, the revised food guide (2007) does recommend a multivitamin for women. Women who could become pregnant and those who are pregnant should take a daily multivitamin with 400 micrograms of folic acid to help prevent serious spinal cord birth defects, such as spina bifida, in newborns.

In my opinion, it's a wise idea for all healthy adults to take a daily multivitamin and mineral pill. A multivitamin helps you meet daily requirements for folate, vitamin B12, vitamin D, and iron, nutrients that can be challenging for some people to consume in adequate quantities from foods alone. Don't get me wrong. A multivitamin and mineral supplement won't make up for a diet that's high in fat and sodium and lacking phytochemical- and nutrient-rich power foods. Rather, a multivitamin is meant to backup a healthy diet by filling nutritional gaps that can affect even the most careful eaters.

Here's a list of important nutrients you should look for in an adult multivitamin and mineral supplement—cited in milligrams (mg), micrograms (mcg), or international units (IU)—and what to avoid:

Vitamin A
Choose a product with 2500 IU or less. Avoid multivitamins that contain more than 5000 IU of vitamin A palmitate or acetate (retinol), since too much may increase the risk of hip fracture and birth defects. You can also choose a multi that contains beta carotene in place of vitamin A.

Beta carotene
Many multivitamins have beta carotene, some of which the body converts to vitamin A. Look for a product with no more than 15,000 IU. Very high doses (more than 30,000 IU) may increase the risk of lung cancer in smokers. As you'll learn in Chapter 2, you're better off eating more beta carotene–rich foods, such as spinach, broccoli, carrots, and sweet potatoes, than getting it from a supplement.

B vitamins
Look for at least 100% of the recommended intakes for B1 (1.2 mg), B2 (1.3 mg), niacin (14–16 mg), B6 (1.3–1.7 mg), B12 (2.4 mcg), and folic acid (0.4 mg).

Vitamin D
Choose a product with 400 IU, especially if you're over the age of 50. I'll tell you more about vitamin D supplements later in this chapter.

Vitamin E

The recommended daily intake is 22 IU. There's no evidence that taking more will ward off heart disease or cancer. In fact, research has linked a daily intake above 100 IU with a greater risk of dying (from any cause). Choose a multi with fewer than 100 IU per day.

Vitamin K

The recommended daily intake is 90 mcg for women and 120 mcg for men, but daily intakes of 150 to 250 mcg may help prevent hip fractures. Until recently, vitamin K was not allowed in multivitamins; now 120 mcg per daily dose is permitted. If you take blood thinners, consult with your doctor before taking a supplement containing vitamin K.

Calcium

This mineral is too bulky to fit a whole day's worth into a one-a-day formula. Get what you can from foods, and take a separate calcium supplement if you need more. Most multivitamins supply 100 to 125 mg.

Iron

If you're a premenopausal woman, choose a multi with 10 to 18 mg; men and postmenopausal women don't need more than 8 mg (though products with 10 mg are fine). If your doctor has told you that your body's iron stores are elevated, choose an iron-free formula.

Magnesium

Men need 420 mg per day; women need 320 mg. Magnesium is found in many power foods described in this book, including legumes, nuts, seeds, whole grains, and leafy greens. To boost your intake, pick a multi with 50 to 100 mg.

Other minerals

Look for 10 mg of zinc, 2 mg of copper, 25 to 35 mcg of chromium, and 55 mcg of selenium.

What you don't need

Extras such as herbs, lutein, and lycopene are not necessary, as the amounts added to a multi are usually too small to be effective. (Lutein and lycopene are best consumed from power foods; I discuss which foods in Chapter 2.) And there's no evidence that "weight loss" multivitamins with green tea extract will help you shed excess pounds. Read Chapter 8 to find out why you should drink your green tea.

WHAT ABOUT VITAMIN D?

Recognizing that vitamin D requirements increase with age (because our skin becomes less efficient at producing it from the sun's UV rays) and that it's challenging, if not impossible, to meet those needs from diet alone, Canada's Food Guide advises adults over the age of 50 to take a 400 IU vitamin D supplement each day. If you followed the news in June 2007, you might recall there was a lot of talk about vitamin D supplements and cancer prevention. Indeed, vitamin D advice for Canadians has changed since the food guide was introduced in February 2007.

Before the revised food guide was launched, numerous studies suggested that vitamin D's benefits extend beyond bone health to the prevention of breast, colon, prostate, and lung cancers. Then, in June 2007, came findings from the first randomized controlled trial to substantiate what earlier observational studies have revealed: Vitamin D is an important tool in fighting cancer. In the 4-year study of 1179 healthy, postmenopausal women, researchers found that those taking 1110 IU of vitamin D per day were 60% less likely to get cancer than their peers taking placebo pills.

(Randomized controlled trials are the gold standard of scientific evidence. In these studies, researchers follow a group of people over a period of time. Half the people are randomly assigned to receive the prescribed diet, food, or nutrient believed to prevent the disease—the intervention—and the others continue with their usual diet or take a look-alike treatment—the placebo. Researchers then wait several years to see if one of the two groups has a higher rate of the disease.)

This new finding—and the fact that Canadians don't produce enough vitamin D from sunlight from October to March—prompted the Canadian Cancer Society to recommend adults consider taking 1000 IU of vitamin D per day in the fall and winter. Older adults, people with dark skin, those who don't go outdoors often, and those who wear clothing that covers most of their skin should take the supplement year-round. The Canadian Cancer Society's vitamin D recommendation does not extend to children, since, so far, research has focused on adults only.

I concur with this advice and recommend 1000 IU of vitamin D year-round to most of my clients. Keep in mind that if you use sunscreen to protect from skin cancer (which is a wise idea), your body makes very little vitamin D. That's because sun protection factor (SPF) blocks the ability of the skin to synthesize vitamin D from sunlight. To determine the dose of vitamin D you need to buy, add up how much you're already getting from your multivitamin and calcium supplements. Choose a supplement that contains vitamin D-3, instead of vitamin D-2, which is less potent.

Phytochemicals

If you follow news stories on diet and health, you've probably heard the word *phytochemical* used. If you're not familiar with phytochemicals, you certainly will be after reading this book. In the chapters that follow, you'll learn how phytochemicals in foods help guard against many diseases and health conditions.

Phytochemicals are not vitamins, minerals, proteins, carbohydrates, or fat. Rather, they're naturally occurring compounds found in plant foods, such as vegetables, fruit, whole grains, legumes, and nuts. (*Phyto* comes from the Greek word for plant.) Although phytochemicals are not classified as nutrients, substances necessary for sustaining life, scientists are learning that these compounds are beneficial to our health.

Plants produce phytochemicals to protect themselves from bacteria, fungi, viruses, and cellular damage. When we consume plant foods, these phytochemicals also defend our bodies from disease. Scientists have identified over one thousand phytochemicals and many more continue to be discovered each day. In fact, there may be more than a hundred different phytochemicals in just one serving of vegetables. Some of the main subgroups of phytochemicals are carotenoids, flavonoids, indoles, and sulphides. Within each subgroup there are many different phytochemicals with disease-fighting properties.

Phytochemicals work in various ways to fight disease. They:

* *Behave as antioxidants.* Most phytochemicals have antioxidant properties, meaning they protect our cells against oxidative damage, thereby reducing the risk of developing chronic disease. Oxidative damage occurs when the production of harmful molecules, called free radicals, overwhelms the body's built-in antioxidant defences.

  As antioxidants, phytochemicals block the process of oxidation by neutralizing free radicals. Phytochemicals with antioxidant powers include sulphur compounds in garlic and onions, polyphenols in green and black tea, and beta carotene in leafy green vegetables and carrots.

- *Act like hormones.* Some phytochemicals, such as isoflavones in soybeans and lignans in flaxseed, mimic the human hormone estrogen and, by doing so, may help reduce the risk of breast cancer and osteoporosis.
- *Stimulate enzymes.* Indoles, phytochemicals found in cabbage and broccoli, can activate enzymes in the body that make estrogen less effective, thereby helping guard against breast cancer.
- *Interfere with DNA replication.* Certain phytochemicals found in legumes can interrupt the replication of DNA, the genetic material of cells, potentially preventing the growth of cancer cells.
- *Fight bacteria and viruses.* Allicin, a phytochemical found in garlic, has been shown to kill harmful bacteria, helping the body fight infection. Other phytochemicals, such as anthocyanins in cranberries, prevent harmful bacteria from attaching to cell walls (this is how cranberries are thought to prevent urinary tract infections). Still others have been demonstrated to boost the body's immune system, helping it fend off disease.

Your body can't make phytochemicals—the only way to get them is by eating a variety of power foods each day. Here's a list of some of the most commonly studied phytochemicals and the foods that provide them:

Food	Phytochemical
Allium vegetables (e.g., garlic, onions, leeks)	Allyl sulphides
Berries Citrus fruit	Anthocyanins Ellagic acid Carotenoids Glucarates Limonene
Cruciferous vegetables (e.g., bok choy, broccoli, Brussels sprouts, cauliflower, cabbage, kale, kohlrabi, turnip)	Indoles/glucosinolates Isothiocynates/thiocynates Sulphoraphane
Leafy greens (e.g., kale, rapini, spinach, Swiss chard)	Beta carotene Lutein and zeaxanthin
Whole grains and legumes (e.g., soybeans, oats, flaxseed, kidney beans, lentils)	Isoflavones Lignans Phytic acid Saponins

Food	Phytochemical
Tea (green, oolong, black)	Catechins
Tomatoes	Lycopene

You'll become better acquainted with these potent disease-fighters, and many more, in the chapters that follow.

What should you eat?

As far as science goes, nutrition is a relatively young field. Although humans have written about food and its effect on the body throughout history, it wasn't discovered until the early 1900s that food contained life-sustaining vitamins. Ever since, scientists have been busy exploring the relationship between the foods we eat and our health. Although we have yet to solve all the mysteries of human nutrition, what we have learned has resulted in dietary guidelines, a national food guide, daily nutrient intake recommendations, nutrition labels, and government-enforced regulations (e.g., trans fat limits for the food industry).

It's only recently that foods, and the nutrients they contain, have been looked upon as a means of preventing disease. When Canada's first food guide—called the Official Food Rules—was introduced in 1942, its purpose was to prevent nutrient deficiencies during a period of wartime food rationing. Forty years and five food guides later, the 1982 "Canada's Food Guide" encouraged Canadians to limit fat, sugar, salt, and alcohol in an attempt to curb the rising rate of diet-related chronic diseases, including heart disease and certain cancers.

In February 2007, Health Canada launched its most recent food guide; it hadn't been updated since 1992. You can imagine that over the course of 15 years much had changed in the world of nutrition. Among the wealth of scientific findings that had emerged, we had learned about the evils of trans fat, the importance of vitamin D, the cardio-protective effects of fish, and the health benefits of whole grains. As well, our daily recommended intakes for almost all vitamins and minerals had been revised since 1992. And the ethnic makeup of the country had changed. The food guide no longer reflected the diversity of foods Canadians were eating.

The latest version of Canada's food guide, "Eating Well with Canada's Food Guide," recommends a pattern of eating that will help persons age 2 and older meet daily nutrient requirements and prevent chronic diseases, such as heart disease, type 2 diabetes, osteoporosis, and certain cancers. I do think our latest food guide is a big improvement. It does a much better job at guiding people on how much food they should eat and in what amounts. It also includes a greater variety of ethnic foods that many Canadians eat. And in terms of fighting disease, the revised food guide offers more direction on what types of foods to choose—many of which you'll learn more about in the chapters of this book.

CANADA'S FOOD GUIDE—FOOD GROUP BY FOOD GROUP

If you were familiar with the previous food guide, you may have noticed some changes. For starters, the food guide has expanded in size; it now consists of six pages instead of two. There's also more detail about the recommended number of servings and serving sizes. There's an emphasis on the importance of reading nutrition labels, physical activity, and special nutrition considerations for women and for older adults. The food guide also gives more directed advice on how to make healthy choices within each food group. In addition to indicating specific foods to eat, the food guide reminds us to make choices that are low in animal fat, sugar, and sodium.

Here's a recap of what's new and improved in each of the four food groups, each represented by a coloured arc in the Canada's Food Guide rainbow.

VEGETABLES AND FRUITS

The 2007 food guide has promoted this food group to the outer, most prominent, arc of the rainbow. (The previous food guide featured grain products as the most dominant food group.) The vegetables and fruits food group was repositioned based on literally hundreds and hundreds of studies linking a produce-packed diet with a lower risk of many cancers and heart disease.

In order for us to consume enough beta carotene and folate, two nutrients linked to disease prevention, the food guide advises eating at least one dark green and one orange vegetable each day. You'll learn all about dark green vegetables—romaine lettuce, spinach, rapini, Swiss chard—and how to add then to your diet in Chapter 2. Ditto for bright orange vegetables, such as carrots, sweet potatoes, and winter squash. And in order to increase our fibre intake, we're told to consume whole veggies and fruit more often than juice.

Adults should eat 7 to 10 servings of vegetables and fruit each day. That might seem like a lot, but it really isn't when you consider that 1 serving is equivalent to 1/2 cup (125 ml) of raw or cooked vegetables, 1 cup (250 ml) of salad greens, one medium-sized fruit, 1/4 cup (50 ml) of dried fruit, or 1/2 cup (125 ml) of 100% juice. If you're stuck repeatedly eating the same old banana at breakfast and salad for dinner, don't be: You'll find plenty of interesting serving suggestions and recipes in the pages that follow.

GRAIN PRODUCTS

Foods such as bread, cereal, rice, and pasta provide energy-yielding carbohydrates that fuel our brain cells and muscles. Yet, not all grains are created equal. Unrefined grains, which have not been stripped of their nutrient-rich bran and germ layers, offer more fibre and magnesium, nutrients that help guard against heart disease, than do refined grains, such as white flour and white rice. The food guide recognizes this by encouraging whole-grain consumption. For the first time, the food guide advises Canadians to eat at least half of their daily grain servings as whole grain.

As you'll read in Chapter 4, whole grains offer more than just fibre and magnesium. They're excellent sources of many nutrients and phytochemicals that their refined counterparts are lacking. Plus, the body can't digest whole grains as quickly as it can refined grains. This helps keep our energy levels sustained longer after eating them. Refined white starchy foods behave much like sugar in the body. They provide few nutrients other than a handful of vitamins that manufacturers add back to them after refining. And the ability of refined starches to spike your blood sugar increases the risk of heart disease and type 2 diabetes.

Eating one-half of your daily grain servings as whole grain is definitely a good start and will help you boost your nutrient, fibre, and phytochemical intake. However, I recommend that you try for even more. Ideally most, if not all, of your grain choices should be whole grain. You'll learn why in Chapter 4.

MILK AND MILK ALTERNATIVES

Building bones and keeping them dense takes calcium, along with vitamin D. Children age 1 to 3 years need 500 milligrams of calcium, kids age 4 to 8 need 800 milligrams, and teens require 1300 milligrams per day. Adults age 19 to 50 must strive for 1000 milligrams, while older adults need 1200 milligrams each day. (Osteoporosis Canada recommends that adults over the age of 50 consume 1500 milligrams of the mineral daily.) For adults, these numbers translate into 3 or 4 servings of milk and alternatives each day. (One serving of milk or yogurt packs roughly 300 milligrams of calcium.)

The food guide has conditioned us to reach for dairy to get our calcium, but I certainly don't think it is the only source. Formerly called the "Milk Products" food group, this newly named group now considers calcium-enriched soy beverages to be nutritionally equivalent to milk (1 serving also packs 300 milligrams of calcium). That's good news for vegetarians and the large number of Canadians who don't drink milk because they are lactose intolerant. (Lactose intolerance is the inability to properly digest lactose, the natural sugar found in milk. Symptoms include abdominal cramping, gas, and sometimes diarrhea.)

If you don't like dairy products and you don't drink much soy beverage, calcium supplements are an easy and inexpensive way to meet your daily calcium needs. Check the ingredient list on the supplement's package label to see how much elemental calcium each pill provides and to determine how many tablets you need to take to get your recommended dose. Choose a formula with vitamin D, since this nutrient works in tandem with calcium to promote bone health. If you need to take more than 500 milligrams from a supplement, split your dose over two or three meals. Finally, don't get more than 2500 milligrams of calcium per day from food and supplements combined.

MEAT AND ALTERNATIVES

The foods in this group supply protein, fats, iron, zinc, magnesium, and B vitamins. Although the same players as before remain in Meats and Alternatives—meat, poultry, fish, legumes, nuts, and soy—I am pleased to see that there is somewhat of a de-emphasis on red meat. By recommending other protein-rich foods, the food guide downplays the role of red meat. That's a good thing, since a high intake of fresh and processed red meat is associated with a greater risk of colon cancer and possibly breast cancer.

In light of the wealth of research that fish can reduce the risk of heart attack, the food guide advises consuming 2 servings of low-mercury fish per week. To reduce saturated fat and boost fibre, you're also told to eat beans, lentils, and tofu more often than meat. If you're like many people I see in my private practice, you're probably unsure how to incorporate these meat alternatives into your family's meals. In Chapter 5, I'll tell you plenty of tasty and easy ways to add legumes—and fish—to your diet.

UNSATURATED OILS

The food guides makes a break from previous versions, where all fats were considered bad. Relegated to the "Other Foods" group, we were told to use added fats such as vegetable oils, salad dressings, margarine, and mayonnaise sparingly, if at all. Times have changed. In keeping with our scientific understanding that some fats are actually beneficial to health, Health Canada now recommends adding 2 to 3 tablespoons (25 to 50 ml) of unsaturated fat to your daily diet. You'll learn more about how these healthy fats fight disease—and which ones are my top picks—in Chapter 7.

Eating the right foods, in the right amounts, will help you maintain a healthy weight and have more energy. You'll look better and feel better, too. But the foods that you eat now can also affect your health later in life. Your risk for developing heart disease, stroke, type 2 diabetes, cataract, Alzheimer's, and many cancers can be reduced if you incorporate the right foods into your meals on a regular basis. On the pages that follow, you'll learn how more than 40 foods can help your body fight disease. Instead of telling you which foods to eat less of, I'll tell you which foods you should be eating more of. And you'll find plenty of tips and recipes that will make eating healthfully a pleasure rather than a chore. Now, it's time to introduce you to the world of disease-fighting power foods.

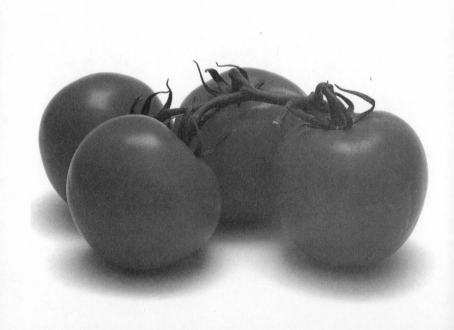

2

Power vegetables

leafy greens

arugula ⋆ beet greens ⋆ collard greens ⋆ dandelion greens ⋆ kale ⋆ mustard greens ⋆ leaf lettuce ⋆ rapini (broccoli raab) ⋆ romaine lettuce ⋆ spinach ⋆ Swiss chard ⋆ turnip greens

cruciferous vegetables

bok choy ⋆ broccoli ⋆ broccoflower ⋆ broccoli sprouts ⋆ broccolini ⋆ Brussels sprouts ⋆ cabbage ⋆ cauliflower ⋆ rutabaga ⋆ turnip

bright orange vegetables

carrots ⋆ sweet potato ⋆ winter squash

tomatoes

ketchup ⋆ fresh red tomatoes ⋆ stewed tomatoes ⋆ tomato juice ⋆ tomato paste ⋆ tomato sauce

allium vegetables

chives ⋆ garlic ⋆ leeks ⋆ onions ⋆ scallions ⋆ shallots

It's no surprise that vegetables are at the top of my list of power foods. Despite all the controversy surrounding the optimal components of a healthy diet, there's little disagreement among scientists regarding the importance of vegetables. Over the past few decades, hundreds of studies have linked eating plenty of vegetables (and fruit) with protection from heart attack, stroke, high blood pressure, type 2 diabetes, certain cancers, and osteoporosis. Research even suggests that boosting your intake of certain vegetables can help preserve your eyesight as you age.

Although eating more vegetables in general is a good thing, some vegetables deserve a special mention. Each of the power vegetables discussed in this chapter has been demonstrated in scientific studies to lower the risk of certain diseases. Each contains unique nutrients and/or phytochemicals believed to help the body ward off disease. In the sections that follow, you'll learn why each power vegetable is an important addition to your family's diet. As well, I'll give you plenty of tips and recipes to help you add them to breakfast, lunch, dinner, and snacks, since, if you're like many Canadians, you're not eating enough of these power foods to reap their health benefits.

According to the latest research, Canadians of most ages eat fewer than 5 servings of vegetables and fruit each day. Fifty percent of adults and 70% of kids age 4 to 8 don't consume 5 daily servings—a habit that's likely to limit your intake of important nutrients, such as folate (a B vitamin), vitamins C and A, potassium, magnesium, and dietary fibre.[1] The new version of Canada's Food Guide advises adults to consume 7 to 10 servings of vegetables and fruit each day. In other words, the daily minimum servings have been raised from 5 to 7.

Despite being told repeatedly the benefits of eating more vegetables, why do so many of us miss the mark? For starters, some people just don't like vegetables. I've met many adults and kids in my private practice whose intake is limited because they don't like the taste or texture of vegetables.

When it comes to children, parents need to start introducing vegetables in the diet early. By the time kids get into preschool and are exposed to the world of junk food, their tastes are already shaped. It's important for parents to lead by example (kids needs to see their parents eating greens too!), and try and try again. Research has demonstrated that a child might have to try a food as many as 15 times before liking it.

That goes for adults, too. If you turn your nose up at spinach yet haven't eaten it for years, it's time to give it another try. Prepare vegetables using different flavourings and cooking methods. For instance, add spinach leaves to an Asian-flavoured stir-fry, toss a handful of baby spinach into pasta sauce, or eat a spinach salad with slices of strawberry or mandarin orange segments. You might be surprised to learn that you actually do enjoy spinach, as long as it's not boiled like your mother used to serve it.

Second, vegetables aren't the most convenient food. Unless you are eating them raw, vegetables need to be washed, peeled, chopped, and then cooked. When you're pressed for time, it's much easier to throw an apple into your lunch bag or briefcase than it is to prepare a baggie of carrot and red pepper sticks. We're more likely to snack on a granola bar than pour a glass of tomato juice or vegetable cocktail.

If you're like many people I know, you probably do a better job of eating vegetables at dinner. Most of my clients manage to include at least 1 vegetable serving in their evening meal, be it a green salad, steamed broccoli, or carrots. But if you forgo vegetables until the end of the day, you won't get enough.

Perhaps the reason your diet is short of vegetables is because you think that 7 to 10 servings is a large amount of food. How is it possible to eat so many vegetables and fruit in a day? In fact, a serving size isn't that large. You're probably eating 2 servings when you think you're only eating 1 serving. One vegetable serving is the equivalent of 1/2 cup (125 ml) of raw or cooked vegetables, 1/2 cup (125 ml) of cooked or 1 cup (250 ml) of raw leafy vegetables, or 1/2 cup (125 ml) 100% of vegetable juice.

Unfortunately, you can't take vitamin supplements to make up for a diet that's lacking vegetables. Although studies provide consistent evidence that diets high in vegetables guard against certain diseases, clinical trials have not shown that using high doses of individual nutrients have the same result. Along with vitamins, minerals, and dietary fibre, vegetables contain thousands of biologically active phytochemicals that are thought to interact with one another in numerous ways to keep you healthy.

The mix of vitamin C, folate, potassium, fibre, and phytochemicals likely contributes to the heart healthy effects of vegetables (and fruit). The fibre and magnesium in produce may enhance your blood sugar control and reduce your future risk of developing type 2 diabetes. The interaction of two phytochemicals in leafy greens, called lutein and zeaxanthin, is thought to guard against age-related eye diseases.

Strategies to increase your daily vegetable intake

PLAN AHEAD

The best way to take advantage of these disease-fighting interactions is to incorporate vegetables into most of your meals. With a little planning and the help of prepared produce in the grocery store, eating your 7 to 10 daily servings of vegetables and fruit is a breeze. The key is mapping out a plan to incorporate vegetables and fruit into all your meals.

You can easily bump up your vegetable intake by eating more—why stop at 1/2 cup (125 ml) of stir-fried vegetables when you can enjoy 1 cup (250 ml) and get 2 vegetable servings? Use the road map below to help you eat more vegetables.

Eat more veggies

Breakfast	Include 1 vegetable serving—optional (e.g., spinach or red pepper in an omelet, a small glass of carrot or other vegetable juice with whole-grain toast).
Snacks	Have raw vegetable sticks handy to munch on between meals. Prepare them in advance to save time during the day. Try baby carrots, red pepper sticks, broccoli florets, zucchini slices, and cherry tomatoes.
Lunch	Include 1 to 2 vegetable servings (e.g., tomato juice, spinach leaves in a sandwich, a handful of baby carrots, a bowl of vegetable soup, green salad).
Dinner	Include at least 2 different vegetables servings (e.g., carrots and broccoli, mixed vegetable stir-fry, tomato sauce with spinach served over pasta).

THINK CONVENIENCE

If scrubbing, peeling, and chopping isn't your thing, take advantage of convenient pre-prepped produce sold at the grocery store. You'll find ready-to-eat salads, carrot sticks, broccoli florets, chopped celery, sliced onions, chopped garlic, stir-fry vegetables, shredded cabbage, grated carrot, triple-washed fresh spinach, even cubed turnip and squash.

Packaged, ready-to-eat vegetables are big time savers. But they can also be potential sources of food poisoning, since these foods are subject to more handling before they make it into your fridge, and because they're often eaten raw (most harmful bacteria are killed by cooking to a high temperature).

Over the past decade, contaminated spinach, cabbage, alfalfa sprouts, lettuce, and parsley have been traced to food poisoning outbreaks. Vegetables and fruits can become contaminated if they're handled by people already infected or if they come into contact with animal manure or contaminated irrigation water or soil. Improper food handling can also cross-contaminate, inadvertently transferring harmful bacteria from one food to another.

Practice safe food handling

You can't see or smell bacteria, so there are no clues to food contaminated with harmful bacteria. The only way to guard against food-borne illness—from any food—is to handle them safely:

- Always wash your hands (for at least 20 seconds), utensils, and cooking surfaces with soap and hot water before handling food, repeatedly while preparing food, and again once you've finished.
- Choose fresh-cut or ready-to-eat produce that is refrigerated or surrounded by ice.
- To prevent cross-contamination, separate fresh produce from raw foods such as meat and poultry in your grocery cart, your shopping bag, and at home in your fridge.
- Thoroughly wash fresh vegetables and fruit under cold running water before eating, preparing, or cutting.
- Scrub produce that has a firm surface (e.g., oranges, potatoes, carrots, squash, and melons) even if you don't intend to eat the skin or rind—

improperly washed produce can become contaminated during cutting. Cut away damaged or bruised areas, since harmful bacteria can thrive in these places.

- Don't eat sprouts—mung bean, alfalfa, broccoli, radish, and clover—raw. Salmonella or E. coli bacteria can lodge into tiny seed cracks; they then flourish in the humid sprouting conditions. Cook sprouts in stir-fries or soups rather than eating them raw in a sandwich or salad.

Which is best: fresh, frozen, or canned vegetables?

Using frozen and canned vegetables are both time-saving ways to incorporate more vegetables into your diet. When I suggest to my clients that they try frozen vegetables, I often get a strange look—how could frozen vegetables possibly be as healthy as fresh? Many people think that fresh vegetables beat out frozen and canned varieties when it comes to nutrition. This may be true regarding sodium, but it's not always the case for vitamins and minerals.

So-called "fresh" produce may not be as fresh as you think. By the time fresh vegetables travel from farm to supermarket to your dinner plate, 2 or 3 weeks may have passed, during which time nutrients are lost. The freshest vegetables are often to be found at your local farmer's market, since the time between harvesting and retailing is reduced.

Research from the University of Illinois found that many canned and frozen vegetables (and fruits) rival or outshine fresh as a source of vitamins and minerals. That's because processing and packaging takes place almost immediately after harvest, locking in more nutrients. And with today's growing trend to convenient meal solutions, there are more frozen and canned vegetable options to choose from in the grocery store. If you've never liked the taste or texture of frozen vegetables, I suggest you try one of the premium brands, such as Europe's Best. If you're like many of my clients, you'll find it hard to believe you're eating vegetables that have been frozen. Their taste and texture is as close to fresh as you'll find.

Canned vegetables do pose a nutritional problem: sodium. For instance, 1/2 cup (125 ml) of canned green peas, drained, has 226 milligrams of sodium, roughly 15% of most people's daily requirement. That might not sound like a lot in the whole scheme of things, but sodium numbers quickly add up. Plus, vegetables weren't intended to come with a dash of salt; they're naturally sodium-free.

Don't get me wrong. It's better to eat canned vegetables than no vegetables at all. And canned produce is easier on your wallet, too. Look for low-sodium or sodium-free brands in the grocery store. With consumers' heightened awareness of diet and health, food manufacturers are slowly starting to decrease the sodium content of processed foods. If you can't find "no salt added" canned vegetables or a low-sodium version, drain and rinse the vegetables before cooking to remove most of the sodium.

Which is best: organic, conventional, or locally grown vegetables?

Many people wonder if organic produce is better for you than conventionally grown vegetables and fruit. Simply stated, for produce to be certified organic, it cannot be grown with synthetic pesticides, fertilizers, food additives, or sewage sludge, and it can't be genetically modified or irradiated.

But whether eating organic food is more nutritious or helps ward off cancer is under debate. Studies have found certain organic crops to contain more vitamin C, iron, magnesium, and phosphorus than their conventional counterparts. But most experts feel the slight increase isn't enough to make a discernible difference to health. Preliminary research also suggests that some organic produce contains higher levels of polyphenols, natural compounds thought to have anti-cancer properties.

Many people choose organic fruits and vegetables as a way of limiting exposure to pesticide residues. The concern is that consuming pesticide residues on conventionally grown produce may increase one's risk of cancer. Studies conducted in the United States have found that organic foods contain fewer and generally lower levels of pesticide residues than conventionally grown foods. (Most of the residues on organic foods are the result of environmental contamination by past pesticide use on the farm or by sprays blown from nearby non-organic farms.) Research has also revealed that adults and children who consume organic foods have lower levels of pesticides in their bodies.

Yet, the potential health risks from consuming pesticide residues from foods have not been established. In 1997, a review from the National Cancer Institute of Canada concluded that pesticide residues from vegetables and fruit do not pose an increased risk of cancer.[2] In fact, as mentioned earlier, hundreds of studies show that eating plenty of vegetables and fruit reduces, rather than increases, the risk of many cancers.

But not everyone needs proof that organic foods are healthier for you to justify buying them. When it comes to synthetic chemical residues in foods—pesticides, hormones, and antibiotics—many people feel it's better to be safe than sorry. It's taken on faith that consuming fewer chemical residues translates into a lower health risk. Some people don't want to wait around to find out if long-term exposure to pesticide residues does in fact increase cancer risk. This is especially true of many women and parents of young children; some scientists and watchdog groups worry that pregnant and breastfeeding women, infants, and young children may be more vulnerable to the harmful effects of pesticide residues, especially during critical periods of development. If you want fewer pesticides in your body—and in the environment—organic foods are a better choice over produce grown by conventional means. There's little argument that organic farming is better for the environment. And in my opinion, that's the underlying point of organic agriculture—to produce foods in a way that encourages soil and water conservation and reduces pollution. Organic farms don't release synthetic chemicals into the environment (some of which harm wildlife), they use less energy, and they produce less waste.

In some cases, organic may not be the best choice, from an environmental perspective. Some people prefer buying locally grown food rather than organic food that's been produced far away. Buying local simply means buying food grown or raised as close to your home as possible. As the distance food travels from the farm to your fork increases, so does the use of fossil fuels to refrigerate and transport that food, and the release of pollutants into the atmosphere. Plus, buying locally grown food usually means you're getting food at its prime—it will be fresher and taste better.

The organic-versus-local debate is certainly gaining momentum among people who consider how their food purchases impact the environment. Depending on what part of the country you live in, or the time of year, it may not be possible to buy organic food that's locally grown. If you're faced with the choice of buying a bag of organic spinach grown in California or non-organic locally grown spinach, you'll need to make a decision. And that decision will depend on what's most important to you.

LEAFY GREENS

arugula ★ beet greens ★ collard greens ★ dandelion greens ★ kale ★ leaf lettuce ★ mustard greens ★ rapini (broccoli raab) ★ romaine lettuce ★ spinach ★ Swiss chard ★ turnip greens

Eat at least 1 serving per day
1 serving = 1/2 cup (125 ml) cooked *or* 1 cup (250 ml) raw

When you hear the phrase *leafy green vegetables,* chances are you picture a head of lettuce. And you're right, some types of lettuce are included in this category, such as romaine and leaf lettuce, but you also need to think kale, Swiss chard, collard greens, mustard greens, and rapini—those strange looking vegetables you never buy because you're not sure how to cook them, let alone eat them. Even many grocery store clerks have a hard time identifying them.

Leafy greens are those plant leaves that we eat as vegetables. With some—for instance, Swiss chard and beet greens—the tender stalks can also be eaten. Although there are many types of leafy greens, most share common nutritional benefits. If you don't regularly include leafy greens in your diet, there are plenty of reasons why you should start eating them more often.

Nutrition powerhouses

When it comes to vitamins, minerals, and disease-fighting chemicals, leafy green vegetables are hard to beat. Leafy greens are low in calories, virtually fat-free, high in fibre, and a good source of vitamins A, C, and K, folate (a B vitamin), iron, calcium, and potassium. What's more, they're an exceptional source of phytochemicals, including beta carotene, lutein, and zeaxanthin.

Consider that 1/2 cup (125 ml) of cooked kale packs more than four times your daily vitamin K and half a day's worth of vitamin A, along with generous amounts of vitamin C and potassium—all for only 18 calories. Here's how leafy greens stack up in terms of their nutrient content.

Notable nutrients in leafy green vegetables

Per 1/2 cup (125 ml) serving, cooked, unless otherwise noted

	Calories	Vit. A (mcg)	Vit. C (mg)	Vit. K (mcg)	Folate (mcg)
Arugula, raw, 1 cup (250 ml)	5	25	3	0	20
Beet, greens	21	291	19	368	11
Beet greens, raw, 1 cup (250 ml)	9	127	12	161	6
Collard greens	26	408	18	442	93
Dandelion greens	18	275	10	108	7
Dandelion greens, raw, 1 cup (250 ml)	26	144	20	159	16
Kale	19	468	28	561	9
Leaf lettuce, raw, 1 cup (250 ml)	9	219	11	103	22
Mustard greens	11	234	19	221.5	54
Rapini	22	150	24.5	169	47
Romaine lettuce, raw, 1 cup (250 ml)	10	172	14	61	80
Spinach	22	498	9.3	469	139
Spinach, raw, 1 cup (250 ml)	7	149	9.0	153	61
Swiss chard	18	283	16.6	303	8
Turnip greens	15	290	21	280	90

	Calcium (mg)	Magnesium (mg)	Iron (mg)	Potassium (mcg)
Arugula, raw, 1 cup (250 ml)	34	10	0.3	78
Beet greens	87	52	1.5	692
Beet greens, raw, 1 cup (250 ml)	47	28	1.0	306
Collard greens	141	20	1.2	116
Dandelion greens	78	13	1.0	129
Dandelion greens, raw, 1 cup (250 ml)	109	21	1.8	231
Kale	49	12	0.6	157
Leaf lettuce, raw, 1 cup (250 ml)	21	8	0.5	115
Mustard greens	55	11	0.6	149
Rapini	78	18	0.85	227
Romaine lettuce, raw, 1 cup (250 ml)	20	8	0.6	146
Spinach	129	83	3.4	443
Spinach, raw, 1 cup (250 ml)	31	25	0.9	177
Swiss chard	54	80	2.1	508
Turnip greens	104	17	0.6	154

Source: Canadian Nutrient File, 2007.

When it comes to cooked vegetables, nutrient databases provide the nutrient numbers after the vegetable has been boiled and drained. I don't know about you, but I rarely boil my vegetables. Nutritional breakdowns are not available for steamed or stir-fried vegetables, they way I prefer to cook my vegetables. Veggies that are steamed, stir-fried, or microwaved will retain more of their vitamin C and folate, meaning these amounts will be higher than those listed above.

Leafy greens and health

LEAFY GREENS AND CANCER PREVENTION

Numerous studies have linked higher intakes of leafy green vegetables with a lower risk of various cancers. The Iowa Women's Health Study followed 41,837 postmenopausal women for 4 years to examine the link between vegetables and fruits and lung cancer. The researchers found that women who consumed the most leafy green vegetables were half as likely to develop lung cancer compared with women whose diets contained the least.[3]

Leafy green vegetables may also guard against gastric (stomach) cancer. In a large study of Swedish men and women, those who consumed at least 3 servings of green leafy vegetables each week were 36% less likely to be diagnosed with gastric cancer than were adults who ate less than half a serving per week.[4]

A steady diet of leafy greens might also offer protection against ovarian cancer. A report from the Iowa Women's Health Study, in which 29,083 women age 55 to 69 years were followed for 10 years, found that, compared with women who consumed few leafy green vegetables, those whose diets provided the most were 56% less likely to develop ovarian cancer.[5]

It's thought that vegetables work best at fighting cancers that involve epithelial cells, the cells that line the body's organs. Greens contain vitamins A and C, both of which may reduce the risk of cancer. Vitamin A is necessary for maintaining healthy body tissues, especially epithelial and mucous tissues, the body's first line of defence against invading organisms and toxins. When our vitamin A levels are low, we are much more susceptible to infection. As one of the best-known immune-enhancing and antioxidant nutrients, vitamin C is vital to a healthy immune system and neutralizing harmful free radicals.

Free radicals are essentially unstable oxygen molecules that our bodies create every day as a consequence of normal metabolism. Pollution and cigarette smoke increase the number of free radicals our bodies are exposed to. If free radical production overwhelms the body's built-in antioxidant system, cellular damage can occur that may lead to cancer.

Researchers have also found that certain phytochemicals in leafy greens called carotenoids (compounds closely related to vitamin A) can inhibit the growth of certain types of breast cancer cells, skin cancer cells, lung cancer, and stomach cancer.

Folate may also play a role in the anti-cancer properties of leafy greens. The body needs folate when it makes DNA (the genetic material of our cells), and folate is also involved in repairing DNA when it develops mistakes. Too little folate may increase the risk of cancers of the colon, rectum, and breast, especially in people who drink alcohol. There's good evidence from animals susceptible to cancer that giving them folate reduces their risk. In humans, populations with high dietary folate intakes seem to be at lower risk of colon cancer.

LEAFY GREENS AND HEART HEALTH

Eating more leafy greens might also ward off heart attack and stroke. A recent report in the *Journal of the National Cancer Institute* revealed that total vegetable and fruit intake was linked with a reduced risk of heart disease, with green leafy vegetables offering the most protection. For every serving of leafy greens consumed per day, risk of heart disease decreased by 11%.[6] Similarly, research from the Harvard School of Public Health revealed that leafy green vegetables are good for the heart. The scientists followed 84,251 women and 42,148 men for 14 and 8 years respectively, and found that eating 1 daily serving of green leafy vegetables reduced the risk of heart disease by 23%.[7]

The same researchers investigated the effect of vegetables and fruit on the risk of ischemic stroke in this large group of men and women. (An ischemic stroke is caused by a blocked blood vessel supplying the brain.) They found that people who averaged 3 to 5 servings of vegetables and fruit per day had a 30% lower risk of ischemic stroke compared with folks who ate fewer than 3 daily servings. What's more, leafy green vegetables offered strong protection: Eating 1 serving per day reduced the risk of stroke by 21%.[8]

LEAFY GREENS AND EYESIGHT

Your eyes can benefit from eating leafy green veggies, too. Leafy greens contain lutein and zeaxanthin, two phytochemicals that when consumed make their way to the eye, where they protect both the retina and the lens from oxidative damage. Studies have found that people who get the most lutein from their diet have a 20% to 50% lower risk of cataract or needing cataract extraction surgery compared with people who consume the least.[9]

A cataract is a clouding of the eye lens, affecting vision. In a healthy eye, light passes through the transparent lens to the retina. Once it reaches the retina, light is changed into nerve signals that are sent to the brain. The lens must be clear for the retina to receive a sharp image. If the lens is cloudy from a cataract, the image will be blurred. Cataracts occur when some of the proteins in the lens clump together in a small area of the lens. Risk factors include cigarette smoking, diabetes, aging, and poor nutrition.

A diet that contains lutein-rich leafy greens might even forestall age-related macular degeneration, the leading cause of blindness in older adults. Age-related macular degeneration (AMD) is a disease that attacks the macula, the central part of the retina that controls fine, detailed vision. The condition results in progressive loss of visual sharpness, making it difficult to drive a car, read a book, and recognize faces. AMD affects more than two million Canadians over the age of 50 and is the leading cause of severe vision loss in older adults.

In the macula, lutein acts as a filter, protecting structures of the eye from the damaging effects of the sun's ultraviolet light. Lutein contributes to the density, or thickness, of the macula—the denser the macula, the better it can absorb incoming light. Indeed, experimental research has shown that adding spinach to one's daily diet can increase the density of the macula within 4 weeks, suggesting it can prevent AMD.[10]

The exact cause of AMD is unclear, but factors such as family history, cigarette smoking, high blood pressure, excessive sunlight exposure, obesity, and a diet low in antioxidants are linked with a greater risk of developing the disease. Antioxidants are thought to protect cells in the retina from the harmful effects of free radicals, unstable molecules formed from cigarette smoke, pollution, and ultraviolet light.

Scientists speculate that an intake of 6 to 15 milligrams of lutein plus zeaxanthin per day is optimal for eye health. Besides leafy greens, you'll also get lutein from green peas, broccoli, Brussels sprouts, nectarines, and oranges. I'm afraid you can't rely on a multivitamin with added lutein to get your daily dose—most provide no more than 0.5 milligrams per daily dose.

Lutein and zeaxanthin content of selected leafy green vegetables (milligrams)

Per 1/2 cup (125 ml) serving, cooked, unless otherwise noted	
Spinach, frozen	14.9
Kale	11.9
Spinach	10.2
Collard greens	7.3
Turnip greens	6.1
Mustard greens	4.2
Dandelion greens	2.5
Spinach, raw, 1 cup (250 ml)	1.8
Beet greens	1.3
Romaine lettuce, raw, 1 cup (250 ml)	1.3
Leaf lettuce, raw, 1 cup (250 ml)	1.0

Source: U.S. Department of Agriculture, Agricultural Research Service. 2006. USDA Nutrient Database for Standard Reference, Release 19. Nutrient Data Laboratory home page, www.ars.usda.gov/nutrientdata.

LEAFY GREENS AND BONE HEALTH

If you need another reason to eat your greens, it's this: They're good for your bones, thanks to their sizeable vitamin K content. Research from the Human Nutrition Center on Aging at Tufts University in Massachusetts revealed that, compared with women who consumed the most vitamin K, those whose diets provided the least had significantly lower bone density in the spine and femoral neck, the upper part of the thigh bone.[11]

Since having a low bone density is a risk factor for osteoporosis and hip fracture, it's logical to suspect that getting too little vitamin K might lead to bone fracture. Sure enough, findings from two studies suggest that this is the case. The Nurses' Health Study (an ongoing study following 121,700 female nurses) found that women who consumed higher amounts of vitamin K (150 to 250 micrograms per day) had a 30% lower risk of hip

fracture compared with their peers who consumed fewer than 109 micrograms daily. What's more, a woman's risk of hip fracture was also tied to
how much lettuce she ate, the food that contributed the most vitamin K in
this study. Compared with women who ate 1 or fewer servings per week,
those who enjoyed lettuce at least once daily were 45% less likely to
experience a hip fracture.[12] A study of elderly men and women also
reported that low vitamin K intakes were associated with a greater risk of
hip fracture.[13]

Most of us don't get enough vitamin K in our diet. The recommended
daily intake of vitamin K is 90 and 120 micrograms, for women and men
respectively. This amount is designed to help our blood clot, not protect
our bones. Scientists speculate it takes about 200 micrograms per day to
protect bones from thinning. As you'll see, all it takes is 1 serving per day
of leafy greens to get plenty of bone-building vitamin K.

Vitamin K content of selected leafy green vegetables (micrograms)

Per 1/2 cup (125 ml) serving, cooked, unless otherwise noted	
Kale	531
Spinach, frozen	514
Spinach	444
Collard greens	418
Beet greens	349
Turnip greens	265
Mustard greens	210
Spinach, raw, 1 cup (250 ml)	144
Dandelion greens	102
Leaf lettuce, raw, 1 cup (250 ml)	97
Romaine lettuce, raw, 1 cup (250 ml)	57

Source: U.S. Department of Agriculture, Agricultural Research Service. 2006. USDA Nutrient
Database for Standard Reference, Release 19. Nutrient Data Laboratory Home Page,
www.ars.usda.gov/nutrientdata.

LEAFY GREENS AND MEMORY

A daily serving of leafy greens might also keep your mind sharp as you age. According to researchers from the Rush Institute for Healthy Aging in Chicago, adding a few servings of vegetables to your dinner plate can help keep your brain young and slow mental decline.

Age-related cognitive decline is considered by many experts to be a normal consequence of getting older—it's the subtle decline over time in memory and thinking processes that affects most people. (For some older adults, however, cognitive declines go beyond what's considered normal and can progress to mild cognitive impairment or dementia.) Risk factors for cognitive decline include hypertension, diabetes, cigarette smoking, and lack of exercise—both physical and mental.

In the Chicago Health and Aging Study, researchers asked 3718 healthy men and women, age 65 years and older, about their diet and tested their short-term and delayed memory three times over a 6-year period. Those who ate more than 2 servings of vegetables each day experienced a 40% decrease in cognitive decline compared with those who ate fewer than 1 serving per day—a result expected in people 5 years younger. The study found all types of vegetables protective, especially zucchini, eggplant, broccoli, lettuce, tossed salad, and—you guessed it—leafy greens, such as kale and collards.[14]

This isn't the first study to link vegetables to improved brainpower. In 2005, researchers from Harvard Medical School reported that, among 13,388 women, those who consumed the most vegetables, especially leafy greens, experienced slower cognitive decline than those who ate the least.[15]

Scientists attribute the protective effect of vegetables to vitamin E, an antioxidant nutrient that's more abundant in vegetables—especially leafy greens—than in fruit. Vegetables are also often cooked or eaten with fats, such as salad dressing, margarine, and vegetable oil, which help the body absorb vitamin E and other antioxidants, including beta carotene and flavonoids.

Vitamin E is thought to protect brain cells from damage caused by free radicals. The brain is especially vulnerable to free radical damage because of its high demand for oxygen, its abundance of easily oxidized cell membranes, and its weak antioxidant defences.

Enjoying leafy green vegetables

Buying

When shopping, select greens that are fresh, tender, and have brightly coloured leaves. There should be no signs of yellowing or browning. Avoid greens with wilted leaves, discoloured edges, blemishes, or slimy spots. Generally, small leaves will be more tender and have a milder flavour than larger leaves. Leafy greens should have a sweet, fresh smell. If they smell sour, don't buy them.

Washing and storing

Once home, remove any rubber bands or ties from the leaves. If you see any discoloured or damaged leaves, remove them. Leafy greens can be stored washed or unwashed, but they must be dried thoroughly before storing. If greens are stored wet, the excess moisture will cause them to deteriorate faster. (Also, wet greens make for a soggy salad and affect the consistency of the dressing when added.)

Greens need to be washed thoroughly. Some greens, including collards and spinach, tend to collect sand and soil. Before washing, trim off the roots and separate the leaves. Place the greens in a sink or large bowl filled with tepid water, swish around, and then lift out. The dirt and sand will have settled to the bottom of the sink or bowl. Empty the sink or bowl, and fill with clean water. Repeat the washing process—usually it will take two or three times—until all the grit is rinsed away.

If you prefer, you can wash the greens in a salad spinner instead of the sink. When spinning greens dry, don't place too many in the spinner at one time, so as to allow the greens to dry faster and prevent them from crushing each other. Larger leaves can be washed by holding under cold running water. Unfold any folded leaves to remove all the dirt.

Once washed, dry greens with a paper towel, blotting excess water. They're now ready to use or be stored in the refrigerator crisper. If you're not going to use them right away, wrap the greens in small batches in dry paper towel and place in resealable plastic bags, or, better yet, perforated vegetable bags, which allow greens to breathe.

Greens will keep anywhere from 3 days to 1 week, depending on the type. Delicate greens such as arugula, spinach, and dandelion will spoil more quickly than kale, collards, and rapini, which have sturdier leaves.

Preparing and cooking

Most leafy greens can be eaten fresh, in salads. Greens with larger leaves, such as romaine lettuce, kale, and collard greens, can be wrapped around other ingredients, similar to a tortilla. All leafy greens can also be cooked, using various methods: blanching, braising, sautéing, steaming, even microwaving. Or add them to stir-fries, pasta sauces, stews, and soups.

Cooking greens actually makes them more nutritious than when raw. That's because leafy greens contain oxalates, natural compounds that bind tightly to calcium and iron. Cooking greens releases their minerals from oxalates, making them more available for absorption in your gastrointestinal tract. Just don't overcook your greens. Overcooking leafy greens will reduce their vitamin C and folate content, not to mention make them taste bitter. Green vegetables are overcooked if they turn an olive green colour. Delicate leafy greens require only a few minutes to cook.

Whichever cooking method you choose, use the liquid that's left over to make sauces or add extra flavour and nutrients to soups, stews, and pasta sauces. Keep in mind that greens shrink considerably when cooked, often to less than half their volume. Three cups (750 ml) of fresh greens can easily be reduced down to 1 or 2 cups (250 to 500 ml) depending on the green.

Here's a guide to cooking leafy greens:

Blanching

A method by which food is plunged into boiling water briefly, then into cold water to stop the cooking process. Blanching is used to soften the texture of some greens and provide a flavour less pungent or bitter than when raw. It's also used to heighten and set colour and flavour before freezing vegetables.

A recipe may call for greens to be blanched before the main cooking method, for example, sautéing. Greens that benefit from blanching include kale, collard greens, mustard greens, turnip greens, and rapini. More delicate greens such as spinach and arugula don't need blanching.

To blanch, bring water to boil in a large pot. Add greens to the boiling water and cooked for 1 to 5 minutes, or until greens have wilted. Remove from heat and drain. Allow greens to cool before squeezing the moisture from them. If they're not going to be used immediately, rinse them under cold running water and squeeze out any excess moisture.

Braising

A method by which food is cooked, tightly covered, in a small amount of liquid at low heat for a lengthy period. The long, slow cooking develops flavour and tenderizes leafy greens by gently breaking down their fibres. Braising can be done on the stovetop or in the oven.

Head-type greens (kale, Swiss chard, collard greens) may benefit from being blanched for 2 minutes before being braised. To braise, placed greens in a skillet and add broth until the greens are almost covered. Add onion, garlic, or your favourite herbs and spices. Cover the skillet and cook at a simmer for 10 to 20 minutes or until tender. To make a sauce to serve with the greens, boil the cooking liquid left in the pan until most of the liquid evaporates.

Sautéing

Using this method, greens are cooked quickly in a small amount of oil in a skillet or sauté pan over direct heat. (Nonstick pans will require less oil than other pans.) To sauté, add greens to heated oil. Other flavourings, such as garlic, onions, and red chili peppers, can be sautéed with the greens. Sauté for 3 to 10 minutes, stirring constantly. Remove from pan and serve while hot.

Steaming

Using this method, greens are cooked with water in a covered pan, or on a rack or in a metal or bamboo steamer basket over boiling or simmering water in a covered pan. Steaming does a better job than boiling of retaining many of the vitamins in greens. Steaming is also superior to microwaving when it comes to preserving antioxidants called flavonoids. To maximize nutrient retention, add vegetables to the steamer basket after the water has started steaming, cover the pot, and then cook until tender crisp, not soft.

If steaming in a pan, wash but do not dry greens. The water that remains on the greens will often be enough to steam them. Place greens in a heavy pan. For larger, firmer greens (kale, collards, Swiss chard), cover bottom of the pan with 1/4 to 1/2 inch (5 mm to 2.5 cm) of water. You could also put the greens in a steamer basket or on a rack. Cover and simmer the water over low heat until the greens are wilted. Cooking time will vary from 2 to 10 minutes, depending on the size and toughness of the greens.

Microwaving

This method cooks with high-frequency radio waves that cause food molecules to vibrate, creating friction that heats and cooks the food. Because microwaves travel so fast, foods cook quickly. To microwave, clean but don't dry the greens. Place wet greens in a microwave-safe dish, add 2 to 4 tablespoons (15 to 50 ml) of water, and cover. Microwave on high for 2 minutes or until tender.

It's easy to make a salad of romaine lettuce, leaf lettuce, or arugula. And you're probably pretty familiar with adding spinach to meals. But it's time to be adventurous and add variety—and nutrition—to your meals. The following tips will help you incorporate those not-so-familiar greens you often pass by in the grocery store. I've also noted the delicious recipes for many of these greens that you'll find in the Recipes That Fight Disease section of this book.

★ COLLARD GREENS

To prepare, remove the leaves from the stalk, then chop the leaves. Collard greens taste best when they're sautéed. But you can also add this green to soups, tomato-based pasta sauces, and stir-fries.

TIPS FOR ADDING COLLARD GREENS TO YOUR MEALS

- Drizzle sautéed collard greens with extra-virgin olive oil and freshly squeezed lemon juice.
- Add blanched collard greens to a chicken and vegetable stir-fry.
- Serve steamed collard greens with black-eyed peas and brown rice for a Southern-inspired dish.
- Sauté collard greens with cubes of firm tofu, garlic, and crushed red chili peppers for a spicy vegetarian meal.
- Add chopped collard greens, along with golden raisins and slivered almonds, to sautéed onion and garlic. Cook for 5 minutes or until tender.

RECIPE
Spicy Sautéed Collard Greens, page 327

★ KALE

Both leaves and stalks can be eaten; however, many recipes call for leaves only. I use a knife to remove the leaves from the stems. Kale leaves are sturdy and hold up well in soups, sauces, and stir-fries.

TIPS FOR ADDING KALE TO YOUR MEALS

- Sauté kale leaves with sliced onion, sliced apple, and a hint of yellow curry paste.
- Sauté kale with fresh garlic and red chili peppers; drizzle with roasted sesame oil just before serving.
- Braise chopped kale and apple. Before serving, sprinkle with balsamic vinegar and chopped walnuts.
- Combine chopped kale (blanched or steamed), pine nuts, sun-dried tomatoes, and feta cheese with whole-wheat pasta. Drizzle with extra-virgin olive oil.
- Stir cooked kale into a pot of garlic mashed potatoes.
- Add raw kale leaves to any soup and simmer until leaves are tender. (I add chopped kale and cubes of firm tofu to hot-and-sour soup from the grocery store, sold fresh in mason jars. When serving, I add a drizzle of Asian hot sauce. It's a tasty—and low calorie—one-dish meal.)
- Toss tender young kale leaves into a salad of mixed greens.
- Add cooked kale to your favourite pasta salad.

RECIPE
Raspberry Grilled Kale, page 324

★ MUSTARD GREENS (CURLY MUSTARD)

In addition to its peppery flavoured leaves, this plant also produces the seeds used to make Dijon mustard. Mustard greens can have either a crumpled or flat texture and may have toothed, scalloped, or frilled edges. To prepare, use a knife to cut the leaves away from the stem. If you're planning to add mustard greens to a soup or stew, keep the leaves intact with the stem.

TIPS FOR ADDING MUSTARD GREENS TO YOUR MEALS

- Add young mustard greens to a mixed green salad.
- Sauté mustard greens with chopped garlic and cashews; serve with a drizzle of roasted sesame oil.
- Add chopped mustard greens to a pasta salad for a peppery kick.
- For a hot pasta dish, add sautéed or steamed mustard greens to cooked pasta along with roasted red peppers, artichoke hearts, pine nuts and goat cheese. Toss with a little extra-virgin olive oil.
- Sauté mustard greens, sweet potatoes, and firm tofu.

★ RAPINI (BROCCOLI RAAB)

The leaves, stems, and flower heads are cooked and eaten just like regular broccoli. Rapini has a flavour similar to broccoli but it is much more pungent and has a slightly bitter taste. Rapini is considered an acquired taste— but once acquired, you'll love it. (Some people prefer to blanch rapini before cooking it or adding it to other dishes.)

To prepare rapini, rinse and trim 1/4 inch (5 mm) from the bottom of the stems. Cut stalks crosswise into 2-inch (5 cm) pieces and drop into salted (optional) boiling water. Blanch for 1 to 2 minutes; remove with a slotted spoon.

TIPS FOR ADDING RAPINI TO YOUR MEALS

- Sauté rapini for 3 to 5 minutes with crushed fresh red chili peppers. Before serving, drizzle with freshly squeezed lemon juice and sprinkle with grated Romano or Parmesan cheese.
- Add sautéed rapini and turkey sausage to a tomato-based pasta sauce.
- Sauté rapini in olive oil and chopped garlic for 3 to 5 minutes until tender. Add crushed dried red pepper flakes to taste. Enjoy as a side dish or add to whole-grain pasta and drizzle with extra-virgin olive oil.
- Sauté rapini with garlic, red chili peppers, and chickpeas for a vegetarian dish.

RECIPE
Pepper and Rapini Sauté, page 323

★ SPINACH

Three types of spinach are commonly available. Smooth-leaf has flat, unwrinkled spade-shaped leaves; Savoy has crisp, creased, curly leaves; while semi-Savoy is similar in texture to Savoy but not as wrinkled. Baby spinach has a slightly sweeter taste than regular spinach and is great for adding to salads. Use spinach leaves in sandwiches or throw into pasta sauces, stir-fries, and soups during the last few minutes of cooking.

TIPS FOR ADDING SPINACH TO YOUR MEALS

- Steam spinach, adding a splash of raspberry vinegar just before serving.
- Add chopped spinach to an omelet for breakfast or for a quick dinner.
- Add layers of steamed spinach to your favourite lasagna.
- Toss fresh baby spinach with walnuts, sliced apples, and red onions for an easy salad.

- Toss fresh spinach with sliced strawberries and mandarin orange segments for a refreshing summer salad. (The vitamin C in the fruit increases the amount of iron your body absorbs from the spinach.)
- For a warm salad, top spinach leaves with sautéed onions and mushrooms. Sprinkle with balsamic vinegar and toasted pine nuts.
- Sauté spinach and top with a drizzle of peanut sauce and crushed peanuts.
- Add spinach leaves to sandwiches and burgers instead of lettuce.
- Top your next homemade or frozen pizza with wilted spinach leaves. (Be sure to squeeze excess moisture from spinach leaves to prevent a soggy crust.)
- Add chopped spinach to pasta sauce at the end of cooking.

RECIPES
Blueberry and Roasted Walnut Spinach Salad, page 288
Garlic Sautéed Spinach, page 318
Spinach with Spicy Peanut Sauce, page 329
Spinach Almond Pesto, page 370

★ SWISS CHARD

This tall leafy green vegetable has thick, crunchy, white, red, or yellow stalks and fanlike green leaves. Both the leaves and the stems are edible, though the stems vary in texture, white stems being the most tender. Red-stemmed chard has a slightly sweeter taste than its white-stemmed cousin.

To prepare, trim the bottom end of the stalk. If you find the stalks too fibrous, make incisions near the base of the stalk and peel away the fibres as you would do with celery. Separate the leaves from the stalks, then chop the stalks. Since the stalks are thicker in texture, they will take longer to cook than the leaves, so starting cooking them a few minutes earlier.

TIPS FOR ADDING SWISS CHARD TO YOUR MEALS
- Stir-fry Swiss chard with canola oil, garlic, and crushed red chili flakes.
- Toss cooked Swiss chard with penne pasta, extra-virgin olive oil, garlic, lemon juice, sun-dried tomatoes, black olives, and grated Parmesan cheese.
- Add steamed Swiss chard to omelets, quiches, and frittatas.
- For variety, use Swiss chard in place of spinach in recipes.
- For a new wave cabbage roll, wrap fresh Swiss chard leaves around your favourite grain and vegetable salad and roll into a small package. Bake at 350°F (180°C) until hot.

RECIPE
Balsamic Swiss Chard, page 313

★ TURNIP GREENS

You've probably eaten turnip root numerous times without giving thought to its leaves. (Turnip, another power vegetable, belongs to the family of cruciferous vegetables, which you'll learn about later in this chapter.) Turnip leaves are smaller and more tender than their cousin, collards. They have a slightly bitter flavour and are a staple of traditional South American cooking.

To prepare, remove the leaves from the stem with a knife. If you plan to cook turnip greens for a length of time, as you would in a soup, there's no need to remove the stem.

TIPS FOR ADDING TURNIP GREENS TO YOUR MEALS

- Season sautéed or steamed turnip greens with freshly squeezed lemon juice and cayenne pepper.
- Sauté turnip greens with cooked lentils (canned, rinsed), onions, and a hint of curry powder.
- Add turnip greens to your favourite vegetable soup.
- Use turnip greens in addition to spinach in any pasta dish.

CRUCIFEROUS VEGETABLES

bok choy ★ broccoflower ★ broccoli ★ broccoli sprouts ★ broccolini ★ Brussels sprouts ★ cabbage ★ cauliflower ★ rutabaga ★ turnip

Eat 3 to 5 servings per week
1 serving = 1/2 cup (125 ml) raw or cooked

Although they differ in colour, size, and shape, broccoli, cauliflower, cabbage, and turnip all come from the same species of plant, *Brassica oleracea*. The cruciferous family of vegetables derives its name from their four-petalled flowers, which looks like a cruciform, or cross. (The word *cruciferous* comes from the Latin word for cross.) Many of the leafy greens I mentioned earlier in this chapter also belong to the cruciferous gang. These include kale, collards, rapini, Swiss chard, turnip greens, mustard greens, and arugula.

Cruciferous vegetables, isothiocynates, and nutrition

Cruciferous vegetables have a strikingly high concentration of the cancer-fighting chemicals known as glucosinolates. When you eat cruciferous vegetables, bacteria in the digestive tract break down the glucosinolates, transforming them into compounds called isothiocynates and indole-3-carbinol. As well, enzymes in cruciferous vegetables convert glucosinolates to isothiocynates and indole-3-carbinol when they're chopped or chewed.

Scientists are learning that isothiocynates are potent protectors against cancer development. They help eliminate cancer-causing substances by regulating the body's detoxification enzymes. Researchers suspect that the various compounds in cruciferous vegetables work together to promote a greater cancer-fighting effect. In other words, taking a supplement that contains just one isothiocynate, like indole-3-carbinol, probably won't do you much good. You're much better off consuming the natural mix of cruciferous chemicals that occurs naturally in vegetables. (Manufacturers' claims that indole-3-carbinol supplements can help prevent breast cancer are based on studies suggesting that indole-3-carbinol in cruciferous vegetables may protect against hormone-responsive tumours, such as breast, ovarian, and prostate cancers.)

Isothiocynates also act as antioxidants by preventing harmful free radicals from damaging the genetic materials of cells—DNA. According to the American Institute for Cancer Research, components of cruciferous vegetables have shown the ability to stop the growth of cancer cells for tumours of the breast, uterine lining (endometrium), cervix, lung, colon, and liver.

You might already be familiar with isothiocynates—one of the best known is sulphoraphane, the phytochemical that's plentiful in broccoli, broccoli sprouts, and kale. More than 125 papers have been published on the anti-cancer properties of sulphoraphane.

Cruciferous vegetables do more than add cancer-fighting isothiocynates to your dinner plate. Many are also exceptional sources of vitamin C and fibre. As an added bonus, cruciferous vegetables also supply vitamin A, folate, calcium, and potassium. Here's a nutrient breakdown of many cruciferous vegetables.

Notable nutrients in selected cruciferous vegetables

Per 1/2 cup (125 ml) serving cooked, unless otherwise noted

	Calories	Vitamin A (mcg)	Vitamin C (mg)	Folate (mcg)	Calcium (mg)	Potassium (mcg)
Bok choy	11	190	23	37	84	333
Broccoli	29	81	54	89	66	241
Brussels sprouts (4 sprouts)	30	33	52	50	30	266
Cabbage, raw	9	3	12	16	17	91
Cauliflower	15	1	29	29	10	93

Source: Canadian Nutrient File, 2007.

Cruciferous vegetables and health

CRUCIFEROUS VEGGIES AND CANCER PREVENTION

Studies suggest that eating more cruciferous vegetables can reduce your risk of several types of cancer. In fact, one review published in 1996 showed that more than 70% of the studies found a link between cruciferous vegetables and protection against cancer.[16] What's more, laboratory research supports this link. A recent Italian study found that juice from different varieties of cauliflower suppressed the growth of cancer cells.[17] Need further convincing before you eat more cruciferous vegetables? Consider these findings:

Breast cancer

Although the results of studies on cruciferous vegetables and breast cancer risk are inconsistent, several case-control studies have revealed that women diagnosed with breast cancer had significantly lower intakes of cruciferous vegetables than their cancer-free controls. (In case-control studies, researchers contact people who have been diagnosed with a disease—the cases—and people who have not—the controls. Both groups are asked about the foods they ate during the years before they were diagnosed with the disease. The objective is to see if the people who are sick were more likely to consume certain foods, or nutrients, than people without the disease.)

Triggered by the observation that breast cancer risk of Polish women rose threefold after they immigrated to the United States, scientists from Michigan State University recently evaluated the diets of Polish immigrant women living in Chicago and Detroit. They found that women who ate at least 3 servings of raw or lightly cooked cabbage and sauerkraut per week had a significantly lower risk of breast cancer compared with those who ate only 1 serving. Interestingly, cabbage cooked a long time had no bearing on breast cancer risk.[18]

Lung cancer

When it comes to lung cancer and cruciferous vegetables, the study findings are mixed. A number of case-control studies have shown that people with lung cancer eat fewer cruciferous vegetables than people without the disease. Two studies that followed large groups of healthy men and women for several years linked a higher cruciferous vegetable intake (3 or more servings per week) with strong protection from lung cancer.[19] Yet, other research has found no protective effects of cruciferous vegetables.

Why the inconsistency? It turns out that your genetic profile might make you more or less likely to reap the cancer-protective effects of cruciferous vegetables. Scientists have determined two genes that eliminate isothiocynates from the body. It stands to reason that people who have inactive forms of these genes would have higher concentrations of isothiocynates because of their reduced elimination capacity. After further investigation, scientists have found that people with inactive forms of the genes are indeed less likely to develop lung cancer. What's more, several studies have found that consumption of cruciferous vegetables had a much more pronounced protective effect against lung cancer in people who have inactive forms of these genes.[20]

Prostate cancer

When the diets of more than 1619 men with prostate cancer were compared with that of 1619 men free of the disease, researchers learned that cruciferous vegetables (and yellow-orange vegetables) were protective against prostate cancer, especially advanced forms of the disease. The study revealed that, compared with men who consumed the least, men whose diets included the most cruciferous vegetables were 39% less likely to have prostate cancer.[21]

Bladder cancer

When asked which types of cancer pose the greatest threat to men's lives, most don't think about bladder cancer. Yet, it's the fourth most commonly diagnosed cancer among Canadian men, after prostate, lung, and colorectal. In a study tracking 47,900 males over a 10-year period, researchers from Harvard School of Public Health found that eating cruciferous vegetables was effective at lowering bladder cancer risk. Just 1/2 cup (125 ml) of cabbage or two 1/2-cup (125 ml) servings of broccoli per week reduced the risk by 44%, compared with those who ate less than 1 serving of either vegetable per week.[22]

Pancreatic cancer

In a study of 81,922 men and women in Sweden, researchers found a significant association between the risk of pancreatic cancer and cruciferous vegetable intake. Compared with those who ate less than 1 serving per week, individuals who consumed cruciferous vegetables at least three times each week were 30% less likely to develop pancreatic cancer. Cabbage was found to be especially protective against pancreatic cancer. Eating at least 1 serving per week versus none reduced the risk by 38%.[23]

Non-Hodgkin lymphoma

It appears that a regular intake of cruciferous vegetables might guard against non-Hodgkin lymphoma, a group of cancers that affect the body's lymphatic system. (The lymphatic system is a network of channels and glands that help the body fight infection and protect it from disease.) When researchers from Harvard School of Public Health in Boston followed 88,410 healthy women for 14 years, they determined that eating more fruits and vegetables in general was clearly linked with protection from the cancer. When it came to cruciferous vegetables, women who consumed at least 5 servings per week were 33% less likely to develop non-Hodgkin lymphoma compared with those who ate fewer than 2 servings per week.[24]

CRUCIFEROUS VEGETABLES AND STROKE PREVENTION

Diets rich in cruciferous vegetables may also help guard against cardiovascular disease. One study that followed 75,596 women and 38,683 men for

8 to 14 years revealed that eating 1 daily 1/2 cup (125 ml) serving of cruciferous vegetables conferred a 32% lower risk of ischemic stroke.[25] (An ischemic stroke occurs when an artery carrying oxygen-rich blood to the brain is blocked. If the artery remains blocked for more than a few minutes, the brain cells may die.)

It's thought that eating plenty of cruciferous vegetables helps lower markers of inflammation in the body. Elevated inflammatory markers signal an elevated risk of cardiovascular disease.

Enjoying cruciferous vegetables

COOKING CRUCIFEROUS VEGETABLES

Steaming, quick sautéing, and stir-frying are the healthiest ways to cook cruciferous vegetables to retain their water-soluble nutrients, including vitamin C and folate. These methods are gentler on nutrients because vegetables don't come in contact with cooking water. Glucosinolates in cruciferous vegetables are also water soluble and will leach into cooking water during heating (glucosinolates are compounds in cruciferous vegetables that are metabolized into isothiocynates when they're eaten; chopping also causes conversion of some glucosinolates to isothiocynates). Boiling cruciferous vegetables results in the loss of 20% to 60% of their isothiocynates. Cooking methods that use less water are best for retaining cancer-fighting isothiocynates.

However, even some cooking methods that use little water can destroy glucosinolates and isothiocynates. A study published in the *Journal of the Science of Food and Agriculture* found that microwaving broccoli on high power destroyed 97%, 74%, and 87% of three types of antioxidants. Steaming, on the other hand, resulted in a loss of only 11%, 0%, and 8% respectively.[26]

The researchers speculate that high temperatures generated by microwave cooking may inactivate the enzyme in cruciferous vegetables that converts glucosinolates to isothiocynates and indoles. Several studies have found, even though bacteria in our gut can break down glucosinolates to some degree, heat inactivation of the enzyme substantially decreases the amount of isothiocynates that's available for absorption. To maximize the amount of isothiocynates and indoles you get from cruciferous vegetables, steam, quickly sauté, or microwave them on low power—or better yet, enjoy them raw. If you do boil cruciferous vegetables, save the leftover cooking liquid to add to soups, sauces, stews, or vegetable juices.

However you decide to cook cruciferous vegetables, don't overcook them. Doing so can produce a strong sulphur odour, one many people find unappealing. Overcooking will also diminish the taste of cruciferous veggies. And if broccoli and cauliflower are cooked too long, they'll become mushy and fall apart.

You'll find more specifics about preparing and cooking specific cruciferous vegetables in the sections below.

★ BROCCOLI

Buying

When you think of broccoli, you probably picture a tree-like green vegetable—the most common variety sold in grocery stores. But there's more than just one type of broccoli to choose from. Each variety offers slightly different tastes and textures:

- *Sprouting broccoli* is the most popular and common type of broccoli.
- *Purple broccoli* is similar to spouting broccoli except, as you probably guessed, its florets are a purplish colour. Despite the different colour, purple broccoli tastes the same as sprouting broccoli.
- *Broccolini* is a cross between broccoli and kale and looks like asparagus with small broccoli buds on top.
- *Broccoflower* is a cross between broccoli and cauliflower. Its looks like cauliflower except it is light, bright green in colour. When cooked, it's tastes very similar to broccoli.
- *Romanesco broccoli* also is a cross between broccoli and cauliflower. It's bright green and has a pointed head consisting of many small, spiral florets that form peaks.
- *Broccoli sprouts* are best known for their high concentration of the anticancer phytochemical sulphoraphane. These sprouts come from germinated broccoli seeds. They can be added to salads and sandwiches or quickly (20 to 30 seconds) sautéed or stir-fried. Although they might add a crispy bite to your sandwich, eating broccoli sprouts raw increases your risk for food poisoning. That's because bacteria can lodge in tiny seed cracks and multiply in the humid sprouting conditions, increasing the risk of salmonella contamination. Heating to high temperatures, as in cooking, kills harmful bacteria. So play it safe and enjoy broccoli sprouts in stir-fries or soups, but not raw.

Choose broccoli with heads of compact, tiny bud clusters that are evenly coloured—either dark green, sage, or purple-green depending on the variety. Broccoli should smell fresh and have firm but tender stalks. Avoid heads that have yellowing florets, a strong odour, or open buds. Yellow flowers are a sign of over-maturity. And avoid broccoli that shows signs of wilting of the florets or the stalk.

Storing

Broccoli can be stored unwashed in a plastic bag in the refrigerator for up to 5 days. Leave the plastic bag open or use a perforated vegetable bag to avoid excess moisture, which encourages mould to grow. (It's for this reason that you should not wash broccoli before refrigerating.) Broccoli is very sensitive to ethylene, a gas given off by other fruits and vegetables as part of the ripening process. If you don't intend to use the broccoli in a day or two, avoid storing it next to apples, apricots, bananas, cantaloupe, kiwi, mango, peaches, pears, or tomatoes.

Broccoli that's been blanched (see page 61) and then frozen can be stored for up to 1 year. Leftover cooked broccoli should be placed in a sealed container and stored in the refrigerator for up to 3 days.

Preparing

Before preparing broccoli, be sure to rinse the head thoroughly in cold water and remove any wilted or damaged leaves. If you're going to use the stalk (it's great steamed or in a stir-fry), cut off the tough bottom end. Then trim off the stalk, leaving about 3 inches (8 cm) below the florets. If you like, remove the tough outer layer from the stalk using a vegetable peeler before cutting the stalk to desired size. Finish trimming the broccoli by cutting each floret off the head, leaving a little stalk on each cluster. If the individual florets are too large, slice them in half lengthwise.

TIPS FOR ADDING BROCCOLI TO YOUR MEALS

- Sprinkle freshly squeezed lemon juice and sesame seeds over lightly steamed broccoli.
- Add sautéed broccoli florets to whole-wheat pasta and toss with extra-virgin olive oil, toasted pine nuts, and sun-dried tomatoes.
- Try puréed broccoli soup. Sauté onion and garlic in a large saucepan. Add 4 to 6 cups (1 to 1.5 L) of low-sodium chicken broth and one bunch of broccoli, chopped (stems and florets). Bring to a boil, then cover and simmer for 15 minutes. Purée in batches, add seasonings, and enjoy.

- Top a baked potato with chopped, steamed broccoli florets.
- Top your next pizza, whether homemade or frozen, with steamed broccoli florets.
- Add raw broccoli florets to your favourite pasta sauce.
- Add chopped broccoli florets and stalks to omelets.
- Use chopped broccoli stems in stir-fries.
- Peel broccoli stems and use in stir-fries or slaws.
- Snack on raw broccoli florets with hummus dip.

RECIPE
Broccoli with Sesame Thai Dressing, page 314

★ BRUSSELS SPROUTS

Buying
Brussels sprouts are available fresh all year-round, but their peak growing season is from fall to early spring. Choose Brussels sprouts with firm, compact bright green heads. (Smaller sprouts will be more tender than larger ones.) They should not have any yellowed or wilted leaves and should not be puffy or soft in texture. Don't buy any Brussels sprouts with perforations in their leaves; this may indicate that there have been aphids living in them.

Storing
Keep unwashed and untrimmed Brussels sprouts in the vegetable crisper of your refrigerator. Stored in a plastic bag, Brussels sprouts can be kept for up to 10 days. Brussels sprouts that have been blanched and then frozen can be stored for up to 1 year.

Preparing
Before washing, remove stems and any yellow or discoloured leaves from the Brussels sprouts. Wash under cold running water or soak in a bowl or sink filled with cold water. If cooking Brussels sprouts whole, lightly score an X on the bottom of the stem to promote even heating throughout the sprout.

TIPS FOR ADDING BRUSSELS SPROUTS TO YOUR MEALS
- Add Brussels sprouts, halved lengthwise, to a stir-fry.
- Braise Brussels sprouts in liquid infused with your herbs and spices. (See page 62 for braising instructions.)

- Try Brussels sprouts roasted with pancetta. Place Brussels sprouts, halved lengthwise, face up in a shallow baking dish. Drizzle with olive oil, season with pepper, and top with chopped pancetta. Bake at 400°F (200°C) for 20 to 25 minutes.
- Combine halved, cooked Brussels sprouts with walnuts and goat cheese for a delicious side dish.
- Grate raw Brussels sprouts and add to soups and stews.
- Eat leftover cooked Brussels sprouts cold as a snack. Just season with a little salt and pepper.

RECIPES
Garlic Roasted Brussels Sprouts, page 317
Hearty Minestrone Soup, page 307

★ CABBAGE

Buying
Like broccoli, there's more than one variety of cabbage to choose from:

- *Green cabbage* is the most common and has a mild flavour. The outer leaves of green cabbage vary from pale green to dark green, and the inner leaves are white to pale green. In general, the darker green the leaves, the more flavour they have.
- *Red or purple cabbage* is sweeter in flavour and its leaves are tougher than that of green cabbage because it takes longer to mature.
- *Savoy cabbage* has crinkled leaves. Its head consists of loose leaves that vary in colour from dark green to light green with lacy patterned veins. Many cooks prefer Savoy cabbage for cooking because of its mild, sweet flavour.
- *Napa cabbage* is more oblong shaped than green, red, and Savoy cabbages. It has a tall, compact head, with pale or dark green leaves. It's often used raw in salads and slaws or cooked in Asian-style stir-fries. Napa cabbage is also called Chinese cabbage, celery cabbage, and Peking cabbage.
- *Bok choy* is also known as Chinese white cabbage. It has dark green ruffled leaves and white celery-like stalks that have a mild, peppery flavour. Both the greens and the stalks are used in salads and stir-fries.

Look for cabbage with heads that are compact and firm and heavy for their size. They should have fresh, shiny, and crispy leaves that aren't marked or browned, which may be an indication of worm damage. A head of cabbage should have just a few outer loose leaves attached to the stem.

If you buy precut cabbage, either halved or shredded, keep in mind that it will have lost some of its vitamin C content, since it starts to degrade once the cabbage is cut.

Storing
Keep cabbage cold to keep it fresh and retain its vitamin C content. Store the whole head, uncut, in a perforated plastic bag in the crisper drawer of your refrigerator. Red and green cabbage will last for 2 weeks; Savoy cabbage will keep for 1 week. Store partial heads covered tightly with plastic wrap, and use within a couple of days.

Preparing
To preserve its vitamin C content, don't cut or wash cabbage until right before cooking or eating it. First remove the wilted, discoloured, and thicker outer leaves, then rinse the cabbage head under cold running water. Even though the inside of a cabbage is usually clean because the outer leaves protect it, you still should clean it. Cut the cabbage head lengthwise in half and then into wedges or quarters. If you see any sign of insects inside the cabbage head, soak the wedges in cold salted water for 15 to 20 minutes to help force the insects out.

Use a stainless steel knife to cut cabbage, since natural compounds in the vegetable react with carbon steel, causing the leaves to turn black. Depending on what dish you're preparing, cabbage can be cut into slices of varying thickness, grated by hand, or shredded in a food processor.

TIPS FOR ADDING CABBAGE TO YOUR MEALS
- Stuff cabbage leaves with a savoury meat-and-herb filling for homemade cabbage rolls.
- Braise red cabbage with chopped apple and red wine. (The alcohol evaporates during cooking, so kids can eat this dish too.)
- Sauté cabbage and chopped onions and serve over a bed of brown rice.
- Use cabbage leaves to wrap your next taco or burrito.
- Wrap up your leftovers—rice, chopped meat or chicken, and veggies—in cabbage leaves and roll into small packages. Bake at 350°F (180°C) for 15 minutes or until hot.
- Add shredded cabbage to sandwiches as a change from lettuce.
- Mix shredded red cabbage into your next green salad for added colour.

- Add chopped or shredded cabbage to soup, whether homemade or store-bought.
- For an Indian-flavoured coleslaw, combine shredded cabbage with freshly squeezed lemon juice, extra-virgin olive oil, chopped scallions, and turmeric, cumin, and coriander.

RECIPES
Hot Apple and Cabbage Salad, page 289
Sesame Coleslaw, page 291

★ CAULIFLOWER

Buying

Unlike other members of the cruciferous family, cauliflower lacks chlorophyll, the molecule that gives plants their distinctive green colour. Choose cauliflower with thick, compact heads of creamy white florets. The florets, or bud clusters, should not be loose or separated. A head of cauliflower should be heavy for its size, and the leaves surrounding it should be bright green and show no signs of wilting.

Avoid cauliflower that is blemished or whose florets have started to turn brown, which is a sign the head is getting old. Check the bottom of cauliflower head—if it is soft, it's no longer fresh. If the florets have started to flower, the cauliflower is overripe. Keep in mind that the size of a cauliflower head is not a sign of quality.

The most commonly used cauliflower is white. But you can also buy purple cauliflower and orange cauliflower. Purple cauliflower cooks faster than white cauliflower and has a milder taste. When cooked, its colour changes from purple to green. Orange cauliflower is a relatively new variety that was first discovered in Canada. Its bright orange colour is a sign that it's a good source of the antioxidant beta carotene.

Storing

Store unwashed cauliflower, stem down, in an open plastic bag or perforated plastic bag in the refrigerator. Storing cauliflower stem down prevents excess moisture from developing in the floret clusters, which causes it to spoil more quickly. Cauliflower will keep in the fridge for 5 to 7 days. Precut cauliflower loses its freshness faster; it will keep for up to 2 days. Cauliflower that has been blanched and then frozen will keep for up to 1 year.

Preparing

Don't wash cauliflower until you're ready to cook or eat it. Remove the outer leaves from the cauliflower head, then remove the stalk from the head by cutting around it with a sharp knife. When the stalk is removed, you'll be left with the core, with the florets attached. Remove the florets by cutting each cluster from the core, leaving a little stem with each cluster. If the florets are larger than needed, cut each into smaller, uniform pieces. Rinse the florets well in cold water. You may also soak them in salt water or vinegar water to help force out any insects that might be lodged within the florets.

TIPS FOR ADDING CAULIFLOWER TO YOUR MEALS

- Serve steamed cauliflower dusted with grated Parmesan cheese or grated part-skim cheddar cheese.
- Add cauliflower florets to curries, pasta sauces, and soups.
- Lightly sauté cauliflower florets with garlic and minced fresh ginger. Or sauté it with a pinch of turmeric or saffron.
- Add raw cauliflower florets to a vegetable platter and serve with a healthy dip.
- Make puréed cauliflower soup. Before serving, add toasted fennel seeds for extra flavour.

RECIPE

Roasted Cauliflower with Red Pepper, page 325

★ TURNIP AND RUTABAGA

Most of the "turnips" you see in the grocery store are actually rutabagas. Both root vegetables belong to the cruciferous family. Turnips are round with a smooth skin that can range in colour from white to yellow, green, or scarlet red. The flesh of a turnip is creamy white and crisp textured. When eaten raw, turnip has a sharp taste; this mellows when the turnip cooked.

A rutabaga looks like a turnip but it's slightly larger and has a coarser texture, which makes it hard to cut. The skin of a rutabaga is pale yellow with hints of purple. The flesh is pale yellow-orange, which turns a brighter orange when cooked. Sound familiar? Rutabagas are also referred to as Canadian turnips.

Buying

When buying turnips, choose those that have smooth skins and are plump and heavy for their size. As with rutabagas, avoid turnips that appear dry or shrivelled, a sign of over-maturity. Turnips may also be coated with a food-grade wax.

When selecting, choose rutabagas that are 3 to 4 inches (8 to 10 cm) in diameter, for the sweetest flavour. They should be firm, smooth skinned, and feel heavy for their size. Most rutabagas found in the grocery store are coated with a food-grade wax that's used to seal in moisture and maintain colour. Avoid rutabagas that appear dry or shrivelled, a sign of over-maturity.

Storing

To store turnips, place in a plastic bag and store in the refrigerator for up to 3 weeks. Rutabagas will keep for 2 to 4 weeks if stored in a cool, dry location.

Preparing

To prepare turnips and rutabagas, wash under cold running water and then peel with a knife or vegetable peeler. Cut the vegetables as desired, trimming away any damaged spots. Very small turnips (also called baby turnips) do not need to be peeled because their skin is tender. Turnips and rutabagas can be baked, roasted, boiled, microwaved, and stir-fried. Shredded or thinly sliced raw turnip make a tasty and nutritious addition to salads.

TIPS FOR ADDING TURNIP AND RUTABAGA TO YOUR MEALS

- Roast cubed rutabagas with maple syrup, salt, and pepper until slightly crispy. Serve as an alterative to hash browns at breakfast.
- Use puréed turnips and rutabagas as the base for hearty, thick soups.
- Stir-fry julienned rutabagas and turnips with fresh ginger, garlic, and snap peas. Top with your favourite low-fat stir-fry sauce.
- Use rutabagas or turnips as the base of a creamy gratin. Use low-fat milk or soy milk instead of heavy cream for a healthier version.
- Purée cooked turnips or rutabagas with potatoes and apples; sprinkle with ground nutmeg. Serve as a side dish with pork tenderloin or ham.
- Boil cubed rutabaga, drain, then mash with pepper and a little butter. Garnish with chopped parsley.
- Peel and wash raw turnip, slice into coins, and enjoy as a snack with your favourite low-fat dip.
- Combine diced turnips and rutabagas with other root vegetables of your choice in a roasting pan. Drizzle with olive oil, dried rosemary, and thyme and bake until tender and slightly crispy.

RECIPE
Oven-Roasted Root Vegetables, page 321

BRIGHT ORANGE VEGETABLES
carrots * sweet potato * winter squash (acorn, butternut, buttercup, Hubbard, pumpkin, spaghetti)

Eat 1 serving a day
1 serving = 1/2 cup (125 ml) raw or cooked

Here's another group of vegetables you should be eating on a regular basis. In fact, the most recent version of Canada's Food Guide (2007) advises that we include 1 serving of bright orange vegetables in our diets every day. That's because adding these foods to your diet helps ensure you're meeting your daily requirement for vitamin A. Vitamin A is essential for growth and development, immune system function, and maintaining normal vision.

Carrots, sweet potatoes, and winter squash are best known for beta carotene, the molecule that gives these foods their bright orange colour. Beta carotene is a phytochemical that belongs to the carotenoid family, a group of over six hundred pigments responsible for the red, orange, and yellow colours of many fruits and vegetables. The deeper the orange colour, the more beta carotene present. (You'll learn about another disease-fighting carotenoid, lycopene, later in this chapter.)

Beta carotene is important for two reasons. First, some of it is converted in the body to retinol, an active form of vitamin A. For this reason, beta carotene is often called "provitamin A." There are about fifty types of carotenoids that the body can convert to vitamin A, but beta carotene is among the most commonly consumed provitamin A in the North American diet. Foods rich in beta carotene can help prevent vitamin A deficiency, which can lead to dry eyes, dry skin, impaired bone growth, susceptibility to respiratory infections, and night blindness. (Night blindness is a condition in which vision is normal in daylight or other strong light but is very weak or completely lost at night or in dim light.)

Beta carotene and health

There's more to beta carotene than its vitamin A activity. This phytochemical is also a powerful antioxidant, protecting cells in the body from damage caused by free radicals. Its antioxidant properties may help in preventing certain cancers and other diseases. Observational studies have revealed that people with low blood levels of beta carotene have a greater risk of lung cancer. When researchers followed 27,000 Finnish male smokers for 14 years, they found that high intakes of total carotenoids from foods—including beta carotene—were very protective against lung cancer.[27]

Carotenoids, including beta carotene, have also shown the ability to stimulate cell communication, which is essential for maintaining properly functioning cells. In cancer, the ability of cells to communicate is impaired, and instead of cells having assigned functions, they proliferate and form tumours. Normally when a cell senses there is something wrong with a neighbouring cell, it sends a message to that cell instructing it to self-destruct. But when cell communication is impaired, this does not occur, and cancerous cells may grow.

A diet rich in beta carotene might also help ward off heart disease. Beta carotene and other carotenoids are fat soluble. That means they circulate in the bloodstream along with cholesterol and other fats. Scientists speculate that these phytochemicals prevent LDL (bad) cholesterol from being oxidized, or damaged, by free radicals (oxidized LDL cholesterol is dangerous because it readily sticks to artery walls). A handful of studies have found that people with higher levels of carotenoids in their bloodstream also have significantly lower levels of carotid artery wall thickness. The thickness of the carotid arteries (the arteries that supply blood to your brain) can be measured using ultrasound technology; increased thickness is a reliable indicator of heart disease. What's more, studies have found that higher intakes of carotenoid-rich produce is linked with a reduced risk of cardiovascular disease.[28]

It's also thought that beta carotene may aid in female reproductive health. Although scientists don't understand the exact role beta carotene plays in reproduction, it is known that the corpus luteum, the area in the ovary where the egg is released at ovulation, has the highest concentration of beta carotene of any organ in the body.

You need to get your beta carotene from food, not supplements. There's no evidence that getting your beta carotene in pill form reduces the risk of heart disease. And when it comes to lung cancer, taking a beta carotene supplement may actually boost your risk for the disease. Two large trials conducted in men at high risk for lung cancer (cigarette smokers, former smokers, or those with a history of occupational asbestos exposure) found that supplemental beta carotene increased lung cancer risk by 16% and 24% respectively.[29]

Even if you never smoked, it's best to get your beta carotene from bright orange vegetables rather than from a supplement. In addition to beta carotene, these foods provide dietary fibre, vitamins, minerals, and other phytochemicals that guard against disease.

HOW MUCH BETA CAROTENE?

To date, no official recommended dietary intake for beta carotene has been established. Experts contend that consuming 3 to 6 milligrams of beta carotene daily will maintain blood levels of beta carotene in the range that's associated with a lower risk of chronic diseases. A diet that provides 7 to 10 servings of fruits and vegetables per day *and* includes one bright orange vegetable daily should provide sufficient beta carotene, as well as other carotenoids.

Beta carotene content of bright orange vegetables (milligrams)

Per 1/2 cup (125 ml) serving, unless otherwise noted	
Sweet potato, baked, 1 medium	16.8
Carrot juice	11.0
Pumpkin, canned	8.5
Pumpkin pie, 1 slice	7.4
Carrots, cooked	6.5
Carrots, raw	4.6
Winter squash	2.9

Source: U.S. Department of Agriculture, Agricultural Research Service. 2006. USDA Nutrient Database for Standard Reference, Release 19. Nutrient Data Laboratory Home Page, www.ars.usda.gov/nutrientdata.

Although the foods listed above deliver significant amounts of beta carotene, carotenoids are fat soluble, which means they're best absorbed in the body if they're eaten with a little fat or oil. Chopping, puréeing, and cooking bright orange vegetables in oil will increase the amount of beta carotene that's available for your body to absorb. All it takes is 3 to 5 grams of fat—roughly 1 teaspoon (5 ml)—in a meal to ensure the beta carotene from your veggies gets absorbed. If you like your carrot sticks raw, serve them with a vinaigrette dip.

You might have noticed from the table above that cooking can improve the availability of beta carotene in foods. One-half cup (125 ml) of cooked carrots has about 40% more beta carotene than the same serving size of raw carrots. However, overcooking can alter the structure of beta carotene, rendering it less easily absorbed in the intestine. To get the most beta carotene—and flavour—from your vegetables, lightly steam or sauté them.

Can you overload on beta carotene? A high intake of beta carotene–rich foods does not have toxic effects. That's because once your body's vitamin A stores are topped up, conversion of beta carotene to vitamin A decreases. But if you eat a couple of bags of baby carrots each day, you might notice the palms of your hands and soles of your feet turn yellow. This condition is called carotenoidemia, but don't worry—it's harmless and reversible.

Enjoying bright orange vegetables

Although there are many interesting ways to add these colourful vegetables to your diet, preparation and cooking methods vary depending on the vegetable. You'll find specifics below.

★ CARROTS

One medium-sized carrot supplies enough beta carotene for a whole day's supply of vitamin A. Carrots are also a good source of fibre, vitamin C, and potassium.

Buying

Choose carrots that are firm, are well formed, and have a deep orange colour. The deeper the orange colour, the more beta carotene is present in the carrot. Avoid carrots that are excessively cracked, split, or forked, as well as those that are limp and rubbery. If green tops are still attached, they should be brightly coloured and not wilted.

Carrots are usually sweeter and more tender the smaller they are. Baby carrots are actually larger carrots that have been trimmed down to "baby" size for sale.

Storing

If stored properly, carrots will maintain their freshness and nutritional value for up to 2 weeks. To maximize their shelf life, it's important to reduce the amount of moisture they lose. Store carrots in a plastic bag or wrapped in paper towel in the coolest part of the refrigerator. Like broccoli, carrots are ethylene-sensitive and should be stored separately from ethylene-producing fruits and vegetables (apples, apricots, bananas, cantaloupe, kiwi, mango, peaches, pears, and tomatoes).

If you buy carrots with green tops attached, cut off the tops before storing in the fridge. Leaving them on will cause carrots to wilt prematurely, since they pull moisture from the carrot.

Baby carrots will keep for at least 1 week in the fridge. Sometimes baby carrots, which are already peeled, will develop a light frosting on their surface. Soaking them in cold water for a while will return them to their bright orange colour.

Preparing

Wash carrots and gently scrub them with a vegetable brush right before cooking or eating. Young and baby carrots need only to be washed. Older carrots, and non-organic carrots, should be peeled. If the stem end is green, it should be cut away, as it will taste bitter. If the carrots are limp, you can restore some of their crispness by placing them in a bowl of ice water for 5 to 10 minutes.

TIPS FOR ADDING CARROTS TO YOUR MEALS

Enjoy carrots raw or cooked. Raw carrots are excellent as snacks and appetizers, and when added to salads. Carrots can be boiled, steamed, sautéed, roasted, and grilled. Cooked carrots can be eaten on their own as a side dish, cooked with other vegetables, or made into savoury dishes, such as stir-fries, casseroles, quiches, omelets, soups, and stews. Carrots can also be baked—their sweet flavour can be enjoyed in cakes, muffins, breads, and cookies.

- Make a batch of healthy, whole-grain carrot muffins, with chopped walnuts for added flavour and healthy fat.
- Add shredded carrot to an omelets, pasta sauce, and green salads.
- Combine shredded carrots and beets with chopped apples for a healthy salad.
- Make a beta carotene–rich soup by puréeing boiled carrots and potatoes (and cooking water) in the blender or food processor. Add herbs and spices to taste.

- Add baby carrots or sliced carrots to curries and stir-fries.
- Eat raw carrots with lunch or as a midday snack. Dip them in a little dressing, since dietary fat enhances beta carotene absorption.
- Enjoy a nutrient-rich shake by combining 1/2 cup (125 ml) of carrot juice, 1 banana, and 3/4 cup (175 ml) of low-fat milk or soy milk in the blender.

RECIPE
Honey Dijon Carrots, page 319

★ SWEET POTATOES

Sweet potatoes are often confused with yams. In most cases, the "yams" sold in grocery stores are actually orange-coloured sweet potatoes. The sweet potato has orange flesh and its skin may be white, yellow, orange, or purple. Sometimes it's shaped like a potato and sometimes it's longer and tapered at both ends.

Yams, on the other hand, have a flesh colour that varies from white to ivory to yellow to purple. Their shape is long and cylindrical and their skin has a rough and scaly texture. Unlike sweet potatoes, yams are not an exceptional source of beta carotene. (They are, however, an excellent source of dietary fibre, vitamin C, potassium, and vitamin B6.)

Buying

Choose firm small to medium-sized sweet potatoes with smooth skin. Avoid sweet potatoes with cracks, soft spots, or blemishes. Don't buy sweet potatoes that are displayed in the refrigerator of the produce section, since cold temperatures changes their taste.

Storing

If kept in a cool, dark place, sweet potatoes will last for 3 to 5 weeks. If kept at room temperature, they should be used within a week of purchase. High temperatures and exposure to sunlight will cause sweet potatoes to sprout. They should be stored loose and not in a plastic bag. Don't store sweet potatoes in the fridge: Doing so will produce a hard core in the centre and an "off" taste. If stored in a spot that is too cool, the natural sugars turn to starch, which affects their flavour.

Cooked sweet potatoes freeze well: They will keep for 8 to 10 months. Wrap unpeeled cooked sweet potatoes individually in aluminum foil or freezer wrap. Place in plastic freezer bags, label, date, and freeze.

Preparing

Organically grown sweet potatoes can be eaten in their entirety—flesh and skin. Just scrub them under cold running water, and they're ready to use in a recipe. If you buy conventionally grown sweet potatoes, you might want to peel them before eating to minimize exposure to pesticide residues. Even though you don't intend to eat the peel, it's still necessary to scrub them under running water before peeling to avoid contamination.

TIPS FOR ADDING SWEET POTATOES TO YOUR MEALS

Use sweet potatoes wherever you would use white potatoes or squash. They're great as a side dish baked, boiled, grilled, or puréed. Or add to soups, stir-fries, risottos, and curries. Their versatility, nutrient content, and sweet flavour make them a popular dish with all family members.

- Add puréed sweet potato to muffin, quick bread, and pancake batters.
- Sauté julienned sweet potato with strips of ham and onion, and add to beaten eggs for an omelet or a frittata.
- Purée cooked sweet potato with bananas, maple syrup, and cinnamon; top with chopped pecans.
- Add diced, cooked sweet potato to a fruit salad. Sweet potatoes pair especially well with pineapple, banana, apples, or pears.
- Substitute grated sweet potatoes for the cabbage in your favourite slaw.
- Add diced sweet potato to any soup, whether homemade or store-bought.
- Toss cooked sweet potato with whole-grain pasta. Toss with extra-virgin olive oil, fresh herbs, and grated Parmesan cheese.
- Mix steamed sweet potato cubes with tofu and broccoli. Top with raisins and serve with a vinaigrette dressing.
- Serve baked sweet potato wedges with roasted meats and poultry dishes.
- Make sweet potato chips. Thinly slice sweet potato, brush with olive oil, and sprinkle with salt, pepper, and spices of your choice—try paprika, cinnamon, cumin, or rosemary. Roast in a 400°F (200°C) oven until golden and crisp.
- Bake a sweet potato and top it with a dash of cinnamon and brown sugar.
- Add raw sweet potatoes to your next veggie platter and enjoy with a healthy dip.

★ WINTER SQUASH

There are many varieties of winter squash to choose from, including acorn, butternut, buttercup, pumpkin, Hubbard, and spaghetti squash. Although they vary in size and shape, they all have thick, hard skins that protect the golden yellow to brilliant orange flesh.

The arrival of the fall and early winter months heralds the peak season for winter squash. But not to worry if you don't get your fill: Because of their hard, thick skins, many winter squashes store well beyond their peak season and are thus available throughout the year.

Buying

In general, look for a dry and uniformly hard surface free of spots and bruises. The squash should feel heavy for its size. The rind should be dull; a shiny rind indicates that the squash was picked too early and will not have reached its full sweetness. The rind should also be firm—a soft rind is a sign of a watery squash that lacks flavour. Choose squash with their stems still attached. The stems should be rounded and dry, not collapsed, blackened, or moist.

Some very large squash, such as Hubbard or calabaza, are sold precut in quarters or chunks and wrapped in plastic. When buying precut squash, look for good interior colour and fine-grained flesh. Acorn squash should have a deep green colour. They may have splashes of orange, but avoid any that has orange on more than half its surface. Butternut rind should be uniformly tan, with no tinge of green.

Storing

Thanks to its hard skin, winter squash can be stored longer than most vegetables. In a cool, dark, dry place, depending on the variety, uncut squash will store well for 1 to 6 months. Be aware that storage below 50°F (10°C), as in the refrigerator, will cause squash to deteriorate more quickly. However, refrigerator storage is acceptable if storing for only a week or two.

Cut squash should be refrigerated and cooked within 1 week; cooked squash can be frozen for up to 2 months. Pumpkins will keep for about 1 month.

Preparing

Rinse off any dirt before using. If you need peeled chunks of squash, cut the squash into pieces first, then peel them with a sturdy, sharp paring knife. Very hard shelled squash is much easier to peel after cooking.

When cutting, first and foremost—be careful. Use a heavy chef's knife or a cleaver, especially for larger squash. Make a shallow cut in the rind to use as a guide and to prevent the knife blade from slipping. Place the blade in the cut and tap the base of the knife (near the handle) with your fist or, if necessary, a mallet or rolling pin until the squash is cut through. If you're not comfortable with this, you might want to use precut or frozen squash instead.

Here's another method if you're not fussy about how the squash is divided. To crack a hard squash, such as Hubbard, wrap it in two plastic grocery bags. Hold it above your head and then drop it onto a cement or tile floor. (Do not drop on hardwood or ceramic.) Some small, very hard shelled squash, such as golden nugget, are often impossible to split before cooking; bake or steam them whole.

For all squash, once split, scoop out the seeds and fibres and cut into smaller chunks, if desired. Peel if required.

TIPS FOR ADDING WINTER SQUASH TO YOUR MEALS

Winter squash is quite versatile and can be incorporated into sweet or savoury dishes. Classic dishes include pumpkin pie, stuffed acorn squash, acorn squash baked with a butter and brown-sugar glaze, and pumpkin or butternut squash soup. But there are plenty more ways to add winter squash to meals.

- For easy cooking, freeze puréed squash in ice cube trays. Once frozen, pop out of trays and store in freezer bags until needed. Use in baking, soups, stews, and casseroles.
- Use squash purée in pancakes, waffles, muffins, and breakfast quick breads.
- Toss cooked, cubed winter squash into pasta primavera, curries, or stews.
- Add cooked, diced squash to homemade or canned vegetable soups.
- Top cooked spaghetti squash with your favourite pasta sauce for a low-carb meal. Once cooked, chill the pasta-like strands of spaghetti squash and toss with a light vinaigrette or serve hot with your favourite pasta sauce.

- Baked halved acorn squash sprinkled with butter and brown sugar or maple syrup for a side dish.
- Enjoy stuffed squash halves. Bake squash halves, then scoop out and mash the flesh with seasonings of your choice. Spoon the mashed squash back into the shells, sprinkling with grated cheese, bread-crumbs, chopped nuts, or sesame seeds, if desired, and return to the oven until heated through.
- Enjoy puréed squash as a side dish. Top with maple syrup and cinnamon or, for a variety of side dishes, add different flavours—honey and ginger, orange and maple (syrup), chives and jalapeño.
- Enjoy a pumpkin cheesecake on special occasions or as a holiday dessert.
- Munch on roasted pumpkin seeds for an addictively good—and healthy—snack.

Recipes
Curried Pumpkin Soup, page 305
Roasted Squash and Garlic Dip, page 362

★ TOMATOES
ketchup ★ fresh red tomatoes ★ stewed tomatoes ★ tomato juice ★ tomato paste ★ tomato sauce

Eat at least 5 servings per week
1 serving = 1 medium tomato or 1/2 cup (125 ml) tomato juice or
2 tablespoons (25 ml) tomato sauce

Botanically, a tomato is a fruit, since it is the ovary of a flowering plant. But from a culinary perspective, tomatoes are not as sweet as other fruits, and they're typically served like other vegetables, as part of the main course of the meal. That's why a tomato is usually considered a vegetable rather than a fruit.

I can't think of many people who don't like tomatoes. What's not to like? Some of our favourite dishes incorporate a healthy dose of tomatoes: spaghetti and meatballs, lasagna, pizza, tomato soup, even chips and salsa. These foods might not seem like nutrition all-stars at first glance. So you might be surprised to learn that they do contain potent disease-fighting nutrients, thanks to their tomato content.

Tomatoes, nutrition, and lycopene

Low in fat and calories, tomatoes are an excellent source of vitamins A and C, and they're a good source of B vitamins and potassium, a mineral that helps regulate blood pressure. Tomatoes also contain vitamin K, a vitamin important for maintaining healthy bones as we age. But it's their lycopene content that's positioned tomatoes as a disease-fighting food. Lycopene is a phytochemical that gives tomatoes their bright red colour. The bright red pigment is also a powerful antioxidant that scientists believe plays an integral role in the health benefits of tomatoes.

As an antioxidant, lycopene neutralizes free radicals that can interfere with normal cell growth and activity. But if you want to get the most lycopene from your tomatoes, there are a few things you need to know. For starters, cooking tomatoes increases the amount of lycopene that's available for absorption in the body. That's because lycopene is tightly bound to fibre in foods; processing breaks down some of the fibre, releasing lycopene. That's why heat-processed tomato products such as tomato paste, tomato juice, tomato sauce, and ketchup (yes, a little bit is healthy) contain the highest concentrations of bioavailable lycopene. (Bioavailability refers to the ability of a substance to be absorbed and used by the body.)

How much lycopene should you consume? Scientists don't know the exact amount needed for optimal health, but studies suggest that a daily intake of 6 to 12 milligrams offers cancer protection. It's not hard to get this much lycopene in your diet when you consider that 1 cup (250 ml) of tomato juice packs 22 milligrams! Here's how tomatoes and common tomato products compare.

Lycopene content of selected tomato products (milligrams)

Per 1/2 cup (125 ml) serving, unless otherwise noted

Tomato paste	37.6
Tomato purée, canned	27.2
Tomato sauce, canned	18.6
Vegetable juice cocktail	11.7
Tomato juice, canned	11.0
Tomato soup, canned	6.3

Lycopene content of selected tomato products (milligrams), cont'd.

Tomatoes, stewed, canned	5.1
Vegetable soup, canned	3.5
Tomatoes, red, raw, 1 medium	3.1
Ketchup, 1 tbsp (15 ml)	2.5

Source: U.S. Department of Agriculture, Agricultural Research Service. 2006. USDA Nutrient Database for Standard Reference, Release 19. Nutrient Data Laboratory Home Page, www.ars.usda.gov/nutrientdata.

Lycopene is fat soluble, so adding a little oil or fat to meals (e.g., to the spaghetti and pizza sauce) aids in its absorption from the digestive tract into the bloodstream.

Tomatoes and health

Tomatoes, and their disease-fighting ingredients, are often mentioned in the news because of the growing number of studies linking tomatoes and tomato products with protection from many types of disease, from cancer to heart disease to macular degeneration.

TOMATOES AND CANCER PREVENTION

When it comes to cancer, tomatoes have received the most attention for their potential to reduce the risk of prostate cancer. Over the past decade, numerous studies have shown that men who eat tomato-based foods frequently are less likely to develop prostate cancer than their peers who seldom eat tomato products.

The first study that made a news splash was published in 1995 and reported the results of a study from Harvard Medical School in which researchers followed 47,894 healthy men from 1986 to 1992. At the end of the follow-up period, men who consumed the most lycopene were 21% less likely to have prostate cancer than were their peers who consumed the least. Of the 46 foods investigated, 4 were significantly associated with protection from prostate cancer: tomato sauce, tomatoes, tomato juice, and pizza. In fact, men who consumed 10 servings of these foods per week had a 35% lower risk of prostate cancer compared with men who ate fewer than 1.5 servings per week.[30]

The researchers followed up again with this large group of men to see if the tomato–prostate cancer relationship persisted. For the period from 1992 to 1998, frequent tomato or lycopene intake was associated with less prostate cancer. When the researchers analyzed the data for the 12-year period from 1986 to 1998, tomato sauce was found to be most protective. Compared with eating tomato sauce less than once per month, eating at least 2 servings each week reduced the risk of disease by 23%.[31]

Men aren't the only ones who can benefit from eating more tomatoes. Observational studies have shown high dietary intakes and high blood levels of lycopene are associated with a lower risk of colon and pancreatic cancers. Preliminary studies also suggest that lycopene-rich vegetables such as tomatoes might guard against cancers of the lung, breast, ovarian, bladder, cervix, and skin.

TOMATOES AND HEART DISEASE

Tomatoes might also have cardio-protective properties. In a 7-year study of almost 40,000 women, higher intakes of lycopene-rich foods were linked with fewer heart attacks and strokes. Compared with women consuming fewer than 1.5 servings of tomato-based products per week, a weekly intake of at least 7 servings reduced the risk of cardiovascular disease by roughly 30%. Among tomato-based foods, tomato sauce and pizza offered the most protection.[32]

It's not just the lycopene in tomatoes that provide health benefits. Researchers are learning that it's the mixture of nutrients and phytochemicals that do the trick, including, but not limited, to lycopene. It appears that all the healthy ingredients in tomatoes work in synergy to confer disease-fighting powers. For instance, tomatoes contain many nutrients linked to heart health, such as potassium, folate, and vitamin B6. Diets rich in potassium have been shown to lower blood pressure. Folate and vitamin B6 are needed to covert a potentially harmful compound, homocysteine, to benign molecules. Homocysteine is an amino acid in the bloodstream that can accumulate and damage blood vessel walls. Numerous studies have linked elevated homocysteine levels with a greater risk of heart attack and stroke.

Enjoying tomatoes and tomato products

Tomatoes are available year-round, so it's easy to enjoy them at any time. But if you want to enjoy the truly delicious flavour of tomatoes, buy them locally during their peak growing season—July through September. They're best when freshly picked off the vine. Since fresh tomatoes are perishable, grocery stores often buy tomatoes that have been picked when green and then forced to ripen. These tomatoes will last longer in the supermarket but will never match the taste and texture of a vine-ripened tomato fresh from the garden or a farmer's market.

Buying

Choose tomatoes that are brightly coloured, plump, and heavy and whose skins have not shrivelled. Don't buy tomatoes with bruises, blemishes, cracks, or soft spots. When buying tomatoes, smell them: A ripe tomato should have a slightly sweet fragrance, especially at the stem end. If you won't be using the tomatoes for a few days, choose ones that have a lighter red colour, and allow them to ripen before using. For smaller tomatoes such as cherry, yellow pear, and currant, look for containers that are not stained. Avoid tomatoes that have gone mouldy or soft.

When buying tomato products such as tomato juice and canned tomatoes, look for brands that are low in sodium.

Storing

Do not store tomatoes in the refrigerator. Cool temperatures can change a tomatoes composition, converting its natural sugars to starch. The end result: a mealy, pulpy, tasteless tomato. Tomatoes are best stored at room temperature, in a single layer, shoulder side up, and away from direct sunlight.

Once they're ripe, use tomatoes within 1 week. If you want to speed up the ripening process, store tomatoes in a plain brown paper bag with an apple or pear. The ethylene gas produced by the fruit will quicken ripening. In fact, the tomatoes you buy in the supermarket may have been ripened by a commercial method that also uses ethylene gas.

Fresh tomatoes don't freeze well. If you want the taste of fresh tomatoes in the winter, cook your tomatoes and make them into a tomato sauce or purée, both of which freeze very well.

Preparing

As with any fresh produce, wash tomatoes well under cool running water before preparing or eating. Drain on a paper towel or clean kitchen towels.

TIPS FOR ADDING TOMATOES TO YOUR MEALS

Tomatoes are one of nature's most versatile vegetables. Whether you are eating them whole and warm straight off the vine or in a classic ratatouille or an ever-popular salsa, tomatoes add great flavour and good nutrition to any meal. Tomato blends perfectly with many seasonings, including garlic, shallot, basil, tarragon, and cumin.

- Enjoy broiled fresh tomatoes as a side dish. Remove tomato core and halve crosswise. Drizzle with olive oil, sprinkle with salt, pepper, bread-crumbs, or other seasonings. Broil until tomatoes are tender and topping is lightly browned. Or bake in a 425°F (220°C) oven for 10 to 15 minutes or until tender.
- Serve bruschetta as an appetizer. Top thick slices of grilled or broiled hearty French stick or Italian bread, rubbed with garlic, with finely diced tomatoes, onion, and basil. Sprinkle with Parmesan cheese and then broil until heated.
- Add chopped fresh tomatoes to omelets, frittatas, and quiches.
- Garnish meat, poultry, fish, and egg dishes with homemade or store-bought tomato salsa.
- Toss diced fresh tomatoes into a three bean salad and serve on crisp lettuce leaves.
- Stuff hollowed-out whole tomato with your favourite meat or seafood salad for a quick cold lunch.
- Add canned tomatoes (chopped, puréed, or whole) to pasta sauces, canned soups, chili, stews, and casseroles.
- Serve Caprese salad. Slice fresh tomatoes, drizzle with extra-virgin olive oil, top with shredded fresh basil leaves and slices of fresh mozzarella or bocconcini cheese, and then sprinkle with salt and freshly ground pepper.
- Enjoy a bowl of gazpacho. Purée tomatoes, cucumbers, bell peppers, and green onions, and a drizzle of extra-virgin olive oil in the food processor. Season with your favourite herbs and spices.
- Add diced tomatoes to guacamole or hummus for extra colour and nutrition.
- Enjoy a fresh in-season tomato out of hand, just as you would an apple.
- Enjoy a glass of lycopene-rich tomato juice or vegetable cocktail with lunch or dinner or as a snack.

RECIPES

Oven-Roasted Tomatoes with Feta Cheese, page 322
Tarragon Sautéed Cherry Tomatoes, page 330
Garden Vegetable Lasagna, page 354
Spaghetti with Olive and Rosemary Sauce, page 356

ALLIUM VEGETABLES
garlic ★ onions ★ leeks ★ chives ★ scallions ★ shallots

Eat two cloves of garlic per week and multiple servings of onions
1 serving onions = 2 tablespoons (25 ml) raw or cooked

Garlic, onions, leeks, chives, scallions (also called green or spring onions), and shallots belong to the lily, or *Allium,* family of vegetables. They're used around the world for their pungent flavour as a seasoning, a condiment, or to enhance the flavour of other ingredients. Garlic and onions are certainly two of my favourite seasonings. I use them to spice up most dishes, including pasta sauces, stir-fries, curries, soups, omelets, casseroles, and marinades. While they're big on flavour, *Allium* family vegetables also deliver considerable health benefits.

Garlic's healing and medicinal properties have long been known. The herb has been used as both food and medicine in many cultures for thousands of years. Its use dates as far back as to the time the Egyptian pyramids were built. In Biblical times, garlic was thought to preserve strength and was given to slaves to increase their fitness. In ancient Greece, athletes took garlic before competing in the Olympic Games to enhance strength and vigour. In 1858, Louis Pasteur—the great scientist who invented the pasteurization process—noted garlic's antibacterial activity, and it was used as an antiseptic to prevent gangrene during World War I and World War II.

Today scientists are praising garlic's potential to help treat or protect against certain cancers, heart disease, arthritis, and even diabetes. The disease-fighting properties of allium vegetables are attributed to a variety of powerful sulphur-containing chemicals, in particular allyl sulphides. (These sulphur compounds are the same chemicals responsible for garlic's distinctive smell and onion's ability to make your eyes water.) Allium vegetables also contain flavonoids, phytochemicals linked to disease prevention. Onions are particularly rich in quercetin, a flavonoid thought to guard against cancer and heart disease.

In addition to phytochemicals, allium vegetables are valuable sources of nutrients you'd normally expect from more colourful vegetables. Garlic offers vitamins C and B6, manganese, and selenium, while onions are notable for their vitamin C, vitamin B6, chromium, and potassium content.

Allium vegetables and health

ALLIUM VEGETABLES AND CANCER PREVENTION

Many studies provide compelling evidence that garlic and its sulphur compounds inhibit the cancer process. Of 37 observational studies in humans using garlic and its related sulphur compounds, 28 showed some cancer-preventative effect. The evidence is particularly strong for digestive tract cancers. A combined analysis of 18 scientific papers concluded people who eat raw or cooked garlic regularly face about half the risk of stomach cancer and two-thirds the risk of colorectal cancer as people who eat little or none.[33]

Another study published in the *International Journal of Cancer* reported that a diet containing 10 grams of garlic and onions (three cloves of garlic or 1 tablespoon/15 ml of chopped onion) per day was associated with a 30% lower risk for a certain type of stomach cancer.[34] Another study revealed that among the 10,000 subjects studied, the more garlic and onions consumed, the lower their risk for a wide range of cancers, including cancers of the oral cavity, larynx, esophagus, colon, ovaries, and kidneys.[35]

Onions might also help keep lung cancer at bay. A study from the Netherlands that followed 120,852 men and women age 55 to 69 years discovered that those who consumed the most onions had a 35% lower risk of lung cancer than those who ate the least.[36] Later, when researchers from the Cancer Research Center of Hawaii investigated the relationship between diet and lung cancer risk in 582 patients with lung cancer and 582 controls free of the disease, they too noted significant cancer protection from onions. Compared with people who seldom ate onions, those whose diets contained the most onions were 50% less likely to develop lung cancer. The researchers also linked a higher intake of the flavonoid quercetin with a lower the risk of lung cancer.[37]

Scientists believe that garlic and onions help fight cancer in several ways. Studies show that garlic's allyl sulphur compounds can slow or prevent the growth of cancer cells. Recently, these compounds proved able to kill leukemia cells in the laboratory. Allyl sulphides may help rid the body of carcinogens by enhancing the action of certain enzymes in the liver and intestinal tract. It's also thought that natural chemicals in garlic and onions have a direct toxic effect on certain types of tumour cells. Sulphur compounds in allium vegetables also stimulate the body's immune system, helping the body combat disease. Finally, onions are a rich source of quercetin, a potent antioxidant that may block carcinogens as well as slow the growth and spread of cancer cells.

When it comes to cancer prevention, you don't need to eat a lot of garlic to reap the benefits. Studies suggest that eating as little as two cloves per week is beneficial.

ALLIUM VEGETABLES AND HEART HEALTH

Interest in garlic's potential to guard against heart disease began when researchers noticed that people living near the Mediterranean—where garlic is a common ingredient in meals—had lower rates of death from cardiovascular disease. Since then, many studies have investigated garlic's effect on risk factors for heart disease, such as blood cholesterol, blood pressure, and blood clot formation.

More than 40 clinical trials have examined the effects of raw garlic and garlic supplements on blood cholesterol. The results of many trials suggest that garlic supplements modestly lower total cholesterol, LDL (bad) cholesterol, and blood fats called triglycerides over the short term (1 to 3 months). However, similar cholesterol-lowering effects have not been found in studies lasting 6 months. A recent randomized clinical trial at Stanford University Medical School enrolled 192 adults with moderately high LDL cholesterol levels for 6 months and found that raw garlic and garlic supplements were no better at lowering cholesterol than placebo pills.[38]

Despite the conflicting findings on garlic's cholesterol-lowering properties, the vegetable might protect the heart in other ways. Most studies show garlic and garlic supplements can significantly impede the ability of platelets in the blood to aggregate, or clump together. Platelet aggregation is one of the first steps in the formation of blood clots that can lead to a heart attack or stroke. Some, but not all, studies also suggest that garlic might help lower blood pressure.

Thanks to their sizeable quercetin content, onions may play a role in heart health, too. Quercetin, which helps vitamin C in its function, has been shown to improve the integrity of blood vessels and decrease inflammation.

When it comes to garlic, more is not better. Eating too much garlic, especially raw garlic, can have side effects, the most common being bad breath and body odour. More uncomfortable and potentially serious adverse effects include irritation of the digestive tract, heartburn, flatulence, nausea, vomiting, and diarrhea. A hefty dose of garlic can also possibly increase the risk of bleeding. If you're planning to have surgery, avoid consuming fresh garlic (and garlic supplements) 7 days before the procedure.

Enjoying allium vegetables

★ GARLIC

To reap maximum flavour, nutrition, and health benefits, buy fresh garlic. Although dried garlic flakes, garlic powder, garlic salt, garlic oil, and garlic purée may be more convenient, you won't be getting the same health benefits from them as fresh garlic provides.

Buying

Fresh garlic is sold in single heads containing 10 to 20 smaller bulbs, or cloves, individually wrapped in papery skins. Choose plump heads of fresh garlic that are firm to the touch and have their paper-like skin intact. There should be no signs of shrivelling, sprouting, soft spots, or other blemishes.

Storing

Store unpeeled garlic in an uncovered or loosely covered container in a cool, dry place away heat, sunlight, and other foods. This will help prevent garlic heads from sprouting, which diminishes its flavour. If stored properly, unbroken garlic heads will keep for 2 to 3 months, but they're best used within a few weeks. Individual cloves will last from 5 to 10 days.

Preparing

Remove the garlic clove from the head. To peel a garlic clove, first cut off the tough piece, or "toenail," at the end (this is where the clove was attached to the garlic head). To separate the skin from the clove, place clove on a cutting board and put the flat side of a chef's knife on top of it. Apply pressure to the blade with your fist to break the skin for easy removal. If you want crushed garlic, press the clove harder to smash it, then remove the peel and continue mincing the garlic.

To peel a clove, you can also twist it between your fingers to loosen the skin. Once loosened, the skin should peel easily.

If you need to remove the skin from a head of garlic cloves, try the microwave method. Please a whole head on a paper plate and microwave on high for 1 minute, rotating the plate at 30 seconds. Let rest in the microwave for 1 minute, then remove. Let stand until cool enough to handle, then peel.

Peeling, chopping, or crushing garlic activates the enzyme allinase, which starts a series of chemical reactions that produce beneficial sulphur compounds. However, if garlic is cooked immediately after it's peeled and chopped, the enzyme is inactivated and the disease-fighting sulphur compounds are lost. That's why scientists recommend that crushed or chopped garlic be left to stand for 10 to 15 minutes before cooking to allow this chemical reaction to occur.

The intensity of garlic's flavour depends on how it's prepared. Whole cloves have the mildest flavour, chopped cloves have a medium-intense flavour, and crushed cloves have the most intense flavour. The smaller you cut garlic (from chopped to minced to crushed), the more juices and oils are released, resulting in a strong aroma and potent flavour.

Garlic can be sautéed, roasted, fried, or added raw to dishes. When sautéing in oil, be careful not to overcook or brown the garlic. Overcooking causes garlic to become bitter and unpleasant tasting. Minced garlic usually cooks in less than 1 minute. If a recipe calls for sautéed garlic and onions, sauté the onions first, then add the garlic.

TIPS FOR ADDING GARLIC TO YOUR MEALS

Garlic is considered by many people an essential ingredient in many dishes, from soups to stews to pasta sauces.

- Marinate pressed garlic in extra-virgin olive oil and use this garlic-infused oil for salad dressings and marinades. Homemade infused oils will not keep as long as commercially processed ones. Store your herb-infused olive oil in the refrigerator and use within 2 months to prevent it from spoiling.
- Sauté steamed spinach with garlic, and sprinkle with freshly squeezed lemon juice.
- Add minced garlic to soups and pasta sauces.
- Add chopped raw garlic to marinades for meat, chicken, and seafood.
- Use crushed garlic as part of spice rubs for grilled meats.
- When roasting lamb or beef, insert slivers of raw garlic into shallow slits in the surface of the meat to impart great flavour.

- Flavour butter with chopped or crushed raw garlic, and make your own delicious garlic bread.
- Make your own tzatziki with non-fat plain yogurt, garlic, and cucumber. Serve as a condiment with grilled chicken or use as a dip with whole-wheat pita bread.
- Make garlic mashed potatoes. Purée roasted garlic, boiled potatoes, and butter or olive oil together.
- Spread roasted garlic on whole-grain crackers as an appetizer.

RECIPE
Roasted Garlic, page 361

★ ONIONS AND LEEKS

There are plenty of varieties of onions to choose from, and some are more suitable for specific uses than others. Sweet onions (vidalia, Walla Walla, yellow Bermuda) are great raw in salads. Hotter brown or white-skinned Spanish varieties are best for soups, stews, and pasta sauces, and for baking, grilling, and roasting. Red onions turn a greyish colour when cooked, so use them in salads or quick-cooking dishes that allow them to maintain their colour.

Shallots contain less water than onions, so their flavour is more intense than that of onions. Use shallots in dishes where you want the flavour of an onion but not the bulk of a whole onion.

Leeks look like large green onions but their flavour is milder and sweeter. Unlike onions, leeks are usually eaten cooked, since they're fibrous when eaten raw. But if finely chopped, raw leeks make a good addition to a salad.

Green onions or scallions are great raw in salads and salsas. They're also suitable for recipes that cook quickly, such as pastas, stir-fries, omelets, and scrambled eggs.

Chives are the mildest members of the *Allium* family. Use them as an herb to flavour eggs, potatoes, smoked fish, and other fish dishes.

Buying

Choose onions and shallots that are firm, heavy for their size, and dry, with bright, smooth outer skins. Onions should not have an opening at the neck. Avoid those that are sprouting or have signs of mould, soft spots, or dark patches.

Scallions should have bright green, fresh-looking tops that appear crisp, and slightly white ends.

Leeks should be firm and straight with dark green leaves and white necks. Avoid leeks that have yellowed or wilted tops. Overly large leeks will be particularly fibrous, so choose leeks that have a diameter no larger than 1 1/2 inch (4 cm).

Storing

Store onions at room temperature in a cool, dark, well-ventilated place. Keep them in a hanging wire basket, mesh bag, or a perforated bowl with a raised base so that air can circulate underneath. Sweet onions are higher in water and sugar content than Spanish onions, so they require more care when storing to avoid bruising. Avoid storing potatoes with onions because they will absorb potatoes' moisture and ethylene gas, causing them to spoil faster. Sweet onions will keep for 4 to 6 weeks or longer. White and brown-skinned Spanish onions will keep for up to 3 months. Unused cut onions should be tightly wrapped in plastic or kept in a sealed container and used within 2 days. The longer that cut onions are exposed to air, the more nutrients they will lose.

Scallions stored in a plastic bag in the crisper of the refrigerator will keep for up to 1 week.

Fresh leeks, stored unwashed and untrimmed in the refrigerator, will keep for 1 to 2 weeks. Wrap them loosely in a plastic bag to prevent them from drying out. Cooked leeks will last only 2 days in the refrigerator.

Preparing

For many people, peeling and cutting onions results in shedding a tear or two. The same chemicals responsible for an onion's health benefits—allyl sulphides—are those that irritate the eyes. To keep tears from flowing while preparing onions, chill onions for 30 to 60 minutes before cutting. Or try slicing onions under running water, although you might end up rinsing away phytochemicals and nutrients.

If you need only a small portion of onion, don't peel the entire onion. Instead, cut off the section you need and peel that. The remaining onion will store longer in the fridge with the skin on it.

To remove the smell of onion on your hands, rub them with a freshly cut lemon.

Leeks must be cleaned thoroughly before eating or cooking to remove any dirt within the vegetable's overlapping leaves. First, trim the root and a portion of the green top and remove the outer layer. Make a lengthwise cut into the leek, fold it open, and run the leek under cold water. If your recipe calls for cross-sections of leek, first cut the leek into pieces, then place in a colander and run under cold water.

TIPS FOR ADDING ONIONS AND LEEKS TO YOUR MEALS

Like garlic, onions are considered by many people an essential ingredient to many dishes. Leeks, a mild-tasting member of the *Allium* family, can be substituted for onions in most dishes using onions for flavouring. Leeks can be sliced and added to salads and stir-fries, used to flavour soups and stocks, or sautéed and paired with grilled fish or poultry. When preparing leeks as a side dish, cook them until tender and slightly firm; overcooking will make leeks mushy and unappetizing.

- Combine chopped onions, tomatoes, avocado, and minced jalapeño for a delicious salsa.
- Add slices of grilled red onion to your next grilled vegetable platter.
- Toss caramelized onions with cooked whole-grain pasta and goat's cheese for a rich-tasting appetizer or side dish. Top with fresh chopped chives.
- Add onions when sautéing other vegetables, for instance, cabbage, leafy greens, carrots, or mushrooms.
- Sprinkle chopped green onions on baked potatoes and brown rice.
- Add finely chopped leeks to salads.
- Add chopped leeks to soups and stews for extra flavour.
- Braise leeks with fennel seeds for a healthy side dish.
- Add sliced leeks to an omelet or a frittata.

RECIPES
French Onion Soup, page 306
Mushroom Leek Soup, page 310

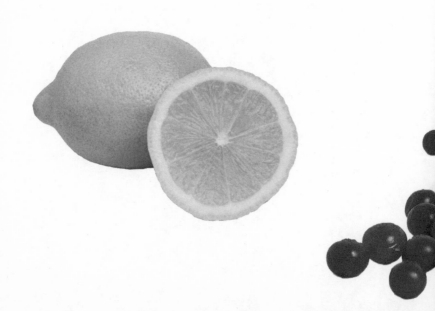

3

Power fruits

berries
blackberries ★ blueberries ★ cranberries ★ raspberries
★ strawberries

citrus fruit
grapefruit ★ lemons ★ limes ★ oranges ★ pummelos
★ tangerines

pomegranate
pomegranate juice ★ pomegranate seeds

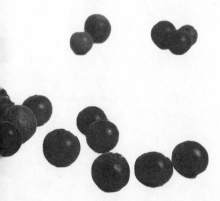

Your mother was right when she encouraged you to snack on fruit. From a nutrition standpoint, fruit is pretty tough to beat. It's an excellent source of dietary fibre, potassium, vitamin C, and folate, nutrients vital for maintaining good health and guarding against disease. Indeed, a diet rich in colourful, nutrient-dense fruit has been linked to lower rates of cancer, heart disease, stroke, cataract, macular degeneration, and type 2 diabetes. Adding fruit to your diet can also help control blood pressure and cholesterol, decrease bone loss, promote weight loss, and prevent a painful intestinal condition called diverticulitis.

It's the combination of healthy ingredients in fruit that act to fight disease:

- Fruit's soluble fibre helps reduce blood cholesterol and may lower the risk of developing heart disease. And as fibre from fruit passes through the digestive tract, it can calm an irritable bowel and relieve or prevent constipation.
- Potassium, a mineral needed to keep our body's fluids in balance, helps maintain a healthy blood pressure.
- Vitamin C is needed for growth and repair of all body tissues, helps heal wounds, and keeps gums, teeth, and bones healthy.
- Folate (a B vitamin) is used to form red blood cells and is needed to repair the genetic material (DNA) in our cells. Consuming enough folate is also an important way for women of child-bearing age to reduce the risk of serious spinal cord birth defects such as spina bifida should they become pregnant.
- The many phytochemicals in fruit help reduce the risk of disease by exerting antioxidant, antibacterial, and immune-boosting powers.

On top of being chockfull of nutrients, fruit lacks those unhealthy ingredients that increase the risk of health problems. It's almost always fat- and cholesterol-free and naturally low in sodium. And let's not forget that fruits are lower in calories than many other foods (think cookies and chocolate bars). In other words, including fruit in your diet can help you cut calories and control your weight. The good news: It's possible to satisfy your sweet tooth without adding inches to your waistline.

There's no need to limit eating fruit for fear of its sugar content. It's true that fruit contains sugars, mainly fructose, which provide a source of energy. But unlike the refined sugars found in candy, baked goods, ice cream, and soft drinks, the sugar in fruit is naturally occurring. They are considered healthy sugars because along with them you also get vitamins, minerals, and fibre, which help make up a healthy balanced diet. Foods rich in refined sugars, such as soft drinks and candy, lack essential nutrients. What's more, almost all fruits have a low glycemic index, meaning their natural sugars are gradually released as sugar into the bloodstream. (Refined sugars produce sharp rises in blood sugar, triggering hunger and overeating. For more on the glycemic index, see Chapter 1, page 14.)

Strategies to increase your daily fruit intake

Canada's Food Guide advises adults to consume 7 to 10 servings of vegetables and fruits combined each day. (Children and teenagers need 4 to 8 daily servings depending on their age and sex.) Although there's no official guidance on how many of these daily servings should be fruit, I recommend you eat at least 4 fruit servings (2 cups/500 ml of fresh fruit) per day.

It's not unusual for me to talk to new clients who eat little or no fruit. It seems that fruit is a food that many people are not in the habit of including in their diets. Some people are stuck in their granola bar–bagel–cookie–chips–candy snack routine. Others satisfy their sweet tooth with ice cream, cake, or a can of pop. And sometimes fruit just isn't available at restaurants, the office, or in vending machines, even if you want it.

These tips will help you increase your fruit intake:

- *Keep fruit at work.* Not all fruits need refrigeration. Keep apples, bananas, pears, and dried fruit in your desk drawer so you'll have a healthy snack handy when you feel hungry.
- *Keep fruit visible.* Decorate your table, kitchen counter, or desk with a bowl of fresh fruit. Keeping fruit visible and within reach will encourage healthy snacking.

- *Include fruit at breakfast.* For a nutritious breakfast, purée milk, soy milk, or yogurt with berries, banana, and a splash of orange juice. Or top a bowl of breakfast cereal with fresh or dried fruit.
- *Serve fruit for dessert.* If you crave a sweet after a meal, reach for fruit instead of a decadent treat. Serve fresh fruit salad, fruit kebabs, fruit crisp, or simply eat a piece of fruit out of your hand.
- *Add fruit to salads.* Who says salads have to contain vegetables only? Dried fruit, berries, orange segments, apple slices, and pineapple chunks add flavour and a boost of nutrition to green salads.
- *Bake with fruit.* Add fruit to pancakes, waffles, muffins, cookies, and pies to increase nutrient and fibre content.
- *Make fruit appealing.* Your family might like fruit better if it's served with a tasty dip. Try vanilla or fruit-flavoured yogurt or even low-fat chocolate pudding.
- *Garnish with fruit.* Sneak fruit into your family's diet by decorating plates or serving dishes with fruit slices or berries.
- *Order fruit when dining out.* Instead of a rich dessert, ask for a bowl of fresh fruit. In fast food restaurants, balance your meal by ordering a fruit cup, sliced apples, or 100% pure fruit juice.
- *Consider convenience.* Buy packages of precut frozen fruit to add to smoothies. Pick up a fresh food salad or precut fresh fruit from the deli section of your grocery store.

Any fruit is good fruit. But there are some fruits that scientists are learning are particularly good for you. So while you strive to boost your daily fruit intake, make a point of adding the power fruits discussed later in this chapter to your diet more often.

Which is best: fresh, frozen, canned, or dried fruit?

Buy locally grown fresh fruit in season for maximum nutrition and taste. Canned, frozen, and dried fruits offer alternatives when fresh fruit is out of season and make for quick meals and snacks. It's pretty easy to throw a box of raisins or a single-serving container of unsweetened applesauce into your briefcase to have as a midday snack.

Generally, canned and frozen fruit provides similar amounts of vitamins and minerals compared with their fresh equivalents. Fruits are usually frozen or canned very soon after harvesting, so the vitamin and mineral content is preserved. Canned fruit will have lower amounts of vitamin C compared with fresh, since the canning process depletes some of the vitamin. However, vitamin C levels remain constant throughout the shelf life of canned fruit.

Canned fruit can have other disadvantages. Canned peaches and pears are lower in fibre than their fresh counterparts because their peel has been removed. And canned fruit packed in syrup has extra sugar and calories that most of us don't need. Buy canned fruit that is unsweetened; look for fruit canned in its own juice or in water.

Like fresh fruit, dried fruit provides fibre, vitamins, and minerals. However, dried fruit delivers smaller amounts of vitamin C and folate than fresh fruit because of losses that occur during drying. For some people, the main drawback to dried fruit is that it contains more calories per serving than fresh fruit. That's because most of its water—which gives fruit its bulk—has been removed. For example, 1 cup (250 ml) of grapes has 110 calories and 29 grams of sugar. The same serving size of raisins (dried grapes) packs in 521 calories and 128 grams of sugar. If you're watching your calorie intake, keep your serving size of dried fruit to 1/4 cup (50 ml).

Dried fruit may be preserved with sulphite, which can trigger an allergic reaction in some people, especially those with asthma. If you're sensitive to sulphites, read the label and avoid foods that contain sulphites and sulphite derivatives. These include products whose ingredient lists warn it "may contain" or "may contain traces of" sulphites and sulphite derivatives.

Is fruit juice healthy?

There's been a lot of talk about the dangers of drinking too much fruit juice. Pediatricians warn that excessive fruit juice contributes to obesity, the development of cavities, diarrhea, excessive gas, bloating, and abdominal pain. Dietitians and doctors also advise overweight adults to limit their fruit juice intake if they want to slim down.

Fruit juice is inherently a healthy food. It supplies vitamins A and C, folate, potassium, and magnesium. Canada's Food Guide counts a 1/2 cup (125 ml) serving as one of the daily 7 to 10 vegetable and fruit servings. Sounds good so far. But fruit juice doesn't have the same benefits as eating whole fruit. Unlike whole fruit, fruit juice lacks fibre and so it doesn't fill you up. It's much easier to drink 1 cup (250 ml) of orange juice than it is to eat two oranges. And with that extra juice comes extra calories in the form of natural sugars. Most fruit juices supply anywhere from 120 calories (orange, grapefruit, apple) to 140 calories (cranberry, pineapple) per 1 cup (250 ml) serving, and some have as many as 190 calories (e.g., prune).

That's fine if you're measuring your portion size. But in the real world, portion control is a challenge, since most single-serve bottles of juice sold in vending machines, convenience stores, and gas stations deliver 16 ounces (473 ml)—almost 4 servings of fruit juice—which most people guzzle as a single serving. That could spell trouble if you're trying to lose weight.

To get the most nutrition from fruit juice, you need to think before you drink. Practice the following tips when buying—and drinking—fruit juice:

- *Read labels.* Look for products that are 100% pure fruit juice. Beware of products labelled "beverage," "cocktail," or "drink." Although some might be fortified with vitamin C, if it's not real juice, it's not as nutritious.
- *Choose nutrient-rich fruit juices.* At the top of the list is orange juice, followed by grapefruit, prune, pineapple, and cranberry. Apple, grape, and pear juices provide the fewest nutrients per serving. Fruit juices rich in colour—pink grapefruit, cranberry, blueberry, pomegranate, and purple grape—are also worth adding to your diet thanks to their sizeable antioxidant content (you'll learn more about these brightly coloured fruits later in the chapter).
- *Control your portion size.* Keep in mind that 1/2 cup (125 ml) of juice counts as 1 fruit serving. If you're watching your weight, dilute the calories by mixing juice with plain or sparkling water.
- *Monitor your child's fruit juice intake.* Children age 1 to 6 years should consume no more than 6 ounces (175 ml) per day. Older kids, age 7 to 18, should limit their daily intake to 12 ounces (375 ml).
- *Eat whole fruit most often.* Get most of your daily fruit servings from whole fruit rather than fruit juice; you'll consume more fibre and fewer calories.

BERRIES
blackberries * blueberries * cranberries * raspberries * strawberries

Eat 1 to 2 servings per day
1 serving = 1/2 cup (125 ml) berries, fresh or frozen

Berries are often referred to as "super fruits," and for good reason. For starters, they're low in calories, contain no fat, and are a great source of vitamin C and dietary fibre. Berries also taste great and require little effort to add to your diet. Just rinse and they're ready to add to smoothies, yogurt, breakfast cereal, and muffin recipes. Or enjoy the delicious taste of berries on their own as a healthy snack or dessert.

Berries' reputation as super fruits comes from their strikingly high antioxidant content. When it comes to antioxidants, berries outshine all other fruits. According to a recent study measuring the antioxidant content of over a thousand commonly eaten foods, blackberries, strawberries, cranberries, raspberries, blueberries, cranberry juice, and blueberry juice were among the top 50 foods containing the most antioxidants per serving.[1] An earlier study that ranked 100 foods for their antioxidant potency listed berries among the top 20 foods, with wild blueberries leading the pack.[2] Not bad at all for such a tiny fruit.

Berries contain a variety of antioxidant phytochemicals shown to have disease-fighting properties. *Ellagic acid,* found in all berries and especially plentiful in strawberries and raspberries, not only acts as an antioxidant but also helps the body deactivate specific carcinogens and it helps slow the reproduction of cancer cells. In laboratory studies, ellagic acid prevented cancers of the skin, bladder, lung, esophagus, and breast.

Anthocyanins are the group of phytochemicals that give berries their deep red-blue colour. They're abundant in blueberries and cranberries and have been shown to inhibit the growth of lung, colon, and leukemia cancer cells in the lab. Anthocyanins also have antibacterial properties in humans.

Yet another powerful berry antioxidant is *pterostilbene,* of which blueberries are an outstanding source. Pterostilbene appears to impact metabolic processes that reduce the risk of cancer and heart disease. Berries also contain flavonoids and phenolic acids, other phytochemicals thought to have anti-cancer properties.

Berries supply *lutein,* a phytochemical that helps guard against cataracts and age-related macular degeneration. Macular degeneration is the leading cause of blindness in older adults. It's a disease that attacks the macula, the central part of the retina that controls fine, detailed vision. Once consumed, lutein makes its way to the eye, where it's thought to protect both the retina and the lens from oxidative damage. Scientists speculate that an intake of 6 to 15 milligrams of lutein per day is optimal for eye health. The darker the berry, the more lutein it contains. Raspberries and blackberries each contain 1.8 milligrams of lutein per 1 cup (250 ml). A similar serving of blueberries has 1.2 milligrams.

Cranberries and blueberries are the most heavily researched berries. Even though blackberries, raspberries, and strawberries have not been the focus of studies, they are packed with many of the same phytochemicals as blueberries and cranberries, and there's no reason to think these delicious fruits won't also keep you healthy.

Here's the lowdown on the many ways in which eating berries can keep you healthy.

★ BLACKBERRIES

These deeply coloured berries are high in cancer-fighting ellagic acid and also contain vitamins C and E, fibre, and potassium. Their dark blue colour makes blackberries an exceptional source of antioxidants. In fact, when it comes to antioxidant levels, blackberries outrank all other berries.

One cup (250 ml) of fresh blackberries has 66 calories, 8 grams of fibre, 38 micrograms of folate (10% of your daily recommended intake), and 32 milligrams of vitamin C.

★ BLUEBERRIES

If you want to boost your brainpower, eat blueberries more often. Researchers from Tufts University found that diets rich in blueberries—the equivalent of 1 cup (250 ml) per day in humans—significantly improved both the learning capacity and the motor skills of aging mice, making them mentally equivalent to much younger ones.[3]

A blueberry-rich diet might also reduce the risk of Alzheimer's disease, if results from animal studies can be extrapolated to humans. Although the exact cause of Alzheimer's is still not clear, evidence points to the buildup of plaque from beta-amyloid deposits in the brain. These deposits of protein are thought to damage and cause the death of brain cells from oxidative stress. It's possible that blueberries' antioxidants can combat some of this oxidative stress and protect against declining brain function.

In one study, researchers fed rats a diet containing a blueberry extract or a control diet for at least 8 weeks. After this, the rats were injected with a solution that causes brain cell loss similar to that experienced by people suffering from Alzheimer's disease. The researchers reported that the blueberry-fed rats showed enhanced performance in a maze. What's more, the rats on the blueberry-enriched diet experienced significantly less brain cell loss.[4] In another study conducted on mice genetically predisposed to develop the same brain plaque that afflicts people with Alzheimer's disease, blueberry anthocyanins were shown to boost the communication between failing brain neurons.[5]

Phytochemicals in blueberries may also keep cancer and heart disease at bay. Laboratory studies show that phenolic acids in blueberries can inhibit colon cancer cell growth and induce cell death. Animal research has demonstrated that blueberry compounds make blood vessels more resistant to oxidative stress and lower blood cholesterol.

One cup (250 ml) of fresh blueberries has 88 calories, 4 grams of fibre, 15 milligrams of vitamin C, and 30 micrograms of vitamin K (one-third of the daily recommended vitamin K intake for women; one-quarter of the daily requirement for men).

★ CRANBERRIES

If you drink cranberry juice to prevent urinary infections, keep drinking it. There's evidence from four well-controlled trials that drinking cranberry juice significantly cuts the number of urinary tract infections over a 12-month period, particularly in women with recurrent infections. Cranberries are an excellent source of anthocyanins, which prevent certain bacteria—including E. coli—from adhering to the bladder wall.[6] (Blueberries may also help prevent urinary tract infections, since they, too, are rich in anthocyanins.)

The anti-adhesion properties of cranberry juice may do more than reduce the risk of E. coli bladder infections. Scientists believe cranberries act as a natural probiotic, supporting the so-called friendly, health-promoting bacteria in the gastrointestinal tract while killing off unhealthy bacteria that cause illness and food poisoning.

Studies suggest that cranberries can block the adhesion of bacteria associated with gum disease and stomach ulcers caused by Helicobacter pylori bacteria. A recent study found that drinking 1 cup (250 ml) of cranberry juice twice daily during and after a 1-week course of antibiotics to treat stomach ulcers enhanced the eradication of H. pylori bacteria in women.[7] By blocking H. pylori from attaching to the stomach, cranberry juice may boost the power of antibiotics. In other words, cranberry juice renders non-adherent bacteria more vulnerable to the effects of antibiotics.

Cranberries might prevent the formation of kidney stones thanks to their quinic acid, an acidic compound that is excreted in the urine. The presence of quinic acid in the urine causes it to be just acidic enough to prevent the binding of substances that form stones. A study in which volunteers drank either 2 cups (500 ml) of cranberry juice diluted with 6 cups (1.5 L) of water or plain water found that drinking cranberry juice altered the chemical composition of the urine for the better. In other words, cranberry juice reduced urinary risk factors for kidney stones.[8]

And finally, cranberries appear to be good for your heart. Experiments in test tubes and on humans have demonstrated the ability of cranberry antioxidants to boost HDL (good) cholesterol and to protect LDL (bad) cholesterol from being oxidized by free radicals. (Oxidized LDL is considered more dangerous because it readily sticks to artery walls.)

One cup (250 ml) of fresh cranberries has 46 calories, 4.6 grams of fibre, and 13.5 milligrams of vitamin C.

★ RASPBERRIES

Their seeds packed with ellagic acid, raspberries help prevent unwanted damage to cell membranes by neutralizing harmful free radicals. But there's a lot more to raspberries than ellagic acid. They're a rich source of anthocyanins, which not only give raspberries their deep red colour but provide antioxidant and antibacterial properties. What's more, research in animals suggests that raspberries have the potential to inhibit cancer cell growth and tumour formation.

Raspberries score well for their nutrient content, too. They're an excellent source of dietary fibre, as well as of vitamin C and manganese, two antioxidants that help protect the body's tissues. Raspberries are also a good source of B vitamins, potassium, and copper.

One cup (250 ml) of fresh raspberries contains 68 calories, 8.5 grams of fibre, 28 micrograms of folate, 34 milligrams of vitamin C, and 0.9 milligrams of manganese (half a day's worth of manganese for women and 40% of the daily intake for men).

★ STRAWBERRIES

As one of the most popular of all berries, strawberries' list of health benefits is impressive. Their unique mix of phytochemicals makes strawberries a fruit that has heart-protective, anti-cancer, and anti-inflammatory properties. Anthocyanins give strawberries their bright red colour and serve as potent antioxidants, protecting cells and tissues in the body from free radical damage. Phytochemicals in strawberries have demonstrated anti-cancer actions, including blocking carcinogen formation and suppressing the growth of tumours.

Along with raspberries, strawberries are one of the richest sources of ellagic acid. The majority of ellagic acid in strawberries is present in the pulp of the fruit, rather than the seeds, as is the case with raspberries. This has led scientists to speculate that ellagic acid in strawberries is more easily absorbed than ellagic acid from raspberries. Ellagic acid in strawberries has been linked with a lower risk of cancer death. In a study of 1271 adults age 66 or older, strawberries topped a list of six foods for their ability to help combat cancer. Compared with people who seldom or never ate strawberries, those who often ate the berries were 70% less likely to die from cancer.[9]

Phytochemicals in strawberries are linked with heart health. As antioxidants, these compounds can inhibit the oxidation of LDL cholesterol, improve the function of blood vessel walls, and help prevent the formation of blood clots. Studies in the lab have also demonstrated the strawberry's ability to reduce inflammation by inhibiting the action of the enzyme cyclo-oxygenase. Overactivity of cyclo-oxygenase contributes to unwanted inflammation in the body, a risk factor for heart disease, not to mention arthritis, asthma, and cancer. Preliminary animal studies have indicated that diets rich in strawberries may also have the potential to provide benefits to the aging brain.

Strawberries have plenty to offer on the nutrition front. They outrank other berries when it comes to their vitamin C and folate content. They're also a good source of fibre, potassium, and manganese. One cup (250 ml) of fresh sliced strawberries has 56 calories, 4 grams of fibre, 42 micrograms of folate, and 103 milligrams of vitamin C (more than a full day's supply of vitamin C).

Enjoying berries

The taste of sweet, juicy strawberries marks the start of summer for me. Every year I look forward to enjoying fresh berries in June, July, and August. Although I can purchase fresh berries all year, there's nothing like the flavour of locally grown seasonal berries. To enjoy fresh berries all year-round, I freeze Ontario wild blueberries, strawberries, and raspberries in the summer.

Buying

Fresh berries are highly perishable, so purchase them as close to when you intend to use them as possible—up to a few days in advance. Choose berries that are firm, plump, and free of mould, with a uniform colour and a good aroma. Avoid overly soft and dull-coloured berries. (The deeper the colour, the higher the concentration of beneficial anthocyanins.) Make sure there is no sign of moisture, which causes berries to decay. When choosing strawberries, avoid ones that have green or yellow patches, as they are likely to taste sour. When buying fresh cranberries, choose very firm berries: Firmness is a primary quality indicator.

If you're buying berries packaged in a container, make sure they're not packed too tightly, as this can crush and damage them. When buying frozen berries, shake the bag gently to ensure the berries move freely. If the berries are clumped together, this might mean they've been thawed and refrozen.

Storing

Before storing berries in the refrigerator, remove any damaged or mouldy berries so they won't contaminate others. Store unwashed berries in their original container, covered with plastic wrap. You can also store raspberries and strawberries spread out on a plate covered with a paper towel and then covered with plastic wrap.

Properly stored in the refrigerator, blueberries will keep for up to 1 week, though they will be freshest within the first few days. Strawberries and raspberries will last for 2 days. Fresh cranberries can be stored in the fridge for several months. Storing berries at room temperature will cause them to spoil faster. Frozen berries will keep for 1 year, except for frozen cranberries, which can last for several years.

Preparing

With the exception of cranberries, fresh berries are fragile and should be handled with care to avoid bruising. Just before using, place berries (cranberries too) in a strainer and briefly rinse under cool running water. That's it—your berries are now ready to eat or add to a recipe.

To freeze berries, rinse in a strainer, drain, and remove any damaged berries. To ensure uniform texture when they're thawed, spread the berries out on a cookie sheet and place in the freezer until frozen. Then put the berries in a sealable plastic freezer bag and store in the freezer. Don't forget to date the packages.

TIPS FOR ADDING BERRIES TO YOUR MEALS

Berries are incredibly versatile fruits that bring colour, juicy flavour, and a strong nutritional punch to dishes. You can add them to a wide variety of sweet or savoury dishes, for breakfast, lunch, or dinner. Of course, they also taste great popped into your mouth, one by one.

Breakfast

- Toss a handful of fresh or dried berries into a bowl of breakfast cereal.
- Mix fresh berries into a bowl of creamy whole-grain hot cereal, such as oatmeal, brown rice, or millet.
- Mix fresh berries with low-fat yogurt and 1/2 cup (125 ml) of 100% bran cereal for an antioxidant-rich, high-fibre breakfast.
- Add berries to muffin, pancake, and waffle batters.
- Mix sliced strawberries and blueberries with cinnamon, lemon juice, and maple syrup, and serve over pancakes or waffles.
- Enjoy a breakfast smoothie made with milk or soy milk, fresh or frozen berries, a scoop of protein powder (optional), and a spoonful of ground flaxseed.
- Make breakfast pizza with whole-wheat pita, light cream cheese, and fresh berries.

RECIPES

Blueberry Walnut Muesli with Rolled Oats and Flaxseed, page 271
Blackberry Shake, page 276
Blueberry Banana Bonanza Smoothie, page 276
Raspberry Kefir Smoothie, page 281

Lunch and dinner

- Add sliced strawberries to a spinach salad for a boost of vitamin C. (The vitamin C will also enhance your body's ability to absorb the iron in the spinach.)
- Add dried cranberries or blueberries to your next green salad.
- Combine 100% pure, unsweetened cranberry juice with equal parts water for an anthocyanin-rich beverage.
- Add dried berries to whole-grain side dishes, such as brown rice, millet, quinoa, and barley. (You'll learn more about cooking whole grains in Chapter 4.)
- Make homemade cranberry sauce with fresh cranberries and orange rind as a condiment for roasted chicken or turkey.

RECIPES
Blueberry and Roasted Walnut Spinach Salad, page 289
Creamy Cold Berry Soup, page 304
Pork Tenderloin with Blackberry Dijon Sauce, page 338

Dessert and snacks

- Enjoy a dish of sliced strawberries sprinkled with a dash of pepper, balsamic vinegar, and orange juice.
- For a nutritious parfait, layer low-fat yogurt with berries in a wine glass, and top with crystallized ginger.
- Make a berry coulis as a sauce over frozen yogurt or angel food cake.
- Purée berries with low-fat milk, yogurt, and ice cubes for a refreshing midday snack.
- Add dried cranberries and blueberries to homemade granola and trail mixes.
- Add dried berries when making your favourite healthy cookie recipe.

RECIPES
Crazy Cranberry Smoothie, page 277
Balsamic Strawberries and Oranges, page 294
Mixed Berry Fruit Salad with Candied Lemon Zest, page 295
Cranberry Orange Flax Quick Bread, page 375
Blueberries Topped with Candied Almonds, page 378
Ginger-Flax Fruit Crisp, page 381
Roasted Fruit Kebabs, page 382

CITRUS FRUITS

grapefruit * lemons * limes * oranges * pummelos * tangerines

Eat 1 serving per day
1 serving = 1 fruit the size of a medium orange or 1/2 grapefruit

For many centuries, oranges were a rare commodity. They were usually made into preserves, used for a table centrepiece or decoration, or presented to guests as a luxury gift. Not so today. Oranges and other citrus fruit—lemons, limes, grapefruit, pummelos, and tangerines—are available to enjoy year-round.

The combination of nutrients and phytochemicals found in citrus fruits has piqued scientists' interest. Researchers have linked a diet high in citrus with protection from certain cancers, heart disease, and stroke. Studies in the lab support these observations. Components of citrus fruit have demonstrated anti-cancer and heart-protective properties. Citrus fruit may also help lower the risk of arthritis, asthma, macular degeneration, cataracts, and cognitive impairment.

Nutrients and phytochemicals in citrus fruits

Citrus, especially oranges, are renowned for their vitamin C, and for good reason. One large orange (3 inches/7.5 cm in diameter) supplies 98 milligrams of vitamin C, more than a full day's requirement. Getting enough vitamin C is essential to building a strong immune system, which helps your body fight illness. Vitamin C also plays an important role in maintaining collagen, a protein that forms a connective tissue supporting the skin, bone, tendons, and cartilage. Vitamin C is a well-known antioxidant, protecting cells and body tissues from oxidative stress. And—especially important if you're a vegetarian—the vitamin C in citrus fruits enhances the body's ability to absorb iron (called non-heme iron) from plant foods.

But citrus fruits have plenty of other nutrients hiding beneath their fragrant peel. Citrus fruit contains generous amounts of folate, potassium, and thiamine, as well as some vitamin A, calcium, magnesium, and fibre. Pink and red grapefruit also contain lycopene, a phytochemical thought to guard against prostate cancer. The chart below illustrates how various citrus fruits rate in terms of nutrition. Nutrients are presented for Canada's Food Guide–serving equivalents, which you'll notice is 1/2 cup (125 ml) for fruit juice. (Also notice the fibre that's missing from juice.)

Notable nutrients in selected citrus fruits

	Calories	Fibre (g)	Vitamin C (mg)	Folate (mcg)	Potassium (mg)
Orange, 1 medium	62	3.1	70	39	237
Orange juice, 1/2 cup (125 ml)	56	0	62	37	248

	Calories	Fibre (g)	Vitamin C (mg)	Folate (mcg)	Potassium (mg)
Grapefruit, pink or red, 1/2	37	1.4	45	11	156
Grapefruit, white, 1/2	39	1.3	39	12	175
Grapefruit juice, 1/2 cup (125 ml)	48	0	47	12	200
Tangerine, 1 medium	47	1.6	23.5	14	146
Lemonade (frozen concentrate, made with water)	49	0	4.8	2	19

Source: Canadian Nutrient File, 2007.

There's far more to citrus than vitamins and minerals. Citrus fruit contains unique phytochemicals that scientists believe play a large role in its ability to fight disease. In fact, an orange contains almost two hundred types of phytochemicals. Of particular interest to scientists are citrus flavanones, including hesperedin and naringenin, and limonoids, which have been the focus of many studies.

Citrus fruits and health

CITRUS FRUITS AND CANCER PREVENTION

Epidemiological studies conducted in various countries suggest that eating plenty of citrus fruit helps reduce the risk of digestive tract cancers, including cancers of the esophagus, mouth, larynx, pharynx, and stomach.[10] Research findings also hint that a citrus-rich diet can help ward off pancreatic, lung, and colon cancer.

Limonoids, found in citrus peel, may protect us from developing skin cancer. Researchers from the University of Arizona examined the link between citrus fruit consumption and squamous cell skin cancer risk among older adults living in the southwestern United States. (Squamous cell skin cancer appears in the upper levels of the epidermis, usually in places that have been exposed to the sun.) Although citrus fruit and citrus juice were not associated with reducing skin cancer risk, the use of citrus peel was protective. People who regularly incorporated citrus peel into their diet (one-third of study participants did) were 34% less likely to develop skin cancer than their peers who consumed very little. The more citrus peel consumed, the greater the protection.[11]

Many animal studies and laboratory tests with human cells have demonstrated the anti-cancer effects of citrus fruit compounds. Limonoids, which the body readily absorbs and utilizes, have been shown to fight cancers of the mouth, breast, stomach, and colon. Studies have demonstrated phytochemicals in citrus block tumour growth by acting directly on cancer cells, impeding their ability to multiply.

Laboratory research has also demonstrated the ability of naringenin, a flavanone concentrated in grapefruit, to repair damaged DNA in human prostate cancer cells. The phytochemical induces two enzymes that repair DNA during the replication phase.[12] Scientists suspect that one of the main anti-cancer properties of citrus fruit is its ability to modulate the body's detoxification systems. Experiments conducted in rats have shown grapefruit juice to significantly increase the activity of liver detoxification enzymes that rid the body of toxic substances.[13]

Folate in citrus fruit is used to make DNA and RNA, the building blocks of cells. As well, it helps prevent changes to DNA that may lead to cancer.

CITRUS FRUITS AND HEART HEALTH

An orange a day may be good for your heart. Studies have linked vitamin C–rich produce, including citrus, with a lower risk of developing coronary heart disease and stroke. In a study involving 75,696 women and 38,683 men, each additional daily serving of citrus fruit or citrus juice was associated with a 19% lower risk of ischemic stroke.[14] (An ischemic stroke results from blockage of the arteries that supply the brain.)

Many components in citrus fruit act synergistically to protect your cardiovascular system. The soluble fibre in citrus fruit helps lower blood cholesterol. The B vitamin folate is essential for the metabolism of homocysteine and helps maintain normal levels of this amino acid. Numerous studies link high homocysteine levels with a greater risk of heart attack and stroke. Potassium helps keep the body's fluids in balance and, as such, can help prevent high blood pressure. In fact, consuming adequate potassium from fruits and vegetables has been shown to lower elevated blood pressure.

Citrus phytochemicals may play a role, too. In animal studies, a diet enriched with hesperedin has been shown to lower high blood pressure and cholesterol. Hesperedin also has strong anti-inflammatory properties and acts to strengthen and tone blood vessel walls. Most of the hesperedin in citrus fruit is found in the peel and inner white pulp. That means you likely get more of this disease-fighting compound by eating citrus fruit whole (but peeled, of course) than you will by processing the flesh into juice.

Grapefruit and medications

If you take certain medications, you'll have to leave grapefruit off your menu. That's because more than thirty commonly prescribed drugs don't mix with grapefruit or grapefruit juice. Compounds in the peel, pulp, and juice of grapefruit interfere with an enzyme in the intestine wall that breaks down drugs, and they can inappropriately raise blood levels of the drug, causing potentially toxic effects.

Medications influenced by grapefruit include certain drugs used to treat high blood pressure, elevated blood cholesterol, migraines, depression, anxiety, sleep disorders, and male impotence. If you take medications for any of these conditions, check with your pharmacist to see if it is affected by grapefruit.

A glass of grapefruit juice or half a grapefruit consumed even 24 hours—and perhaps as long as 48 hours—before or after taking certain drugs can interact with the drug. Some people, especially older adults, are more sensitive than others to grapefruit's effects. It seems to depend on the amount of enzyme in the digestive tract, which varies greatly from person to person. Since the effect of increased blood drug levels can last for 3 days or more, it's recommended that you avoid all grapefruit products if taking medications that are affected. You should also avoid Seville oranges and tangelos, as they may have a similar effect.

Enjoying citrus fruits

Fresh citrus fruit from California, Florida, and Arizona is available in Canada throughout the year. Uncertain about which type of citrus is best for a snack or recipe? Are navel or Valencia oranges better for juicing? Are Meyer lemons best for baking? Here's a guide to the many varieties of citrus fruit available at produce markets and grocery stores:

• *Navel oranges* are easy to identify—they're the ones with the button formation opposite their stem end. Navel oranges are seedless, have a thick skin, and their flesh is juicy and sweet. Navel oranges are great for making juice, for fruit salads, and for snacking, since they peel and segment easily.

- *Valencia oranges* are small to medium sized, usually with a thin skin that is difficult to peel. But doing so is worth it: The flesh is juicy and sweet. The Valencia orange is well suited for juicing because its flesh contains a great amount of juice and its thin skin makes it is easy to hand-squeeze. It's also a good eating orange, containing few or no seeds.

- *Blood oranges* have a bright red to deep maroon interior colour (thanks to their anthocyanins) and an orange-red skin. Their distinctive, strong citrus flavour is sweeter and less acidic than other varieties of oranges. Blood oranges can be used like any other orange but are best used when colour is important. They tend to be small in size, are fairly easy to peel, and have few if any seeds.

- *Seville oranges* have a flattened appearance and a rough, thick skin. The flesh contains a lot of seeds. Seville oranges are bitter tasting and generally not eaten out of hand; they are more often used for cooking because of their strong orange flavour. They're popular for making marmalades, jellies, and jams, and well suited for marinades. They are mostly grown in the Mediterranean regions and have a short growing season, so they are not always readily available.

- *Minneola tangelos* are easily spotted by the knob-like formation at their stem end. This fruit has a deep red-orange skin and a sweet-tart flavour. Minneolas peel very easily and have few if any seeds.

- *Mandarin oranges* are loose skinned and easy to peel. A mandarin's size, shape, colour, and flavour will vary with the variety. In general, mandarins are sweet tasting and juicy.

- *Tangerines* are sometimes mistakenly referred to as mandarins, but they are actually a subgroup of mandarins. The tangerine is a cross between a mandarin and the bitter orange. There are many varieties of tangerines; most are smaller in size than an orange and have a slightly flattened shape. Their skins are generally deep reddish-orange, slightly textured, loose fitting, and easy to peel. They contain 8 to 15 segments, which are easily separated.

- *Pummelos,* sometimes referred to as Chinese grapefruit, are the largest citrus fruit. They grow to be as big or bigger than a grapefruit, have a thick green to yellow skin, and firm flesh. Interior colour varies from white to deep pink. Pummelos commonly have from 16 to 18 firm, juicy segments, whereas most grapefruit have 12 segments. The taste of pummelo is sweeter and less acidic than grapefruit.

- *Meyer lemons* are favourites of chefs and food lovers, as they are sweeter than regular lemons (e.g., Eureka and Lisbon). When a Meyer lemon's flesh or juice is added to a dish, it adds a sweet and only slightly tart flavour. It has a soft skin that develops an orange hue when the fruit is fully ripe. Its distinctive flavour hints at tangerine; indeed, the Meyer lemon is actually a cross between a lemon and another citrus fruit— possibly an orange or a mandarin. It was introduced to North America from China in 1908 by Frank N. Meyer, a U.S. government employee. As they require more care when shipping and storing, they are not widely grown on a commercial basis but are occasionally available in specialty food stores.

Buying

Choose citrus fruit that is firm and heavy for its size, which indicates it contains a fair amount of juice. Avoid any fruit that is damaged, shrivelled, or has mouldy or soft spots.

When selecting oranges, look for skins that are relatively smooth. They may have a hint of green: This does not indicate inferior quality but is caused by warm growing temperatures at night, which deprive the crop of the cool temperatures that contribute to the orange colour. As the fruit ripens, it remains slightly green on the outside, though developing perfectly on the inside.

Choose mandarins with a glossy, bright orange skin. Mandarins should feel soft and puffy compared with oranges because of their loose skin.

Buy grapefruits that are firm but slightly springy when pressed. A grapefruit doesn't have to look perfect to be good quality. Skin discolouration, scratches, or scales will not effect the fruit's interior. Avoid grapefruits that have an overly rough or wrinkled skin; these tend to be thick skinned and will have less juice.

Choose lemons with as thin a skin as possible, since thicker skinned lemons are less juicy. Lemons should be bright yellow in colour and have skin with a finely grained texture. Avoid lemons with green-tinged spots— an indication that the lemon is not fully ripened and will be more acidic.

Limes at the peak of their flavour will have a deep green colour. Brown spots, or scald, on the skin won't affect the taste, but avoid limes that have a hard or shrivelled skin.

Storing

Citrus fruit will keep at room temperature for 1 week if kept out of direct sunlight. When stored at room temperature, citrus fruit will be juicier than if kept in the fridge. However, if you are not planning to use the fruit within 1 week of purchase, store it in the refrigerator crisper, for up to 2 to 3 weeks. If storing citrus fruit in a plastic bag, make sure the bag is perforated to allow air circulation.

Preparing

There's not much to say here. Just peel, then section, cut or juice, and enjoy. Or, to make citrus zest, remove the coloured part of the rind only (avoid the white pith). For strips of citrus peel, use a vegetable peeler. For grated zest, use a zester.

TIPS FOR ADDING CITRUS FRUITS TO YOUR MEALS

Citrus fruits are incredibly versatile. Oranges, grapefruits, tangerines, and pummelos can be eaten as snacks or desserts, juiced, grilled, puréed, or added to myriad dishes, from fruit salad to chicken to soup. They also come with their own protective package, making them perfect for the lunch bag, briefcase, or knapsack. Although you probably won't snack on a lemon or lime, these citrus fruits enhance the flavour of many dishes.

Breakfast

- Start the day with a glass of freshly squeezed orange or grapefruit juice.
- Add citrus fruit segments to a fruit salad.
- Add orange segments and orange juice to smoothies.
- Mix citrus segments with low-fat yogurt for a light but flavourful breakfast.
- Add lemon zest to your favourite muffin or pancake recipe.
- Add 1 teaspoon (5 ml) citrus zest to black or herbal tea for an infusion of limonoids.

RECIPES

Lemon Ginger Infusion, page 278
Low-Fat Lemon Millet Muffins, page 377

Lunch and dinner

- Toss segments of citrus fruit into green salads for a boost of vitamin C.
- Add citrus segments to a mixed bean salad for a dash of colour and flavour.

- Use freshly squeezed citrus juice in vinaigrettes and other salad dressings.
- Top low-fat cottage cheese with orange or grapefruit segments and toasted walnuts for a light and healthy lunch. Drizzle freshly squeezed orange juice on top.
- Toss orange segments into sweet-and-sour stir-fries near the end of cooking.
- Place thinly sliced lemons, peel and all, underneath and around fish before baking. Baking will soften the lemon slices, so they can be eaten along with the fish.
- Use freshly squeezed citrus juice and citrus zest in marinades for chicken, beef, or fish.
- Toss cooked brown rice with chickpeas, scallions, lime juice, and lime zest for a tasty side dish.
- Sauté sliced cooked beets with freshly squeezed orange juice and orange zest for a healthy vegetable dish.
- Combine diced grapefruit with cilantro, chopped red peppers, and red onion for a refreshing fruit salsa.
- Squeeze a wedge of lemon or lime over vegetables to add flavour without sodium.
- Include orange segments in fruit compotes to be spooned over ice cream or frozen yogurt for a flavourful dessert.

RECIPES
Spinach and Grapefruit Salad, page 292
Avocado Citrus Salad, page 293

Dessert and snacks

- Peel an orange and enjoy nature at its best.
- Skewer orange segments, chunks of cantaloupe, grapes, strawberries, and pineapple for festive fruit kebabs. Serve with orange-yogurt dip.
- Include orange or grapefruit segments in fruit compotes, to be spooned over low-fat frozen yogurt for a flavourful dessert.

RECIPES
Balsamic Strawberries and Oranges, page 294
Lemon Ginger Fruit Dip, page 359
Cranberry Orange Flax Quick Bread, page 375
Roasted Fruit Kebabs, page 382

★ POMEGRANATE
pomegranate juice ★ pomegranate seeds
Eat 3 servings per week

1 serving = 1/2 cup (125 ml) pomegranate seeds *or*
 1/2 cup (125 ml) 100% pomegranate juice *or*
 1/4 cup (50 ml) dried berries

The pomegranate has been valued for its medicinal properties since ancient times. But it has only been in recent years that North Americans have come to regard pomegranate as a superfood. It's the juice of the pomegranate that has sparked the interest of nutrition scientists and health enthusiasts.

Inside a pomegranate's rosy red outer shell you'll find individual cells, separated by membranes, containing glistening red seeds. Each seed is surrounded by a juice-filled sac, called an aril, which is pressed during processing. Pomegranate juice contains potent antioxidants, in particular, polyphenols. Research conducted by the manufacturers of POM Wonderful pomegranate juice concluded that the antioxidant level in pomegranate juice was higher than that found in other fruit juices, including blueberry, cranberry, and orange, and even red wine.

Scientists suspect pomegranate's polyphenols may benefit the heart. In a study of 45 patients with coronary heart disease, those who drank 1 cup (250 ml) of POM Wonderful pomegranate juice daily for 3 months had improved blood flow to the heart. Another study found that drinking pomegranate juice each day for 1 year reduced blood pressure, decreased the oxidation of LDL (bad) cholesterol, and reduced clogging of the arteries that supply the brain.[15] Another study demonstrated the ability of daily pomegranate juice consumption to lower total and LDL cholesterol and increase HDL (good) cholesterol levels in patients with type 2 diabetes.[16] Pomegranate juice also appears to stimulate the production of nitric oxide, a chemical that helps blood vessels relax.

Pomegranate juice may slow the progression of prostate cancer. A preliminary study found that after treatment for prostate cancer, the length of time it took for prostate specific antigen (a substance made by the prostate and found in elevated levels when there are prostate abnormalities) to double was significantly longer in men who drank 1 cup (250 ml) of pomegranate juice daily for up to 2 years.[17] Studies in the lab also suggest that pomegranate polyphenols might guard against lung cancer.

These research findings do sound promising. But keep in mind these studies are based on very small numbers of people. Although it's too soon to say that drinking pomegranate juice prevents disease, it's certainly a healthy and nutritious addition to your diet, as pomegranates are a good source of potassium and provide some vitamin C.

If you want to add pomegranate juice to your diet, be prepared to open your pocketbook. A 16 ounce (473 ml) bottle of POM sells for around five dollars—more than four times the price of orange juice. You'll also have to factor in a few extra calories. One cup (250 ml) of pomegranate juice supplies roughly 160 calories, whereas the same serving of orange juice has 110 calories. One-half of a whole pomegranate—a food guide serving—has 53 calories.

Enjoying pomegranate

When late fall arrives and other locally grown fresh fruits begin to disappear from the grocery store shelves, it's time to look for vibrant red pomegranates. Their wonderful shape and beautiful colour make pomegranates a perfect fruit for special holiday meals.

Buying

Pomegranates range in colour from a pale reddish yellow to a deep crimson red. Unlike many other fruits and vegetables, the colour of a pomegranate is not an indication of the quality inside the shell. Even the presence of few external blemishes doesn't mean the fruit is poor in quality. That's because a pomegranate's thick skin protects the inner fruit. When shopping, choose a pomegranate heavy for its size. The heavier the fruit, the more juice inside.

Storing

Fresh, unopened pomegranates will keep at room temperature, out of direct sunlight, for 1 to 2 weeks. If you store them in the vegetable drawer of your refrigerator, they'll last for up to 3 months. Store cut pomegranates in a tightly sealed plastic bag in the refrigerator for up to 1 week.

Fresh arils (the juice-filled sacs that contain the edible seeds) should be stored in an airtight container in the refrigerator, where they'll keep for a few days. You can also freeze arils so that you can enjoy the goodness of pomegranate seeds all year-round. Keep arils in a tightly sealed plastic bag in the freezer for up to 1 year.

Preparing

Before you can enjoy pomegranate seeds, you have to get inside the thick shell. Start by cutting off the crown, then scoring the outer layer of skin into sections. In a large bowl of water, break apart the sections along the score lines. Roll out the arils with your fingers. The arils will sink to the bottom while the white membrane floats to the top of the water. After skimming off the membrane, drain the water from the bowl or pour through a sieve. You can eat the arils whole, seeds and all. Or you might want to add seeds to dishes. To obtain the juice, push the arils through a sieve.

TIPS FOR ADDING POMEGRANATE TO YOUR MEALS

The best way to enjoy the taste and nutrition of pomegranates is to dig in and eat out of hand. And there are many other ways to enjoy pomegranate that require no cooking at all. Of course, I've included a few tasty recipes that do require cooking just to show you how versatile this fruit is. I'm sure that once you start enjoying the sweet-tart taste of pomegranates, you'll find many creative ways to add it to meals and snacks.

Fresh pomegranates

- Try a breakfast smoothie made with pomegranate seeds, banana, ground flaxseed, and low-fat milk or soy milk.
- Toss pomegranate seeds into your green salad for an infusion of antioxidants and vibrant colour.
- Top a bowl of yogurt with pomegranate seeds for a healthy dessert or snack.
- Sprinkle pomegranate seeds over cold breakfast cereal or stir them into a bowl of whole-grain oatmeal.
- Add pomegranate seeds to muffin, pancake, and waffle batters.
- Garnish steamed brown rice and other whole grains with pomegranate seeds. Or add pomegranate seeds to a rice pilaf.
- Mix pomegranate seeds with plain yogurt to make a tasty dipping sauce for skewers of grilled chicken, pork, or lamb.

RECIPES

Pomegranate juice

- Add pomegranate juice, fresh or store-bought, to vinaigrettes for a fruity salad dressing.
- Warm pomegranate juice with honey in a pot over low heat, then brush the glaze over chicken, lamb, or beef during roasting.
- Add a splash of pomegranate juice to sparkling water, or even champagne, for an antioxidant boost.

RECIPE

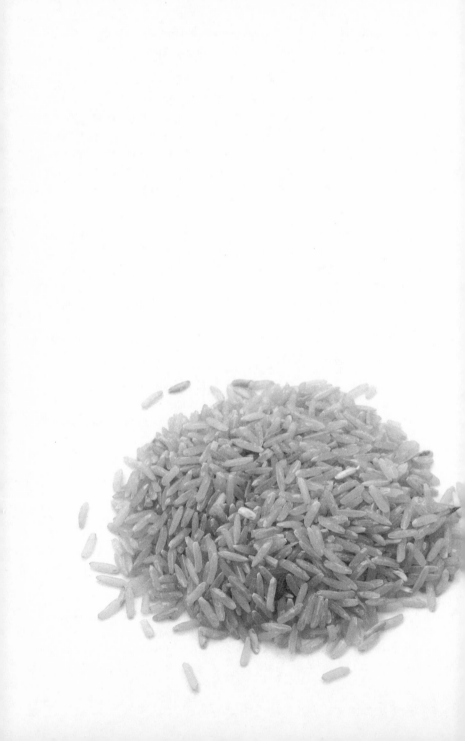

4

Power grains

★ amaranth   ★ oats

★ barley   ★ quinoa

★ brown rice   ★ rye

★ buckwheat   ★ spelt

★ flaxseed   ★ whole wheat

★ kamut   ★ wild rice

★ millet

Judging by the grocery store shelves, the low-carbohydrate diet fad is over. No longer are people shunning bread, pasta, and rice in an effort to lose weight. Bored with bunless burgers and countless cheese sticks and concerned about their health, it appears that weight-conscious Canadians have welcomed carbohydrates back into their meals. But not just any type of carbohydrates. Today the carbohydrates of choice are whole grain.

Growing consumer interest in the link between foods and disease prevention has prompted food manufacturers to add more whole-grain foods to grocery store shelves. You no longer have to rely on cooking a pot of oatmeal or brown rice to get your whole grains. Today you can find a wide variety of breads, crackers, pasta, breakfast cereals, even energy bars made from whole grains. You can even find "whole grain" added to sugary breakfast cereals. (But don't be fooled. You'll learn later in this chapter that all whole-grain products are not created equal.)

When it comes to health—and weight control—scientists are learning that what's most important is the *quality* of the carbohydrate-rich foods you eat. A wealth of scientific evidence shows that people who choose whole grains over their refined counterparts have better health outcomes. Studies consistently link a diet rich in whole-grain foods with protection from heart disease, stroke, type 2 diabetes, certain cancers, and obesity.

The bottom line is that whole-grain foods help fight disease and are a key component of a healthy diet. The sections below will help you choose, prepare, and enjoy nutritious whole grains.

What are whole grains?

All grains—be it wheat, rye, oats, or spelt—start out as whole-grain kernels composed of three layers: the outer bran layer where nearly all the fibre is; the inner germ layer that's rich in nutrients, antioxidants, and healthy fats; and the endosperm, which contains most of the starch. Eating foods made from whole grains means you're getting *all* parts of the grain kernel and all the nutrients, phytochemicals, and fibre they contain. In fact, the fibre content of whole grains can be four times that of refined grains. The reason whole grains are darker and chewier than refined grains is because they contain all three components of the grain kernel.

When whole grains are refined, milled, scraped, and heat processed into flakes, puffs, or white flour, the bran and germ are removed and all that's left is the starchy endosperm. Without bran and germ, about 25% of a grain's protein is lost along with at least 17 nutrients. In addition to having less protein, refined grains contain less fibre, vitamins, and minerals, and 75% fewer phytochemicals. Refined grains are enriched with some, but not all, vitamins and minerals lost through processing. However, disease-fighting phytochemicals are not added back to refined grains.

Whole grains can be eaten whole (e.g., wheat berries, oats), cracked, split, flaked, or ground. Often they're milled into flour and used to make breads, cereals, pastas, and crackers. A whole grain can be a single food, such as oatmeal, brown rice, flaxseed, kamut, millet, or quinoa, or it can be an ingredient in another food, for example, bread, crackers, and ready-to-eat breakfast cereal.

Whole-grain nutrition

All grains are naturally low in fat and good sources of energy-yielding carbohydrate and various vitamins and minerals. But grains that haven't been refined are much better for you thanks to their sizeable nutrient content. It's this package of nutrients—vitamins, minerals, fibre, antioxidants, and phytochemicals—that's thought to exert health benefits. Scientists suspect the individual components of whole grains work together to guard against disease.

Whole grains are particularly good sources of fibre, folate, vitamin E, magnesium, and selenium. The main phytochemicals found in whole grains include compounds called lignans and phytosterols (*phytosterols* is a collective term for plant-derived compounds called sterols and stanols). The chart below outlines important disease-fighting compounds found in whole grains and what they do in the body.

Key nutrients and phytochemicals in whole grains

Nutrient	What it does	Good sources
Insoluble fibre	Adds bulk to stool and helps prevent constipation, hemorrhoids, and diverticulosis and possibly colon cancer.	Whole wheat Brown rice
Soluble fibre	Lowers cholesterol and helps reduce the risk of heart disease and stroke. Helps stabilize blood sugar by slowing the absorption of glucose from the gut. Increases the feeling of fullness after eating and may help prevent weight gain.	Barley Oats, oat bran Rye
Resistant starch	Encourages growth of beneficial bacteria to help keep the bowel healthy.	All whole grains
Folate	Helps produce and maintain new cells, is needed to make DNA, and helps prevent changes to DNA that may lead to cancer.	Fortified whole-grain ready-to-eat cereals
Vitamin E	Protects cells against harmful effects of free radicals (antioxidant), enhances immune function, helps repair DNA.	All whole grains
Magnesium	Helps regulate blood sugar, promotes normal blood pressure, is involved in energy metabolism and bone health.	100% bran Oat bran Brown rice
Selenium	Used to make enzymes in body that act as antioxidants, enhance immune system function, and help regulate thyroid function.	Brown rice Whole wheat
Lignans	Lower LDL cholesterol levels and may help prevent heart disease. May reduce risk of breast, ovarian, endometrial, and prostate cancers.	Flaxseed
Phytosterols	Lower LDL cholesterol levels and may help prevent coronary heart disease.	Whole wheat

Whole grains and health

As you'll read below, there are plenty of reasons to trade in your white bread for whole-wheat, your white rice for brown, and your Special K for Cheerios.

Studies consistently show that people who eat their grains whole instead of refined have better health outcomes. Researchers have linked a high intake of total whole grains, as well as specific whole grains, with a lower risk of many diseases. Scientists have also demonstrated how whole grains act in the body, adding support for their ability to help ward off disease.

WHOLE GRAINS AND HEART DISEASE

When it comes to the beneficial health effects of whole grains, the evidence is the strongest for protection against heart disease. Large studies have reported that people who eat more whole grains have a lower risk for heart attack and stroke. In general, those with the highest intakes of whole grains (about 3 servings per day) had a risk of heart disease that was 20% to 30% lower than those with the lowest intakes. Whole-grain foods consumed in these studies included dark bread, whole-grain breakfast cereals, popcorn, cooked oatmeal, brown rice, bran, barley, bulgur, and kasha.

A combined analysis of seven studies that examined the link between whole-grain intake and cardiovascular disease concluded there indeed was a consistent protective effect from whole grains. Compared with people who ate less than half a serving each day, those whose diets contained 2.5 servings per day were 21% less likely to develop heart disease or stroke.[1]

A steady intake of whole grains may also delay the progression of heart disease by slowing the buildup of plaque in the arteries. A study from Tufts University in Boston found that among postmenopausal women with established heart disease, those who consumed more than 6 servings of whole grains each week had decreased narrowing of the coronary arteries compared with women whose diets contained fewer whole grains.[2]

There are many ways in which whole grains can protect the heart. For starters, they're good sources of nutrients that are linked to protection from heart disease: folate, vitamin E, magnesium, and potassium. Soluble fibre in oats, barley, and flaxseed can also help keep LDL cholesterol levels in the healthy range, thereby reducing heart disease risk. In fact, in a study of 3588 older adults, only fibre from cereal grains (not fibre from vegetables and fruit) was found protective from heart attack and stroke. The most protective fibre came from dark breads, such as wheat, rye, and pumpernickel.[3] Phytosterols in whole grains have also been shown to help reduce elevated blood cholesterol levels.

Compounds in whole grains seem to keep blood vessel walls healthy as well. One study found that among 1178 men and women, whole-grain eaters had carotid arteries that were less thick.[4] (The carotid arteries supply your head and neck with oxygen-rich blood.) The thickness of carotid arteries is a sign of atherosclerosis or hardening of the arteries, a risk factor for heart attack and stroke.

WHOLE GRAINS AND TYPE 2 DIABETES

The incidence of type 2 diabetes is on the rise in Canada, largely because we're getting older and heavier. With type 2 diabetes, the body's cells become resistant to the effects of insulin, the hormone that clears sugar from the bloodstream. As a result, blood levels of glucose rise above what's considered normal. There have been many scientific reports linking a higher intake of whole grain and fibre from cereals with a lower diabetes risk. Research suggests that eating whole grains often (3 servings per day), compared with rarely or not at all, can lower the risk of type 2 diabetes by as much as 30%. In countries where whole-grain intake is high, for example, Finland, the risk of diabetes is reduced by 20% to 35%.

Whole grains are thought to guard against type 2 diabetes by preventing the onset of metabolic risk factors that lead to diabetes. Many studies show that men and women who consume at least 3 servings of whole grains per day are much less likely to develop metabolic syndrome and insulin resistance (when the body can't properly use insulin or blood glucose).[5] Metabolic syndrome is a precursor to type 2 diabetes and heart disease. It's characterized by a cluster of risk factors in one person, including abdominal obesity, high LDL cholesterol, low HDL cholesterol, elevated blood pressure, insulin resistance, and a high level of an inflammatory compound in the blood called C-reactive protein.

The fibre in whole grains is thought to play an important role in helping lower the risk of diabetes. Fibre, especially soluble fibre, dampens the rise in blood sugar after eating by slowing the absorption of glucose from the gut. Another recent study that followed 9702 men and 15,365 women for 7 years found that getting more fibre from grains (but not fruits and vegetables) reduced the onset of type 2 diabetes. Persons who ate the most cereal fibre, 17 grams per day, were almost 30% less likely to develop diabetes than those who averaged only 7 grams per day.[6]

In addition to fibre, magnesium may play a role in protection from type 2 diabetes. Researchers have learned that the mineral helps improve the body's capacity to use insulin. A pooled analysis of 13 studies concluded that a greater magnesium intake was associated with a reduced diabetes risk.[7]

That whole-grain foods have a lower glycemic index (GI) than refined grains may also explain why they have been shown to reduce the risk of diabetes. Because low GI foods raise your blood glucose more slowly and to a less dramatic peak than higher GI foods, your pancreas does not need to produce excessive amounts of insulin to return your blood glucose to the normal range. In other words, low GI whole grains put less wear and tear on your pancreas and can help prevent you from developing type 2 diabetes. (See Chapter 1, page 14, for more information on the glycemic index.)

WHOLE GRAINS AND CANCER

Even though some studies suggest that a diet containing plenty of whole grains can protect against cancer, the science isn't as solid as it is for heart disease and type 2 diabetes. In 1998, researchers pooled the results of 40 case-control studies examining the link between whole-grain intake and different types of cancer and concluded that people who consumed the most whole grains (especially whole-grain bread) were 34% less likely to develop cancer than were those who consumed less. Whole grains appeared to protect the most from digestive tract cancers, including colon and stomach (gastric) cancers.[8]

In case-control studies, researchers contact people who have been diagnosed with a disease (cases), and people who have not (controls). Both groups are asked about the foods they ate during the years before they were diagnosed with the disease. The objective in these studies was to see if the people who were diagnosed with cancer were more likely to consume whole grains than people without the disease. Although this analysis certainly suggests that whole grains guard against digestive tract cancers, results from case-control studies have limitations. People with illnesses often report diets differently from healthy people. For instance, it is possible that when asked about their history, people who have a particular disease recall certain behaviours or exposures differently from people who do not have the disease. Women with breast cancer who are asked what they ate may be more likely to recall certain things they ate because they know diet may be related to their disease. However, if you ask women without breast cancer what they ate, they may be less likely to remember eating these same foods or nutrients. This is because they don't have the disease, so they don't think about their diet in as much detail as do women with breast cancer. This is called recall bias. And on top of this, it's not always easy to recall what you ate 10 or 20 years ago, resulting in inaccuracies.

That's one reason why the evidence for whole grains and cancer prevention is not as strong as it is for heart disease and diabetes. The evidence for whole grains' protective effects on the latter come mainly from prospective, or cohort, studies. In these types of studies, researchers follow a large group of healthy people (the cohort) over a long period—typically 10 years or more—and gather diet, lifestyle, weight, and medical information at regular intervals. After a specified amount of time, researchers observe who develops a certain disease and determine if those who became ill ate more or less of a certain food, or nutrient, than the people who remained healthy. Prospective studies generally provide more reliable results than case-control studies do because prospective studies don't rely on information from the past.

Colorectal cancer

A few prospective studies do, however, suggest that eating your whole grains can help reduce the risk of colon cancer. One such study followed 61,433 Swedish women for almost 15 years and found that those who ate the most whole grains—at least 4.5 daily servings versus fewer than 1.5— were 35% less likely to develop colon cancer.[9]

Scientists have long speculated that it's the fibre in whole grains that helps keep the colon free of cancer. The theory holds that since insoluble fibre in whole grains speeds the passage of food through the digestive tract, there's less time for the colon to be exposed to toxic substances that could potentially promote cancer cell growth. And because fibre adds bulk to stool, it may also dilute cancer-causing substances that could come into contact with the colon. Yet, findings from two randomized clinical trials concluded that fibre supplements did not prevent the recurrence of adenomas, polyps in the colon that have the potential to become cancerous.

I mentioned earlier that scientists believe it's the package of nutrients and phytochemicals in whole grains that's responsible for their health benefits. Perhaps fibre supplements don't reduce colon cancer risk because they lack all the other disease-fighting components found in whole grains. That is certainly what the results from a recent large prospective study suggest. In the study, involving over 291,988 men and 197,623 women age 50 to 71, researchers analyzed fibre intake from many food sources. Interestingly, only fibre from whole grains was associated with a lower risk of colorectal cancer. Participants who ate the most whole grain were one-fifth as likely to develop colorectal cancer as those who ate the least.[10]

Breast cancer

Increasing your intake of high-fibre whole grains may help guard against breast cancer, since a high-fibre diet has been shown to reduce the amount of circulating estrogen in a woman's body. High levels of circulating estrogen have been linked positively to cancer tumour development. Sprinkling ground flaxseed, a whole grain, over your bowl of breakfast cereal might also lower the odds of breast cancer. Flaxseed is particularly high in lignans, phytochemicals that appear to decrease estrogen production and inhibit the growth of some breast cancers. As phytoestrogens (plant estrogens), active substances that have a weak estrogen-like action in the body, lignans can bind to breast cells, thereby blocking the ability of a woman's own estrogen to take the spot. (It's believed that the longer breast tissue is exposed to estrogen that's made in the body, the greater the chance for cells to become cancerous.) Researchers have demonstrated that women who consume 1 or 2 tablespoons (15 to 25 ml) of ground flaxseed each day had significantly lowered circulating estrogen levels.[11] Lignans in whole grains may also inhibit the action of enzymes that are involved in the body's production of estrogen. To date, research on flaxseed has focused on estrogen-receptor-negative breast cancers. The effect of flaxseed on estrogen-receptor-positive breast cancer is unknown.

Other components of whole grains shown to have anti-cancer properties include folate, selenium, and resistant starch. The resistant starch in whole grains, which isn't metabolized until it reaches the large intestine, is used by bacteria to form butyrate and other compounds called short chain fatty acids that are thought to be protective against the formation of cancerous tumours.

Prostate cancer

It's not only women who benefit from flaxseed in their diets. Studies conducted in animals and men suggest that a flaxseed-enriched diet can prevent prostate cancer. To reap the benefits of flaxseed, you need to grind it before you eat it. Grinding flaxseed releases its lignans, as well as omega-3 fatty acids, making them available for absorption.

Adding ground flaxseed to your diet might guard against other cancers as well. In several laboratory studies, flaxseed has inhibited the formation of colon, skin, and lung tumours.

WHOLE GRAINS AND WEIGHT CONTROL

Substituting whole grains for refined grains can also help you control your weight. A study from Harvard Medical School that followed over 74,000 women for 12 years concluded that those who consumed the most whole-grain foods consistently weighed less than those who ate less. What's more, whole-grain eaters were half as likely to become obese over the study period.[12]

A diet based on whole grains is more filling than one consisting of fluffy, processed grains. Fibre-rich whole grains stay in your stomach longer, slowing down the rate of digestion and helping you feel full longer. That's why a single slice of whole-grain bread is more filling—and more satisfying—than two slices of white bread. And the fibre content of whole grains may affect the secretion of intestinal hormones that may increase satiety.

The weight-control effects of whole grains may also be because of their lower glycemic load. Eating foods with a high glycemic index, such as white bread and potatoes, causes blood glucose and insulin levels to rise higher than when you eat those with a low glycemic index. In response to excess insulin secretion, your blood glucose (sugar) level drops lower over the next few hours, which can trigger hunger and overeating. Intact whole grains, on the other hand, are digested more slowly and gradually released as glucose in the bloodstream. As a result, you don't experience an outpouring of insulin, so your blood sugar remains stable and your hunger is kept at bay.

WHOLE GRAINS AND INFLAMMATION

Today, there's much talk among scientists about the role of inflammation—the process by which the body responds to infection or injury—in the development and progression of disease. Inflammation, which can be triggered by environmental factors or genetic influences, is thought to be a risk factor for several diseases, including heart attack, stroke, diabetes, cancer, and Alzheimer's.

It seems that adding whole grains to your diet may actually reduce inflammation in the body. In a study of 41,836 postmenopausal women age 55 to 69, inflammation-related death was inversely linked with whole-grain intake. Compared with women who rarely or never ate whole grains, those who consumed 4 to 7 servings per week were 31% less likely to die from an inflammation-related disease. Because inflammatory responses in the body cause oxidative stress and produce cell-damaging free radicals, it's thought that components of whole grains lessen these harmful effects.[13]

Identifying whole grains—reading labels

It's easy to spot packages of single whole grains such as brown rice, quinoa, and oatmeal in the grocery stores. It can be trickier, however, to find 100% whole-grain breads, crackers, and breakfast cereals. For instance, you might be hard-pressed to know if Kellogg's Special K cereal is refined (yes), a bread labelled "multi-grain" is whole grain (not always), or if unbleached wheat flour is white flour in disguise (always). And what about that pumpernickel bagel—is it whole grain? Is the bran muffin from the bakery made with 100% whole-grain flour?

Food manufacturers are making it easier for you to shop for whole-grain products. In addition to new product offerings, companies are educating consumers about whole-grain benefits and how to identify them in the grocery store. General Mills now stamps cereal boxes with "whole grain" in bright letters. Weston Bakeries has added a "made with 100% whole grains" banner to loaves of Country Harvest breads. Boxes of Triscuit crackers state "made with 100% whole-wheat."

But just because a food has "whole grain" boldly stamped on its package does not mean it's jam-packed with whole grains. Although some products add a significant amount of whole grain to your diet, others provide very little. And not all are nutritionally equal. If you fill your cereal bowl with General Mills' Whole Grain Lucky Charms (made from whole-grain oats), don't be fooled into thinking you're starting your day with the goodness of cooked oatmeal. You may not find any refined grain in a bowl of Lucky Charms, but you will find plenty of sugar and very little fibre. One serving (1 cup/250 ml) delivers 3 teaspoons (15 ml) of sugar and only 1 gram of fibre. (The same size serving of oatmeal provides 4 grams of fibre and no sugar.) Don't get me wrong. A sugary whole-grain cereal is better for you than a sugary refined cereal. I'm just not sure it ranks as a health food.

Similarly, labels that state "multi-grain," "seven grain," and "prairie bran" don't guarantee a food contains whole grains. Colour isn't a good indicator either, since foods may be darker because of the addition of molasses or caramel colouring. Some whole grains, such as oats, aren't brown in colour, so foods made from them may be lighter in colour.

And it turns out that you can't always count on your 100% whole-wheat bread to be a whole grain. That's because under current Canadian regulations, products labelled "whole wheat" can actually have as much as 70% of the germ removed: Manufacturers are allowed to remove a substantial portion of the nutrient-rich germ and still call their product 100% whole wheat. In fact, most whole-wheat products contain only 30% of the nutrient-rich germ. Removing the germ from flour removes unsaturated fats that can turn rancid. As a result, whole-wheat flour and breads made with whole-wheat flour will keep longer on store shelves. What's in the best interest of the manufacturer is not always what's best for your health.

At the time of writing, the Heart and Stroke Foundation of Canada, Dietitians of Canada, and the Canadian Diabetes Association are urging Health Canada to ensure that products labelled "whole wheat" are made from the *entire* grain. While you wait for the government to revise its labelling regulations, read labels. Look for the phrase "whole-grain whole wheat flour including germ." If your favourite bread lists only "whole wheat flour," call the manufacturer to ask if its whole-wheat product is truly whole grain (e.g., it contains 100% of the germ).

The only way to know for sure if a packaged food is 100% whole grain is to read the label. You may need to look past the front of the package and check the ingredient list on the side or back to find out if a product is completely or predominately whole grain.

Look for "100% whole grain" claims on food packages. The greater the percentage of whole grain, the greater the health benefit. Be skeptical if you see only the phrases "whole grain" or "made with whole grains," as these products may contain only tiny amounts of whole grain. Here's what you need to look for on food packages:

Words that always mean whole grain
(These ingredients contain all parts of the grain.)

whole-grain whole wheat
whole [name of grain]
stoneground whole [name of grain]
brown rice
oatmeal
oats
wheat berries

Words that may not mean whole grain

(These ingredients may be missing part of the grain.)

durum wheat
multigrain
organic flour
semolina
whole wheat

Words that mean refined grain

(These ingredients may be missing part of the grain.)

corn meal
unbleached wheat flour
wheat flour
wheat germ

Choose products that list whole grains first in the ingredient list (e.g., whole-grain whole wheat, whole rye, whole spelt, brown rice, oats, flaxseed). If the whole grain is listed second, maybe only a little or nearly half of the product is whole grain, especially if there are only a few ingredients in the product. (Ingredients are listed by weight from most to least.)

How much whole grain do you need?

After reading about the various studies I discussed above, you're probably thinking that 3 daily servings is a pretty good bet. You're right. The 2007 Canada's Food Guide recommends that Canadians eat at least half of their daily grain products as whole grain. For adults, that translates into 3 to 4 servings per day. School-age kids and teenagers should eat 2 to 3 whole-grain servings each day. This advice is in line with the many research findings suggesting you need to eat at least 3 servings of whole grains each day to reap their health benefits. Three servings isn't a lot when you consider what counts as a serving. Take a look:

Children, 5–19 years: Eat 2 to 3 servings per day
Adults: Eat 3 to 4 servings per day

Serving = 1 ounce (30 g) slice of 100% whole-grain bread *or*
1 ounce (30 g) whole-grain breakfast cereal *or*
1/2 cup (125 ml) cooked grain (e.g., brown rice *or* quinoa) *or*
1/2 cup (125 ml) cooked whole-grain pasta *or*
2 tablespoons (25 ml) ground flaxseed

There is more to the world of whole grains than whole-wheat bread and brown rice. Although these are certainly healthy whole-grain foods to include in your diet, there are many other whole grains that will also add flavour, texture, and interest to your meals. Many of the whole grains listed below can be purchased in grocery stores. For some, however, you may need to visit a natural food store or specialty food shop. Here's a quick guide to whole grains. You'll find cooking instructions for most of these whole grains later in this chapter.

★ AMARANTH

This gluten-free grain originates from South America, where it's a staple foodstuff. Amaranth is gaining popularity in North America for its versatility and unusually high protein content. It's also a good source of dietary fibre, iron, calcium, magnesium, copper, and manganese. Amaranth can be cooked as a cereal, popped like popcorn, sprouted, or toasted. It's very high in protein and contains high levels of calcium and iron when compared with other cereal grains. Amaranth seeds can also be ground into flour and used in baked goods and pasta.

Per 1/2 cup (125 ml) cooked: 144 calories, 5.6 grams protein, 5.6 grams fibre.

★ BARLEY (HULLED OR DEHULLED)

Barley is reportedly the oldest cultivated cereal and is thought to even predate the cultivation of rice in the Far East. Barley is a versatile grain with a rich nutty flavour and chewy, pasta-like texture. It's an excellent source of fibre and selenium and a good source of phosphorus, copper, and manganese. Hulled barley (sometimes called dehulled barley) is the whole-grain version; only the outermost hull of the grain is removed, preserving its nutrient content. Because it's been processed to a lesser degree than pearl barley or pot barley, hulled barley is chewier and requires more soaking and cooking.

Per 1/2 cup (125 ml) cooked: 136 calories, 4.8 grams protein, 6.4 grams fibre.

★ BROWN RICE

A staple food for two-thirds of the world's population, rice is a wholesome and nutritious cereal grain that can be made into myriad sweet and savoury dishes. Brown rice, with only the outer layer removed, is a good source of many vitamins and minerals, including fibre, niacin (a B vitamin), vitamin B6, magnesium, manganese, phosphorus, and selenium.

Per 1/2 cup (125 ml) cooked: 108 calories, 2.5 grams protein, 1.5 grams fibre.

★ BUCKWHEAT

Eaten as a staple in many part of Europe, this whole grain is eaten widely in the form of kasha, whole groats, and soba noodles. Buckwheat is actually not a grain seed, even though that's how it's classified in the culinary world. Rather, it's the seed of a fruit that is related to rhubarb and sorrel. That's why buckwheat is a great substitute for people with wheat allergy or gluten intolerance. Buckwheat is sold both unroasted and roasted (kasha). Unroasted buckwheat has a soft, subtle flavour, while roasted buckwheat has an earthy, nutty taste. You can also buy buckwheat ground into flour for baking.

Per 1/2 cup (125 ml) cooked: 77 calories, 2.5 grams protein, 1.5 grams fibre.

★ FLAXSEED

Flax is a blue-flowering crop grown on the Canadian prairies for its oil-rich seeds, which are tiny, smooth, and flat and range in colour from golden to reddish brown. Flaxseed is a good source of soluble fibre and alpha-linolenic acid (ALA), an omega-3 fatty acid linked to heart health. Flaxseed also contains phytochemicals called lignans, compounds thought to help guard against breast cancer.

Grind flaxseed in a coffee grinder before eating or using in cooking. Otherwise, whole flaxseed may pass through your intestine undigested, which means you won't reap their health benefits. You can purchase flaxseed in bulk—whole or ground—at many grocery stores and natural food stores. Ground flaxseed can be stored in an airtight container for several months, and added to many foods and recipes.

Per 2 tablespoons (25 ml), ground: 60 calories, 3 grams protein, 4 grams fibre, 2.4 grams ALA (women need 1.1 grams of ALA per day; men require 1.6 grams).

★ KAMUT

Kamut is an ancient relative of modern wheat, durum wheat to be exact. In fact, *kamut* is an ancient word for wheat. Modern wheat has been altered over the years through breeding to increase its yield and raise its gluten content for commercial baking. Such alterations have made modern wheat more difficult to digest. Because kamut has not been in our food supply long, it has retained many of its original traits and may be easier to digest by some people (but it is not gluten-free). Compared with common wheat, kamut wheat is higher in protein, vitamin E, magnesium, selenium, and zinc. Cooked kamut berries have a buttery flavour. You can also find kamut flour and breakfast cereals made with kamut.

Kamut berries: Per 1/2 cup (125 ml) cooked: 140 calories, 6 grams protein, 5 grams fibre.

★ MILLET (HULLED)

This grain has a long history of cultivation: It was an important food in Europe in the Middle Ages. Today millet continues to be a staple in the diet of many African and Asian countries. This tasty, fluffy grain is rich in B vitamins, iron, and copper. The tiny, pale yellow or reddish orange beads can be cooked like any other grain and served with many types of food. The most common type you'll find in stores is hulled millet. Occasionally, you may find cracked millet sold as couscous, though couscous is most often made from semolina. Millet is also available as flour in natural food stores.

Per 1/2 cup (125 ml) cooked: 104 calories, 3 grams protein, 1.1 grams fibre.

★ OATS

Oats are an excellent source of soluble fibre, the type that lowers elevated blood cholesterol and helps stabilize blood sugar. In addition, oats are a good source of vitamin B1 (thiamine), vitamin B2 (riboflavin), and vitamin E. Oats are available in various forms, from instant to old-fashioned to steel-cut, lending to their versatility. Oats can be cooked and enjoyed as porridge or incorporated into many recipes. All oats start out as oat groats, the whole grain of the oat, with only the outer hard husk removed. The degree to which oats have been processed determines how long they need to be cooked.

- *Steel-cut oats* are whole-oat groats that have been chopped into two or three pieces. Also known as Scotch oats or Irish porridge, steel-cut oats require longer than other oats to cook and remain very chewy (which many people like).
- *Rolled oats* (old-fashioned oats) are oat groats that have been steamed, rolled, and flaked for easier cooking.
- *Quick cooking oats* are rolled oats that have been chopped into small flakes and take only 3 to 4 minutes to cook.
- *Instant oats* are basically powdered oats. Instant oats cannot be used for cooking or baking. Although they're convenient, most packages of instant oats have added salt and sugar. Choose an instant oatmeal that's

low in sugar (ideally unflavoured or no added sugar) and low in salt. Choose brands that contain fewer than 8 grams of sugar and no more than 250 milligrams of sodium per serving.

- *Oat bran* is not truly a whole grain, but you can consider it as a whole grain, since it's a concentrated source of bran that's missing from refined grains. Oat bran is the outer layer of the oat grain, so it's very high in soluble fibre. It can be cooked to make a nutritious hot breakfast cereal.
- *Oat flour* is available at specialty and natural food stores. It's made from oat groats and can be used in baking.

Oats: Per 1/2 cup (125 ml) cooked: 74 calories, 3 grams protein, 2 grams fibre.

Oat bran: Per 1/2 cup (125 ml) cooked: 44 calories, 3.5 grams protein, 2.8 grams fibre.

★ QUINOA

Cultivated in the mountain regions of Peru and Chile for over 5000 years, quinoa was long a staple in the native Indian diet. Commonly considered a grain, quinoa is actually a relative of leafy green vegetables (spinach and Swiss chard). Quinoa is protein-rich and also a good source of calcium and iron. It's fluffy, slightly crunchy, and has a somewhat nutty flavour when cooked. It can be eaten plain as a side dish or used as a substitute for rice in casseroles, stuffed peppers, soups, salads, and stews. Quinoa can also be eaten as a hot breakfast cereal.

Per 1/2 cup (125 ml) cooked: 127 calories, 4.5 grams protein, 2 grams fibre.

★ RYE

The fact that this grain is hardy enough to grow in very cold climates has made it a staple of Northern Europeans, who use it to make breads, crackers, even whisky. Rye is a high-protein, high-fibre grain of at least equal nutritional quality to wheat flour. It has a distinctive, rich, hearty flavour. Soaked and cooked rye berries are sometimes added to breads for extra texture, or used to make pilafs or hot breakfast cereals. Rye flakes are often combined with other grains, then cooked to make a hot breakfast cereal.

Rye berries: Per 1/2 cup (125 ml) cooked: 150 calories, 6 grams protein, 6 grams fibre.

Rye flakes: Per 1/2 cup (125 ml) cooked: 100 calories, 4 grams protein, 4 grams fibre.

★ SPELT

This distant cousin to modern wheat was originally grown in Iran around 5000 to 6000 BC. Spelt has been grown in North America for just over a hundred years, and thanks to its nutty flavour and high nutrient content, it's gaining popularity. Spelt contains more protein than does wheat, and the protein in spelt is easier to digest. This means that some people who are allergic to wheat may be able to tolerate spelt. However, spelt contains gluten, so it is not suitable for a gluten-free diet. Spelt berries can be cooked and served as a whole-grain side dish or hot cereal. Spelt flour is available for baking; it has a somewhat nuttier and slightly sweeter flavour than regular whole-wheat flour. You can also find spelt products such as bread and pasta in most natural food stores. Be sure to choose products that are made with "whole" spelt.

Spelt berries: Per 1/2 cup (125 ml) cooked: 130 calories, 5 grams protein, 6 grams fibre.

★ WHOLE WHEAT

In its unrefined state, wheat is a good source of fibre and many vitamins and minerals. Whole wheat comes in many forms besides a loaf of bread. *Wheat berries* are wheat kernels that have been stripped only of their inedible outer hulls. They're a nutritious whole-grain side dish, but they take a long time to cook. Hard wheat berries can be cooked as a cereal, sprouted for salads, or milled into flour if you have a home grinder.

If you don't have time to prepare the whole berries, cracked wheat, bulgur, or wheat flakes are more convenient alternatives. *Cracked wheat,* as the name implies, is cracked whole-wheat kernels. Cracked wheat cooks faster than wheat berries, but not as fast as bulgur. *Bulgur* is made from whole wheat that's been soaked and baked to speed up the cooking time. It's especially popular in the Middle East, where it's used to make tabbouleh and pilafs. Bulgur comes either whole, or cracked into fine, medium, or coarse grains.

Wheat berries: Per 1/2 cup (125 ml) cooked: 136 calories, 5.5 grams protein, 4 grams fibre.

Cracked wheat: Per 1/2 cup (125 ml) cooked: 140 calories, 5 grams protein, 5 grams fibre.

Bulgur: Per 1/2 cup (125 ml) cooked: 76 calories, 2.8 grams protein, 4.1 grams fibre.

★ WILD RICE

This grain isn't actually related to rice at all but is the seed of an aquatic grass. However, this plant is similar to rice in that both grow in water and produce a grain. Wild rice is the only cereal grain that's native to North America. In its finished form, wild rice is a long, slender, coffee-coloured kernel that butterflies open during cooking to reveal a cream-coloured interior. It has a woodsy flavour and chewy texture. Compared with brown rice, wild rice is higher in protein, iron, potassium, and zinc. Wild rice can be eaten on its own or used in combination with other rices.

Per 1/2 cup (125 ml) serving: 130 calories, 5 grams protein, 1.4 grams fibre.

Enjoying whole grains

Buying

Whole grains are generally available packaged, as well as in bulk-food bins. When buying whole grains in bulk, make sure the bins are covered and that the store has a good product turnover to ensure freshness. Make sure there is no sign of moistness in the grain.

Read labels when choosing whole-grain bread, crackers, and ready-to-eat breakfast cereals. Make sure a whole grain is listed as the first ingredient. Ideally, whole-grain breads should provide 2 grams of fibre per 1 ounce (30 g) slice. Healthier whole-grain breakfast cereals should have at least 5 grams of fibre and no more than 8 grams of sugar per serving. Look for whole-grain crackers that are free of trans fat; compare brands to choose crackers with less sodium.

Storing

Keep whole grains in an airtight container in a cool, dark, dry cupboard or shelf in your pantry. Whole grains should keep for up to 6 months (not years!), so buy only the amount you will use in that period. Whole grains will keep longer if stored in the fridge.

Store whole-grain flours in the refrigerator to best preserve their nutrient content. Whole-wheat products such as bulgur, wheat flakes, wheat bran, and wheat germ should also be refrigerated to prevent their natural fats from turning rancid.

Preparing

With the exception of oats, thoroughly rinse all grains under running water before cooking to remove any dirt or debris. Rinsing quinoa also helps remove the natural seed coating called saponin, which acts as an insect repellent. (Processing methods used in commercial cultivation of quinoa remove most of the saponins, but it's still a good idea to rinse it.) Use water or low-sodium broth as the cooking liquid. To add flavour to cooked grains, add a bay leaf to simmering grains.

Kamut berries, spelt berries, rye berries, and wheat berries must be soaked before cooking. Soaking softens the grain kernel, so cooking time is reduced. To soak, place rinsed berries in a bowl and cover with 2 inches (5 cm) of water. Let soak for 8 hours or overnight. Once soaked, berries are ready to cook according to the instructions below.

Guide to cooking whole grains

Type of grain	Grain to liquid ratio	Cooking time (approx.)
Amaranth	1 part rice to 3 part liquid Bring amaranth and liquid to a boil in a saucepan. Reduce heat and simmer, covered, until cooked. 1 cup (250 ml) dry yields 2 1/2 cups (625 ml) cooked.	20 to 25 minutes
Barley (hulled)	1 part barley to 3.5 parts liquid Bring barley and liquid to a boil in a saucepan. Reduce heat and simmer, covered, until cooked. 1 cup (250 ml) dry yields 3 cups (750 ml) cooked.	60 to 90 minutes
Brown rice (long-grain)	1 part rice to 2 parts liquid Bring rice and liquid to a boil in a saucepan. Reduce heat and simmer, covered, until cooked. For brown basmati rice, wash it in a bowl of cool water before cooking, stirring frequently and replacing the water four times or until the water no longer has a milky appearance. 1 cup (250 ml) dry yields 3 cups (750 ml) cooked.	40 to 45 minutes

Type of grain	Grain to liquid ratio	Cooking time (approx.)
Buckwheat groats (kasha)	1 part buckwheat to 2 parts liquid. Add buckwheat to boiling liquid. Return to a boil; reduce heat and simmer, covered, until tender. 1 cup (250 ml) dry yields 3 1/2 cups (875 ml) cooked.	30 minutes
Bulgur	1 part bulgur to 2 parts liquid. Bring bulgur and cold water to a boil. Reduce heat and simmer, covered, until tender. 1 cup dry yields 2 1/2 cups (625 ml) cooked.	12 to 15 minutes
Kamut berries	1 part kamut to 3 parts liquid. Add soaked and drained kamut berries to boiling liquid. Readuce heat, and simmer, covered, until tender but chewy. 1 cup (250 ml) dry yields 4 cups (1 L) cooked.	30 to 40 minutes. If grains were not soaked, allow 45 to 60 minutes
Millet (hulled)	1 part millet to 2.5 parts liquid. Bring millet and liquid to a boil in a saucepan. Reduce heat and simmer, covered, until tender and fluffy. 1 cup (250 ml) dry yields 4 cups (1 L) cooked.	25 minutes
Oats (old-fashioned)	1 part oats to 2 parts liquid. Bring water and salt to a boil. Add rolled oats, reduce heat, and cook to desired consistency, stirring occasionally. Cover, remove from heat, and let stand 5 minutes before serving. 1 cup (250 ml) dry yields 2 cups (500 ml) cooked.	10 to 20 minutes
Oats (steel-cut)	1 part oats to 4 parts liquid. Add steel-cut oats to boiling water. When the porridge is smooth and beginning to thicken, reduce heat and simmer, uncovered, stirring occasionally, until cooked. 1 cup (250 ml) dry yields 3 cups (750 ml) cooked.	30 minutes

Type of grain	Grain to liquid ratio	Cooking time (approx.)
Quinoa	1 part quinoa to 2 parts liquid Bring quinoa and liquid to a boil in a saucepan. Reduce heat and simmer, covered, until grains are tender and translucent. 1 cup (250 ml) dry yields 3 cups (750 ml) cooked.	15 minutes
Rye berries*	1 part rye to 2.5 parts liquid Add rinsed rye berries to boiling water. Reduce heat and simmer, covered, until tender. 1 cup (250 ml) dry yields 3 cups (750 ml) cooked.	90 minutes Cooking time will be shorter if grains are soaked overnight.
Rye flakes	1 part rye flakes to 2.5 parts liquid Add rye flakes to boiling water. Reduce heat and simmer, covered, until cooked. 1 cup (250 ml) dry yields 2.5 cups (625 ml) cooked.	30 minutes
Spelt berries*	1 part spelt to 3 parts liquid Bring rinsed spelt berries and liquid to a boil in a saucepan. Reduce heat and simmer, covered, until tender but chewy. 1 cup (250 ml) dry yields 3 cups (750 ml) cooked	50 to 60 minutes Cooking time will shorten if grains are soaked overnight.
Wheat berries*	1 part wheat berries to 5 parts liquid Add rinsed wheat berries to boiling water and return to a boil. Reduce heat and simmer, covered, stirring occasionally, until tender but still chewy, adding more water if needed. 1 cup (250 ml) dry yields 3 cups (750 ml) cooked.	60 to 90 minutes Cooking time will shorten if grains are soaked overnight.
Wild rice	1 part rice to 3 1/2 parts liquid Bring rice and liquid to a boil in a saucepan. Cover, reduce heat, and cook until the rice grains have butterflied (split open and curled). Turn off the heat and let stand, covered, for 5 minutes. 1 cup (250 ml) dry yields 3 to 4 cups (750 ml to 1 L) cooked.	40 to 60 minutes

* Whole-grain berries can also be cooked in a slower cooker. Combine berries and liquid in slow cooker and cook on Low for 8 to 10 hours.

Many of my clients complain they don't have time in their hectic morning to cook a pot of steel-cut oats for breakfast. Or that taking 30 to 45 minutes to cook brown or wild rice just isn't conducive to getting dinner on the table in a hurry. One solution: Cook a batch of whole grains on the weekend when you have more time. Refrigerate and then reheat in the microwave or steamer to enjoy them over the next few days. Or freeze in small portions to use in other recipes. Some of my clients will cook a pot of steel-cut oats overnight in the crock pot on the low setting. Rice cookers are handy, too, as you can put the rice on to cook, then ignore it while preparing the rest of your meal or even doing something else altogether; the rice cooker will turn off automatically when the rice is cooked.

TIPS FOR ADDING WHOLE GRAINS TO YOUR MEALS

Whole grains are incredibly versatile. You can enjoy their nutty flavour and chewy texture on their own as a side dish or breakfast cereal or you can enjoy them in soups, stews, casseroles, and salads. Try the serving suggestions and recipes below to add variety and nutrition to your meals. Keep in mind that many grains can be used interchangeably.

Breakfast

- Instead of oatmeal, try another cooked grain as your morning hot cereal. Top with a few nuts, dried or fresh fruit, and a spoonful of yogurt.
- Stir cooked grain or ground flaxseed into muffin, pancake, and waffle batters.
- Sprinkle ground flaxseed on hot and cold breakfast cereals.

RECIPES
Banana Flax Pancakes, page 270
Blueberry Walnut Muesli with Rolled Oats and Flaxseed, page 271
Cinnamon Orange Quinoa Hot Cereal, page 272
Quick Pomegranate Flax Porridge, page 273
Whole-Grain Millet Waffles with Orange and Raspberries, page 275

Lunch and dinner

- Create a whole-grain entree salad by tossing cooked and chilled whole grain with a vinaigrette dressing, chopped vegetables, and diced cooked chicken, firm tofu, or chickpeas.
- Use whole-grain bread for sandwiches and French toast.

- Mix a little ground flaxseed into mustard or mayonnaise for a healthy sandwich spread.
- Make homemade pizzas on whole-wheat tortillas or pita pockets.
- Make a whole-grain pilaf by tossing a hot, cooked grain with cooked brown rice, parsley, herbs, and a little butter.
- Make a whole-grain stuffing for turkey by combining cooked whole grain with chopped onion and celery, and poultry seasoning.
- Add cooked whole grains to stews for a heartier flavour and deeper texture.
- Mix some cooked grain or ground flaxseed into lean ground beef or turkey when making burgers, meat balls, or meatloaf.
- Include a whole grain uncooked to your favourite soup recipe. Increase the amount of water as needed.
- Sprinkle ground flaxseed over salads and soups.
- Toss chilled cooked bulgur with a vinaigrette dressing and chopped fresh mint, cucumber, and tomato for a tabbouleh salad. Or substitute another grain for new wave tabbouleh.
- Toss cooked grain with grated part-skim cheese and a little melted butter for a casserole topping.
- Combine hot, cooked grain and a spoonful of homemade or prepared pesto for a tasty side dish.
- Mix 1/2 cup (125 ml) of cooked whole grain into a bowl of chili or ready-to-serve soup.
- Top cooked whole grain with your favourite Bolognese sauce for a change from the usual pasta.

RECIPES

Hot Apple and Cabbage Salad, page 289
Barley Salad, page 298
Cajun Breaded Trout, page 331
Kasha, Walnut, and Apple Salad with Mint, page 300
Wheat Berry Salad with Smoked Trout and Gingered Squash, page 303
Hearty Minestrone Soup, page 307
Mushroom Barley Casserole, page 311
Quinoa-Stuffed Peppers, page 312
Ginger-Orange Vegetable Stir-Fry with Chicken and Brown Rice, page 339
Kasha Cabbage Rolls, page 341
Wild Rice and Lentil Curry, page 353

Snacks and dessert

- Make a whole-grain pudding by cooking your favourite whole grain in low-fat milk or soy milk. Add cinnamon, nutmeg, raisins, and honey.
- Use ground flaxseed as a topping for fruit crisps.
- Substitute one-half all-purpose flour with a whole-grain flour in muffin, loaf, pancake, waffle, and cookie recipes.
- Add ground flaxseed to homemade smoothies, yogurt, and applesauce.

RECIPES
Pomegranate Power Shake, page 280
Low-Fat Lemon Millet Muffins, page 377
Cranberry Orange Flax Quick Bread, page 375
Flax Bean Brownies, page 379
Ginger-Flax Fruit Crisp, page 381

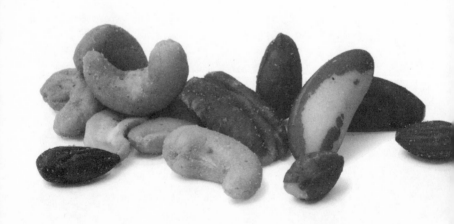

5
Power protein foods

fish and seafood
arctic char ★ clams ★ haddock ★ halibut ★ herring ★ mackerel ★ mussels ★ oysters ★ rainbow trout ★ salmon ★ sardines ★ scallops ★ shrimp ★ squid ★ striped bass ★ tilapia

legumes and soy foods
black beans ★ black-eyed peas ★ chickpeas ★ fava beans ★ kidney beans ★ lentils ★ lima beans ★ navy beans ★ pinto beans ★ soybeans ★ soy beverages ★ split peas ★ tempeh ★ texturized vegetable protein ★ tofu

nuts and seeds
almonds ★ Brazil nuts ★ cashews ★ hazelnuts ★ macadamia nuts ★ peanuts ★ pecans ★ pine nuts ★ pistachios ★ pumpkin seeds ★ sesame seeds ★ sunflower seeds ★ walnuts

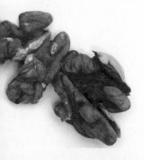

Protein-rich foods, such as fish, legumes, and nuts—as well as meat, poultry, and eggs—supply the body with amino acids, the building blocks of protein that are vital to developing and maintaining muscles and synthesizing hormones, enzymes, and immune compounds that fight infection. Protein-packed foods are also excellent sources of key nutrients, including B vitamins, iron, and zinc.

Protein foods play another important role in your diet: They help keep you feeling satiated longer after eating. That's because protein takes longer to be digested and emptied from your stomach into your small intestine than does carbohydrate in starchy foods, fruit, and vegetables. In other words, if you add a little protein to your lunch, your energy level will be sustained longer after eating. You'll be mentally and physically prepared to tackle all the activities of a busy afternoon.

Although meat, poultry, fish, eggs, legumes, nuts, and soy foods are all excellent sources of dietary protein, I have chosen to highlight fish, legumes, and nuts in this chapter because their health benefits go beyond their high protein content. You'll learn the many ways in which these three power protein foods help fight disease and the role their omega-3 fatty acids, soluble fibre, and phytochemicals play.

That said, I don't want you to think that meat, poultry, and eggs should be avoided. Quite the contrary. Unless you are a vegetarian, these are healthy protein foods to include in your diet provided you choose wisely. In the section below, I share with you tips that will help you make healthful choices when it comes to selecting meat, poultry, and eggs.

Meat, poultry, and eggs

1 serving = 3 ounces (90 g) cooked meat or poultry *or* 2 eggs

Choose lean cuts

The nutritional drawback to animal protein foods is their saturated fat content, the type of fat that raises LDL cholesterol in the blood. When buying meat, be sure to select lean cuts, such as sirloin, flank steak, eye of the round, beef tenderloin, lean and extra-lean ground beef, pork tenderloin, and centre-cut pork chops. Keep in mind that any cut of meat that comes from an animal's stomach area, for example, rib eye steak, rib chops, and spareribs, will be high in saturated fat. Lean poultry choices include chicken breast, turkey breast, and lean and extra-lean ground chicken and turkey.

Limit portion size

When it comes to red meat—beef, veal, pork, lamb—portion size is also an important consideration. Many studies show that people who eat the most red meat (beef, veal, pork, lamb) and/or processed meat (luncheon meat, bacon, hot dogs, sausages) are more likely to get colon cancer than those who eat these foods only once in a while.

Meat might boost colon cancer risk in a few ways. In lab animals, compounds formed when meat is cooked have been shown to cause colon tumours. The form of iron in red meat, heme iron, may also damage colon cells and trigger cancer growth. And it's thought that nitrites in some processed meats may form cancer-causing compounds.

If red meat is eaten at all, limit your serving size to no more than three ounces (90 grams) per day. To help reduce your portion size, enjoy small amounts of red meat in stir-fries and pastas. Serve thin slices of steak rather than a whole piece.

Consider buying organic

If you're like an increasing number of Canadians, you might be concerned about eating growth-hormone beef. In Canada and the United States, hormones are routinely used to speed up the growth of beef cattle, ensuring they gain more muscle and less fat. (Hormones are *not* used in chickens or dairy cattle.) Some scientists have expressed concern that trace residues of hormones in meat could potentially disrupt the hormonal balance and immune systems of pregnant women and pre-pubertal children. Some worry that eating hormone-treated beef may cause girls to reach puberty earlier, increasing their risk for breast cancer.

Conventionally raised beef cattle, hogs, and chickens are also given antibiotics—many of the same ones used to treat disease in people—in their feed to prevent infection. The question debated is whether residues of antibiotic-resistant bacteria from the animal foods we consume can make human illness more difficult to treat. Antibiotic resistance is the ability of certain bacteria to survive exposure to an antibiotic, which is normally able to destroy or limit their growth.

Although these concerns remain theoretical, many people prefer to play it safe and opt for organically raised meat. Organic animals raised for meat, poultry, eggs (and dairy) by law cannot be treated with growth hormones or antibiotics and must be given organic feed and access to sufficient space and the outdoors. Organic meat and poultry is sold in natural food stores, many butcher stores, and an increasing number of grocery stores.

Consider buying grass-fed meat

With more people questioning how their food is grown, grass-fed beef is becoming popular. Traditionally, all beef cattle were left to forage in pastures of grass and fatten naturally; grass fed cattle were typically 4 or 5 years old at slaughter. Today, however, almost all beef in grocery stores is feedlot beef. In order to produce meat faster—feedlot cows are ready for slaughter at 14 to 16 months—the animals are fattened up with corn and soy diets supplemented with growth hormones and antibiotics.

Meat produced from cows that graze on grass is lower in total fat and artery-clogging saturated fat and slightly higher in omega-3 fats than grain-fed beef. Some experts think that grass-fed beef might even have advantages from a food safety standpoint. The reason? A steady diet of grain raises the acidity of a cow's intestinal tract. This favours the growth of acid-resistant E. coli bacteria, which can spread from feces-contaminated carcasses to meat. Eating improperly cooked E. coli–contaminated hamburger can lead to severe, even deadly, food poisoning. (Regardless of what type of beef you buy, always cook burgers to an internal temperature of 160°F/71°C to kill disease-causing E. coli.)

The flavour of grass-fed beef differs according to the breed of cattle and the grass it was raised on. Some people enjoy the nutty flavour, whereas others prefer the flavour of grain-fed beef. Like organic beef (which is usually feedlot beef fed grains free of pesticide residues, growth hormones, and antibiotics), grass-fed beef is more expensive than conventionally raised meat. Ask for it in your local butcher store.

Look for omega-3 eggs

If you're willing to spend a bit more money, I recommend that you buy whole eggs enriched with omega-3 fatty acids, either ALA or DHA. As you'll learn in Chapter 7, omega-3 fats can help guard against heart attack, stroke, dementia, and inflammatory conditions, such as rheumatoid arthritis, colitis, and possibly even type 1 diabetes (the type that occurs mainly in children and young teenagers).

Omega-3 eggs from hens that were fed flaxseed are an excellent source of ALA. The egg yolk will contain more of these omega-3 fats and less saturated fat than a regular egg. Hens fed a diet containing flaxseed (a source of ALA) and fish oil (a source of DHA) are also a good choice, as they contain both of these omega-3 fatty acids. You'll also find liquid eggs enriched with omega-3 fatty acids.

★ FISH AND SEAFOOD

Arctic char* ★ clams ★ haddock ★ halibut (Pacific) ★ herring* ★ mackerel (Atlantic)* ★ mussels ★ oysters ★ rainbow trout* ★ salmon* ★ sardines* ★ scallops ★ shrimp ★ squid ★ striped bass ★ tilapia

*Good source of heart healthy omega-3 fatty acids

Eat at least 2 servings per week
1 serving = 3 ounces (90 g) cooked fish

Fish is an excellent source of protein that's low in cholesterol-raising saturated fat. And fish is certainly one protein-rich food that has been long been praised for its health benefits. Ever since studies demonstrated lower rates of dying from heart disease among Greenland Inuit, North Americans have been told by their national health agencies repeatedly to eat more fish. The cardio-protective benefits of eating fish are so clear that the Heart and Stroke Foundation of Canada advises people to consume fish, especially fatty fish, at least two times per week. The 2007 Canada's Food Guide also advises, for the first time, that Canadians eat fish at least twice weekly.

If your diet doesn't adhere to these guidelines, it's time to consider the following reasons why you should add fish to your meals.

Fish and health

FISH AND HEART HEALTH

The cardiovascular benefits of fish have been documented in several prospective studies and randomized clinical trials. A 2006 report published in the *Journal of the American Medical Association* concluded that eating 1 to 2 servings of fish per week is enough to reduce the risk of dying from heart attack by 36%. Researchers from Harvard School of Public Health and Harvard Medical School based their conclusions on a review of hundreds of studies about fish and health.[1]

Scientists attribute the heart healthy properties of fish to their omega-3 fat content. Omega-3 fatty acids belong to the family of polyunsaturated fats. Polyunsaturated fats are liquid at room temperature and in the refrigerator. Cold water fish such as salmon, trout, sardines, mackerel, and herring are particularly high in two omega-3 fats, DHA (docosahexaenoic acid) and EPA (eicosapentaenoic acid). Once EPA is consumed, the body converts it to DHA.

Studies have demonstrated the ability of omega-3 fats in fish to make the blood less likely to form clots and to protect against irregular heartbeats that cause sudden cardiac death. One trial, which enrolled 11,323 subjects who survived their first heart attack, demonstrated that even a small amount of omega-3 fatty acids (1000 milligrams per day) was effective at reducing overall death and the risk of sudden cardiac death by 20% and 45% respectively.[2]

Omega-3 fish oils can also reduce elevated blood fats called triglycerides. Many people are familiar with blood cholesterol, but they may not have heard much about blood triglycerides. When you eat, any extra calories your body doesn't need for immediate energy are turned into triglycerides and stored in fat cells for later use. Later, triglycerides are released in the blood for energy between meals. If you regularly eat more calories than you burn, you may have high triglycerides.

Although the exact mechanism is unclear, high triglycerides are thought to contribute to hardening of the arteries, which increases the risk of stroke, heart attack, and heart disease. High triglycerides often accompany other conditions known to increase the risk of heart disease and stroke, for example, obesity and metabolic syndrome—a cluster of conditions that includes abdominal obesity, high blood pressure, high blood sugar, and abnormal cholesterol levels.

People with poorly controlled diabetes often have high triglycerides in their bloodstream—one reason why people with diabetes are at increased risk for heart attack. A pooled analysis of 18 randomized trials including 823 people with type 2 diabetes concluded fish oils significantly lowered blood triglycerides.[3]

FISH AND BRAIN HEALTH

There's truth to the saying that fish is brain food. Omega-3 fatty acids, especially DHA found in fish, make up 60% of the communicating membranes of the brain. These fats help keep the lining of brain cells flexible so memory messages can pass easily between cells. All brain cell membranes continuously need to refresh themselves with a new supply of fatty acids.

Omega-3 fatty acids in fish are needed for the development and maintenance of the brain, eye, and nervous tissue throughout life, beginning in the final trimester of pregnancy. DHA is naturally found in breast milk and has been shown to support the visual and cognitive development of infants.[4] An adequate supply of DHA is vital to a fetus during its periods of rapid brain development in the womb, as well as to a child during infancy and childhood. Since the amount of DHA a developing fetus or breastfed infant receives is dependent on a mother's diet, it's important for pregnant and breastfeeding women to include fish in their diet or take a fish oil supplement.

Eating fish may keep our brain healthy as we age. A study that followed 815 adults, age 65 to 94 years, for almost 4 years revealed that those who ate fish at least once per week were 60% less likely to develop Alzheimer's disease compared with people who rarely or never ate fish. Total polyunsaturated fat intake and DHA intake were both associated with a lower risk of the disease.[5] Another study of 5386 healthy adults age 55 years or older found fish consumption was linked with a 60% lower risk of vascular dementia, in particular Alzheimer's disease.[6] (Vascular dementia is a common form of dementia caused by narrowing and blockage of the arteries that supply blood to the brain.)

Fish may help fend off dementia in ways other than through DHA's special role in helping brain cells communicate properly. Omega-3 fatty acids in fish have a protective effect on the vascular system, and as such they can reduce inflammation and prevent the hardening of arteries in the brain.

FISH AND VISION

Numerous studies suggest that eating fish, especially fatty fish, one to four times per week guards against age-related macular degeneration and reduces the risk of the disease progressing to an advanced form. Studies have found higher intakes of fish and omega-3 fatty acids lower the risk by 30% to 60%.[7]

Age-related macular degeneration is a disease that attacks the macula, the central part of the retina, resulting in progressive loss of visual sharpness and making it difficult to drive a vehicle, read a book, and even recognize faces. Macular degeneration affects more than two million Canadians over the age of 50 and is the leading cause of severe vision loss in older adults.

It's been suggested that hardening of the blood vessels that supply the retina contributes to the risk of macular degeneration, the same mechanism that increases the risk of heart disease. Not only do omega-3 fats have a special role in the function of the retina (DHA is a key fatty acid found in the retina), their anti-inflammatory, anti-blood clotting, and triglyceride lowering effects may help keep blood vessels in the eye healthy.

FISH AND PROSTATE CANCER PREVENTION

Although the evidence isn't as strong as it is for cardiovascular health, studies do suggest that eating fish can help prevent prostate cancer. In a study of 47,882 healthy men living in the United States, eating fish more than three times per week versus less than twice per month was associated with a 44% reduced risk of prostate cancer. The strongest association was for metastatic cancer (prostate cancer that spreads to other parts of the body).[8] Another study from Harvard School of Public Health compared blood levels of polyunsaturated fatty acids, including DHA and EPA, in 476 men diagnosed with prostate cancer and the same number of healthy controls. Men with the highest blood levels were 41% less likely to have prostate cancer.[9]

Animal studies have found that omega-3 fatty acids suppress cancer formation or slow cancer progression. Lab studies have also demonstrated omega-3 fatty acids to have anti-tumour effects on prostate cancer cells.

OMEGA-3 FAT CONTENT OF FISH

The health benefits of fish are due, in large part, to their content of omega-3 fatty acids. It's estimated that Canadian children, age 2 to 3, consume

19 milligrams of DHA each day and adults get, on average, 78 milligrams. There are no official recommended intakes of DHA and EPA for Canadians, as the ideal intake is unclear at this time. However, many experts advise we aim to consume at least 500 milligrams of DHA plus EPA per day to help ward off heart disease. The American Heart Association recommends that people with existing coronary heart disease boost their daily intake to 1000 milligrams of DHA and EPA combined.

It's not surprising that our intake of DHA is low when you consider that food sources of the omega-3 fat are limited. The best source is fish, but there's also a small amount in eggs and some meats. Plant foods contain no DHA. Manufacturers have started fortifying food products with DHA. If don't like fish, you can get DHA from designer foods, such as Neilson Dairy Oh! milk or Black Diamond DHA Omega 3 cheese, both produced from cows fed a diet enriched with DHA. Naturegg Omega Pro liquid eggs have been enriched with fish oil (menhaden oil).

Combined DHA and EPA content of selected fish and other foods (milligrams)

Per 3 ounces (90 g) cooked portion	
Haddock	203
Halibut, Atlantic and Pacific	395
Herring, Atlantic	1712
Mackerel, Atlantic	1022
Salmon, Atlantic	1825
Salmon, chinook	1476
Salmon, sockeye, canned	982
Salmon, coho	900
Sardines, Atlantic	835
Shrimp	267
Tilapia	115
Trout, rainbow	981
Tuna, skipjack	733
Fish oil capsule, 1000 milligrams	300–600

Combined DHA and EPA content of selected fish and other foods (milligrams), cont'd.

Fortified foods

Naturegg Omega Pro liquid eggs, 1/4 cup (50 ml)	293
Naturegg Omega Pro, 1 whole egg	125
Naturegg Break Free Omega-3 liquid eggs, 1/4 cup (50 ml)	250
Neilson Dairy Oh! homogenized milk, 1 cup (250 ml)	20
Neilson Dairy Oh! 2% milk, 1 cup (250 ml)	10
Silk Plus Omega-3 DHA Soy Beverage, 1 cup (250 ml)	25
PC Blue Menu Oh Mega J Orange Juice, 1 cup (250 ml)	50
Tropicana Essentials Omega-3 Orange Juice, 1 cup (250 ml)	50
Black Diamond DHA Omega 3 cheese, 1 oz (30 g)	20

Source: Food manufacturers and USDA National Nutrient Database for Standard Reference, Release 17.

Although some types of fish provide a greater amount of heart healthy nutrients, other species contain high levels of chemical contaminants and should be limited, or better yet, avoided.

FISH AND MERCURY

Concerns over potential harm from chemical contaminants in fish have left many people confused about what type of fish is safe to eat—or if they should steer clear of it altogether. Of concern to many people, especially women, is the mercury content of certain fish.

Mercury is naturally occurring at very low levels in the air, soil, lakes, and oceans. It also makes its way into the environment from industry, including pulp and paper processing and mining operations. When mercury enters streams and water, it's converted by bacteria to methylmercury, which is then absorbed by fish and stored in their muscles. When we talk about mercury in fish, we are actually referring to methylmercury. Larger, longer-living predators (shark, swordfish, tuna) have higher concentrations of methylmercury than smaller fish (shellfish, salmon). Unfortunately, cooking has little impact on the mercury content, since the chemical is in the protein (muscle) tissue.

The concern is that mercury can accumulate in the body and affect the developing nervous system, especially the brain, of infants and young children. If women consume too much mercury before and during their pregnancy, it may increase the risk of birth defects and learning disabilities in their child. Some, but not all, studies have found associations between women's mercury exposure during pregnancy and their children's neurologic test scores.

In May 2002, Health Canada issued an advisory recommending that people limit their intake of swordfish, shark, king mackerel, and fresh and frozen tuna—large predatory fish that live long and accumulate mercury in their tissues. Canned tuna was considered safe to eat and exempted from the advisory. Health Canada maintained that canned tuna had lower mercury levels than tuna steaks, for instance, because smaller species of tuna are used for canning.

In March 2007, Health Canada issued an updated advisory after completing a comprehensive review of the science on mercury and fish. The list of high-mercury fish was expanded and now includes fresh and frozen tuna, shark, swordfish, marlin, orange roughy, and escolar. The government now advises women and children age 1 to 11 to limit their intake of these fish to a small portion once per month. Others should consume no more than about 5 ounces (150 g) once per week.

For the first time, the advisory also mentioned canned albacore (white) tuna. On the heels of independent research that found 13% of canned albacore tuna exceeded the government's guidance levels of 0.5 parts per million for mercury, Health Canada now advises women of child-bearing age to consume no more than 4 food guide servings per week. One food guide serving is 2.5 ounces (75 g), slightly less than the smaller 3 ounce (85 g) tin of tuna. This means that women should limit their intake to no more than 10 ounces (285 g) or 2.25 large cans per week. Children age 1 to 4 years can eat up to 1 food guide serving, or 1/2 cup (125 ml) per week. Older children, age 5 to 11, can eat up to 2 food guide servings, or 1 cup (150 g)—basically one standard 4 1/2 ounce (133 g) can of tuna.

Keep in mind that this advisory applies only to albacore—or white—tuna. Canned albacore tuna is generally larger, older fish that has accumulated more mercury. Light canned tuna contains species of tuna, such as skipjack, yellowfin, and tongol, which are smaller and lower in mercury.

Health Canada's Fish Consumption Advice (maximum intake)

	Women*	Children, 1–4 years	Children, 5–11 years
Fresh and frozen tuna, shark, swordfish, marlin, orange roughy, escolar	150 g/month	75 g/month	125 g/month
Canned albacore tuna	4 servings/week (10 oz/280 g)	1 serving/week (2 1/2 oz/75 g)	2 servings/week (5 oz/150 g)

* This fish consumption advice applies only to women who could become pregnant, who are pregnant, or who are breastfeeding.

Some agencies are stricter about its fish advice. The Toronto Public Health Department and the U.S. government advise women of child-bearing age and young children to completely avoid high-mercury swordfish, shark, and king mackerel. When it comes to canned albacore tuna, the U.S. advisory acknowledges that it is higher in mercury than light tuna and advises women and kids to limit their intake to 6 ounces (170 g) per week—a smaller amount for women than Health Canada advises.

It's hard to know what—or how much—to eat when you read such conflicting advice. I advise women and children to avoid high-mercury fish altogether. There are plenty of other low-mercury fish to choose from. If canned tuna is a staple part of your diet (eaten more than once per week), minimize your intake of mercury by avoiding canned albacore tuna and eating only canned light tuna (which is also less expensive).

You might be wondering if the potential harm from consuming mercury in fish diminishes its heart healthy effects. Some people worry mercury accumulation in the body can increase the risk of heart attack. The link between high mercury intakes and the risk of heart disease remains inconclusive. According to the *Journal of the American Medical Association* review I mentioned earlier in this chapter, mercury in fish may lessen the natural benefits from fish, but the overall benefit is still positive. The Harvard researchers concluded the benefits of eating fish far outweigh the potential risks.

Low-mercury fish and seafood
Catfish
Clams

Crab
Haddock
Herring
Mackerel (except king mackerel)
Oysters
Pollock
Salmon, canned
Salmon, wild and farmed
Sardines
Scallops
Shrimp
Tilapia
Trout

FISH AND DIOXINS

Another concern when it comes to fish, especially salmon, relates to contaminants called dioxins. Dioxins refer to a group of several hundred
chemical compounds that share certain chemical structures and biological
characteristics. On the list of dioxins are PCBs (polychlorinated biphenyls)
and PBDEs (polybrominated diphenyl ethers). Dioxins enter the environment as by-products of waste incineration, paper bleaching, and the production of some plastics.

Consumers became leery of eating salmon in January 2004 when a
report published by researchers at Indiana University revealed that farm-
raised salmon harbour significantly higher levels of PCBs than their ocean-
swimming (wild) cousins.[10] Then, in October 2004, the same researchers
reported trace levels of PBDEs in farmed and wild salmon.[11] After reading
all the media stories about toxins in salmon, many of my clients asked me
if they should give up eating salmon. You might be wondering too as you
read this. But before you decide to give up salmon, let me put the study
findings into perspective.

PBDEs are used as flame-retardants in many products, for example,
furniture stuffing, carpet backings, and computer and television casings.
These chemicals are gaining attention because of their increasing levels in
the environment and their potential for accumulation in the body and tox-
icity. PBDEs make their way into the environment during production, use,
or disposal and end up in humans through food, breast milk, and dust.
They enter the food chain because they are stored in the fat of animals.
Meat, poultry, and fish all contribute PBDEs to our diets.

The Indiana University researchers analyzed 700 species of uncooked salmon from around the world and determined that, as a group, farm-raised salmon—especially those from Europe—have higher levels of PBDEs than do wild salmon. When salmon species were compared by location, the highest levels were actually found in wild BC chinook salmon.

Previous studies, including one from Health Canada, have found very low PBDE levels in farmed salmon (1 to 4 parts per billion) and slightly lower levels in wild salmon. In contrast, household dust contains PBDEs at parts per million—one thousand times greater than parts per billion. PBDEs have not been demonstrated to be carcinogenic in animal studies. Limited data in mice suggest harmful effects on the nervous system and thyroid hormone function. According to Health Canada, the extremely low levels of PBDEs in our food do not pose a health risk.

What about PCBs in farmed salmon? These chemicals were widely used for industrial purposes until 1977, when their use was banned in North America. Like PBDEs, PCBs stick around in the environment and accumulate in the fat of animals and fish. PCBs enter the bodies of fish from water, sediment, and through eating prey that have PCBs in their bodies. PCBs build up in fish and can reach levels hundreds of thousands of times higher than the levels in water. Farmed salmon are raised in ocean pens, where they're given feed and antibiotics to make them grow quickly. These salmon are fed from a global supply of fishmeal and fish oil that's manufactured from small open-sea fish. Studies show that commercial fish feeds are the source of PCBs found in farmed salmon.

Excessive exposure to PCBs may cause a wide variety of adverse health effects. Our knowledge about the effects of PCBs comes from studies of people exposed to them in the workplace or who ate contaminated food, as well as from experimental animal studies. Of particular concern are the effects on the development of infants whose mothers have been exposed to these chemicals before and during pregnancy. PCBs are known to increase the risk of cancer, depress the immune system, and cause learning disabilities in children.

Over the past decade, a growing body of research suggests that infants and children with higher PCB exposures during developmental periods score lower on many measures of neurological function, including decreased IQ scores and reduced hearing sensitivity. Some of these effects have even been observed at low levels of PCB exposure. PCB exposure also appears to impair the immune system. Exposure early in life may make people more susceptible to chicken pox or inner ear and respiratory tract infections.

The Indiana University study found an average PCB content of 36.6 parts per billion (ppb) in farmed salmon, as opposed to 3 ppb in wild salmon. A difference, yes, but not that different when you consider the bigger picture. Health Canada, the U.S. Food and Drug Administration, and the World Health Organization have set the acceptable limit of PCBs at 2000 ppb. The trace PCB levels found in farmed salmon represent 2% of the acceptable limit.

Despite this, the Indiana researchers concluded that eating farmed salmon more than once per month could increase the risk of cancer. That risk is theoretical, primarily based on animal studies. To date, there is no credible evidence that eating farmed salmon increases the risk of cancer in humans. There is, however, a mountain of evidence that eating fish rich in omega-3 fats protects against heart disease. In my opinion, one study is not enough to dismiss the long-standing research that demonstrates the health benefits of salmon.

When the researchers from Harvard School of Public Health and Harvard Medical School evaluated the cancer risks and heart benefits associated with eating fish, they found the heart benefits outweighed cancer risks by 100- to 370-fold for farmed salmon and by 300- to 1000-fold for wild salmon.[12]

PCBs are found throughout the environment, not just in farmed salmon. The major dietary contributors of PCBs and dioxins are beef, chicken, and pork (34%), dairy products (30%), vegetables (22%), fish and shellfish (9%), and eggs (5%).[13] Cooking methods that allow the fat to cook off (e.g., baking, broiling, and grilling, versus frying) will lower the amount of PCBs and dioxins in foods.

Ideally, no food should contain contaminants. Unfortunately, we don't live in an ideal world. That's why it is important to take measures to minimize our intake of food contaminants and choose foods that offer the greatest health benefits. The following strategies will help you minimize your intake of PCBs and PBDEs from all foods, including salmon:

- Trim fatty areas from fish, meat, and poultry before cooking.
- Choose broiling, baking, or grilling over frying, as these cooking methods allow the fat (which contains the PCBs and PBDEs) to cook off.
- If you eat salmon frequently during the week, include a mix of wild and farmed. Wild salmon is in season only 4 months of the year: May to August.

- When dining in a restaurant, ask if the salmon is farmed or wild. If salmon is a standard menu item, it's probably farmed. Wild salmon species include chum, coho, chinook, and pink. Canned salmon may also be wild salmon.

Fish and the environment

There's more to consider when choosing fish than chemical contaminants. These days, many people are considering how their food choices impact the environment. Some methods of food production are linked with soil degradation, water and air pollution, depletion of non-renewable resources, and the use of artificial chemicals. Commercial fishing and fish farming are no exception. Certain fishing practices are creating serious pressures on ocean resources and threatening the ocean's health and the wildlife it contains.

Overfishing, the practice of catching fish faster than they can reproduce, pushes the fish population lower and lower. Slow-growing fish such as Chilean sea bass and Pacific rockfish are especially vulnerable to overfishing. Other overfished species are Atlantic cod, orange roughy, Atlantic swordfish, Atlantic bluefin tuna, monkfish, and shark. Today, nearly 70% of the world's fisheries are fully fished or overfished.

Fishing practices can also damage the sea floor, which fish depend on for their survival. Nooks, boulders, and special burrows that fish create provide important hiding and feeding places for young fish and other sea animals. Bottom trawling, in which nets are dragged across the bottom of the ocean, pulls up nearly all plants, animals, and rocks. Once the sea floor is damaged, it takes hundreds and hundreds of years to return to its previous state. Longlining, hook-and-line fishing, and trap fishing do much less damage to the ocean's habitat.

Bycatch also depletes ocean life. Bycatch refers to the unwanted or unintentional animals caught in fishing gear. Dolphins, sea turtles, seals, whales, sharks, swordfish, and red snapper all get caught by accident and are either harmed or killed and then discarded, or retained and sold. Young fish that could otherwise rebuild depleted populations are also harmed by accidental kills. It's estimated that one-quarter of world catch is wasted.

Although farmed fish can supplement our fish supply, industrial-scale fish farming (aquaculture) can have negative effects on the environment. Fish farms generate pollution from feces, uneaten feed, pesticides, and antibiotics that leak into the surrounding environment. Farmed fish can escape from their net pens and spread disease to local wild fish and take over habitat from wild fish. For this reason, farms that raise the fish inland, away from coastal waters where wild fish feed and breed, are more ecologically sound.

To help consumers make smart seafood choices, the Monterey Bay Aquarium in California has developed a program called Seafood Watch. The program recommends which seafood to buy or avoid, helping consumers become advocates for environmentally friendly seafood. At the time of writing, the program has pocket guides for Hawaii and the west coast, mid-west, southwest, southeast, and northeast regions of the United States. These guides target those items most commonly found in the marketplace both at a regional and at a national level.

A guide to choosing sustainable seafood

BEST CHOICES are species that rank well against all criteria for sustainability. The wild population is abundant and well managed, with low levels of wasted catch (bycatch), and the fish are caught or farmed in ways not harmful to the environment.

Arctic char (farmed)
Catfish (farmed)
Clams (wild and farmed)
Crab (Dungeness, snow, Canada)
Halibut (Pacific)
Herring (Atlantic)
Lobster (spiny, U.S.)
Mussels (farmed)
Oysters (farmed)
Salmon (wild, Alaska)
Sardines (Atlantic)
Scallops (bay, farmed)
Striped bass (wild or farmed)
Sturgeon caviar (farmed)
Tilapia (farmed, U.S.)
Trout (rainbow, farmed)
Tuna (skipjack, troll/pole caught)

GOOD ALTERNATIVES are better choices than seafood on the Avoid list, but there are some concerns with the way they are caught or farmed.

Black sea bass
Clams (Atlantic, wild)
Crab (imitation/surimi)
Haddock (hook-and-line caught)
Lobster (American/Maine)
Mahi mahi (U.S.)
Oysters (wild)
Scallops (sea, Canada and Northeast)
Shrimp (U.S. farmed or wild)
Squid
Tuna (bigeye/yellowfin, troll/pole caught)
Tuna (canned light)
Tuna (canned white/albacore)

FISH TO AVOID are those that, at least for now, are not sustainable. These fish rank poorly on many of the Seafood Watch program's criteria.

Chilean sea bass
Cod (Atlantic)
Crab (king, imported, except from U.S.)
Flounder, Sole (Atlantic)
Haddock (trawled)
Halibut (Atlantic)
Mahi mahi (imported, except from U.S.)
Monkfish
Orange roughy
Salmon (farmed, including Atlantic)
Shark
Shrimp (imported, farmed or wild)
Snapper, red
Swordfish (imported, except from U.S.)
Tuna (bluefin)
Tuna (albacore, bigeye, and yellowfin, longline-caught)

Source: Seafood Watch/Monteray Bay Aquarium. www.seafoodwatch.org. Reprinted with permission.

As a consumer faced with so many choices in the grocery store and restaurants, it's often difficult to know where the seafood is coming from. If such information is not available in a store or on a restaurant menu, ask the server or grocer if he or she knows where the seafood comes from, or if it's wild or farmed.

Enjoying fish and seafood

There are health benefits to eating fish and seafood on a regular basis, wild or farmed. To reap the most benefits from fish, choose species that are high in omega-3 fatty acids and low in mercury. If you are an environmentally friendly shopper, you'll want to narrow down your choices to seafood that's caught or raised in ways not harmful to the environment.

Buying

When buying fresh fish and seafood, always buy from a source that maintains high standards and is knowledgeable about fish. I am fortunate to have an excellent fishmonger in Toronto very close to my home, so I can buy fresh fish every week. If you don't have access to high-quality fresh fish, check out your grocery store's frozen fish. You might be surprised by the variety that's increasingly available and equally acceptable in terms of flavour, texture, and appearance. Fresh and frozen fish have the same nutritional value.

Fish is sold in various forms. *Whole fish* is just as it comes from the water, head and fins included, and yields 2 to 3 servings per pound (4 to 6 servings per kg). When buying whole fish, look for full, clear, bright eyes. The gills should be red or pink and clean. Fresh fish should not smell fishy; it should have a mild, fresh odour. The skin should be brightly coloured with tightly adhering scales and feel firm but slightly elastic to the touch. Very importantly, fresh fish—whole or not—should be displayed on ice in a refrigerated case.

Fish steaks are cross-sections of large fish (e.g., salmon, halibut) and include bones. Steaks also yield 2 to 3 servings per pound (4 to 6 servings per kg). *Fish fillets* are the meaty sides of fish and yield 3 to 4 servings per pound (6 to 8 servings per kg). Fish steaks and fillets should appear glossy and freshly cut and have a firm texture. Avoid fish with any signs of browning, discolouration, or drying around the edges.

When buying *frozen fish,* look for solidly frozen products. If the fish is wrapped in clear plastic, look for undamaged, sealed wrapping with little or no air trapped inside the package. Make sure there are no coloured spots on the surface of the fish or ice crystals inside the wrapping. Choose plain uncooked fish fillets, or those that have been grilled or baked instead of fried.

When it comes to breaded and battered frozen fish, the healthier choices are less abundant. But they do exist. Look for products that have no trans fat and contain no more than 10 grams of fat and 500 milligrams of sodium per 3 to 4 ounce (85 to 113 g) serving. If the stated serving size is larger, sodium numbers may be slightly higher.

Tap bivalve shellfish (mussels, clams, oysters) to ensure they are alive when purchased. When alive, the shellfish will be closed or will close when tapped lightly.

Storing

Wrap fresh fish and seafood in plastic wrap or store in an airtight container in the refrigerator. As a general rule, keep fresh seafood for no longer than 1 or 2 days before cooking. Fish can be stored in the freezer for 3 to 10 months depending on its size, but it's best used within 2 months to ensure maximum flavour.

Keep live shellfish (bivalves, lobster) refrigerated in a well-ventilated container, covered with a damp paper towel or clean cloth.

Preparing

Many frozen fish fillets and steaks can be cooked without thawing if additional cooking time is allowed. If you thaw them in the refrigerator before cooking, plan for 18 hours thawing time per pound. It takes only 30 minutes per pound to thaw if submerged in cold water. Proper cooking is important not only to ensure a tender and tasty result but also to destroy any parasites and harmful bacteria present. For whole fish and fish fillets and steaks, cook at 450°F (230°C) and allow for 10 minutes per 1 inch (2.5 cm) of thickness. Turn the fish over halfway through cooking time, unless the fish is less than a 1/2 inch (1 cm) thick. If you're cooking the fish wrapped in foil or in a sauce, add 5 minutes to the cooking time. Properly cooked fish will flake easily with a fork and should be opaque and firm.

Before cooking mussels, rinse several times to remove any sand. Remove the beard (the fibrous threads sticking out the end of the mussel) by sharply tugging it toward the hinge end. To steam mussels, add them to a few cups of boiling liquid of your choice in a large pot or Dutch oven. Steam for about 8 minutes over medium heat, turning the mussels carefully after 4 or 5 minutes. Discard any that do not open during cooking.

If you plan to serve uncooked fresh seafood—sushi, ceviche, or smoked fish—take extra care to prevent food poisoning. Before and after handling seafood, wash your hands with hot soapy water and use safe handling practices. Do not let fish sit at room temperature for more than 2 hours.

TIPS FOR ADDING FISH AND SEAFOOD TO YOUR MEALS

I enjoy cooking with fish not only because I know eating fish is good for me but also because it's so quick and easy to prepare. Whether it's baked, broiled, grilled, poached, or steamed, I can have a healthy and delicious meal ready in less than 30 minutes. Fish and seafood are versatile, too. They can be enjoyed as appetizers, spreads, salads, or as a main course. Here's a sampling of a few ways to enjoy fish and seafood.

Breakfast

- For a twist on scrambled eggs, combine eggs with smoked trout, chopped onions, and red bell pepper.
- Enjoy a whole-grain bagel topped with smoked salmon or smoked trout, light cream cheese, and a few capers.
- Substitute smoked salmon for peameal (back) bacon the next time you make eggs Benedict.

Lunch and dinner

- Serve a grilled or baked salmon fillet over a bed of whole-grain pasta tossed with extra-virgin olive oil, fresh chopped dill, chopped scallions, and freshly ground black pepper.
- For a light meal, simmer a fillet of white fish in vegetable broth with fresh herbs.
- Wrap pieces of sautéed halibut or tilapia, shredded cabbage, guacamole, and salsa in soft whole-wheat tortillas for tasty fish tacos.
- Skewer marinated chunks of fresh fish, scallops, or shrimp and your favourite vegetables and broil or grill on the barbecue.
- Grill or bake an extra fish fillet or steak and serve over a bed of greens for lunch the next day.
- Add cooked shrimp to vegetable soups and stir-fries (add at the end of cooking).
- Combine cooked shrimp with chopped scallions and tomatoes, diced bell peppers, minced garlic, freshly squeezed lemon juice, and extra-virgin olive oil. Season to taste and serve over a bed of romaine lettuce.

- Make your own version of salad niçoise by combining canned light tuna with chilled cooked green beans, halved baby new potatoes, a sliced hard-boiled egg, capers, and black olives. Season to taste and drizzle with a lemon vinaigrette.

RECIPES
Cajun Breaded Trout, page 331
Coconut Curry Tilapia, page 332
Easy Baked Pesto Salmon, page 333
Hoisin Chili Halibut, page 334
Lemon Dill Salmon, page 335
Miso-Glazed Trout, page 336
Spicy Sesame Salmon, page 337

Snacks
- Try slices of smoked salmon or smoked trout on mini rye or pumpernickel bread slices.
- Enjoy a 3 ounce (85 g) can of flavoured light tuna with raw vegetable sticks for a midday energy boost.
- Serve chilled cooked shrimp with seafood sauce or salsa for a light and refreshing snack.

★ LEGUMES AND SOY FOODS
black beans * black-eyed peas * chickpeas (garbanzo beans) * fava beans * kidney beans * lentils * lima beans * navy beans * pinto beans * soybeans * soy beverages (fortified) * split peas * tempeh * tofu

Eat 3 servings per week
1 serving = 3/4 cup (175 ml) legumes or tofu *or* 1 cup (250 ml) soy beverage

Beans, beans the magical fruit … I'm sure you've heard the rest. When I talk about beans, I'm not talking about fresh green beans. Although green beans do belong to the legume family, it's their older cousins that are the real nutritional winners: dried beans, peas, and lentils. Beans develop in three stages, and the maturity of the bean dictates how it is used. The first stage is when beans are very young and tender, and both the beans and the pods are eaten (e.g., snap beans, wax beans). During the second stage, beans begin to mature and the pod becomes tough. At this stage, you must remove the beans from their pods before eating them (e.g., green peas, fresh shelled beans). As the beans mature, the pod and its beans dry on the stalk—it's at this stage you have dried beans, or as I will refer to them throughout this section, legumes.

With so much nutrition packed inside, it's a wonder why we don't eat legumes more often. They're one of the most versatile, nutritious, and inexpensive foods available. Most of my clients tell me it's not that they dislike legumes but that they don't know what to do with them. Aside from making a pot of chili or opening a can of beans in tomato sauce, many people are unsure how to incorporate legumes into meals.

Nutritional benefits of legumes

Legumes are low in fat and an excellent source of protein—1 cup (250 ml) of cooked dried beans provides as much as 21 grams of protein per food guide serving (3/4 cup/175 ml). Not bad at all when you consider a 3 ounce (90 g) chicken breast delivers the same amount of protein. That's why legumes are highlighted as an alternative to meat in the 2007 revised Canada's Food Guide. The food guide advises Canadians to eat beans, lentils, and tofu in place of meat more often to help reduce saturated fat and increase fibre intake. The protein in soybeans is considered complete because it provides all the essential amino acids in the amounts required for growth and development. For more information about protein, see Chapter 1, page 15.

Legumes are a source of low glycemic carbohydrate, the type that helps sustain your energy level longer after eating. The carbohydrate in beans is digested slowly and, as a result, gradually released as blood sugar, fending off sharp rises and dips in energy. (For more information about the glycemic index, see Chapter 1, page 14.)

When it comes to vitamins and minerals, legumes really shine. They're an excellent source of folate, a B vitamin that prevents spinal cord defects in newborns and helps guard against heart disease and certain cancers. For instance, 1 serving of lentils (cooked) supplies two-thirds of your daily folate requirement. Legumes also provide calcium, magnesium, and potassium, minerals that help prevent high blood pressure. And they're a good source of iron for vegetarians.

Like other plant foods, legumes contain disease-fighting phytochemicals, including saponins, protease inhibitors, and phytic acid, compounds that appear to protect cells from genetic damage that can lead to cancer. In the next section, you'll learn more about how adding beans to your diet can prevent cancer and heart disease.

Notable macronutrients in legumes

Per 3/4 cup (175 ml) serving, cooked

	Calories	Carbohydrate (g)	Protein (g)	Fat (g)	Fibre (g)
Black beans	170	30	11.4	0.7	8.9
Chickpeas (garbanzo beans)	202	34	11.0	3.1	9.3
Kidney beans	169	30	11.5	0.7	8.5
Lentils	172	30	13.4	0.5	11.7
Lima beans	162	29	11.0	0.5	10.0
Navy beans	191	35.5	11.2	0.8	14.3
Pinto beans	183	33.6	11.6	0.8	11.5
Soybeans	223	12.8	21.5	11.6	7.7
Edamame (young green soybeans)	142	11.5	12.6	1.4	6.0

Source: Canadian Nutrient File, 2007.

Notable micronutrients in legumes

Per 3/4 cup (175 ml) serving, cooked

	Folate (mcg)	Calcium (mg)	Magnesium (mg)	Iron (mg)
Black beans	192	35	90	2.7
Chickpeas (garbanzo beans)	212	60	59	3.6

	Folate (mcg)	Calcium (mg)	Magnesium (mg)	Iron (mg)
Kidney beans	173	46	56	3.0
Lentils	269	28	53	5.0
Lima beans	117	24	61	3.4
Navy beans	191	94	72	3.2
Pinto beans	221	59	64	2.7
Soybeans	70	132	111	6.6
Edamame (young green soybeans)	362	73	74	2.6

Source: Canadian Nutrient File, 2007.

Legumes and health

LEGUMES AND HEART DISEASE

There's good evidence that adding legumes to your meals can help keep your heart healthy. When researchers at Tulane University School of Public Health in New Orleans followed 9632 healthy men and women for 19 years, they found that those who ate dry beans, peas, or peanuts at least four times weekly had a risk of coronary heart disease that was 22% lower than people who ate these foods less than once weekly.[14] Harvard researchers also found that compared with a typical Western diet (one high in red meat, processed meat, refined grains, and sweets), eating legumes as part of a healthy diet that included fruits, vegetables, whole grains, fish, and poultry was linked with a 30% lower risk of heart disease in men.[15]

Legumes can help ward off heart disease by modifying two risk factors for the disease: high blood cholesterol and high blood pressure. A pooled analysis of 11 studies that examined the effect of legumes (not including soybeans) on blood cholesterol found eating legumes significantly lowered total cholesterol, LDL cholesterol, and blood triglyceride levels. The researchers attributed the cholesterol-lowering properties of beans to many of their healthy components, including soluble fibre, vegetable protein, and phytochemicals.[16] Numerous studies have also demonstrated the ability of soybeans to lower elevated blood cholesterol levels.

Legumes also help lower elevated blood pressure thanks to their high magnesium content. Researchers have known for some time that foods rich in magnesium can help lower blood pressure. The well-known randomized clinical trial Dietary Approaches to Stop Hypertension (DASH) showed that a diet that includes legumes four times per week has a potent blood pressure lowering effect. Persons on the DASH diet who had mild hypertension achieved a reduction in blood pressure similar to that obtained by drug treatment. What's more, blood pressure reductions occurred within 2 weeks of starting the plan. (The DASH diet is low in saturated fat and refined carbohydrates and includes fruit, vegetables, legumes, and low-fat dairy products.)[17]

LEGUMES AND PROSTATE CANCER

Research suggests that eating legumes can lower the risk of prostate cancer. Some, but not all, studies have linked high intakes of soybeans with protection from the disease. In a 6-year study of more than 12,000 Seventh Day Adventists living in the United States, drinking soy milk more than once daily compared with never drinking it was linked with a 70% lower risk of prostate cancer.[18]

A study involving 1619 men diagnosed with prostate cancer and 1618 healthy men found that those who consumed the most legumes were 38% less likely to develop prostate cancer. It's not only soybeans that offer protection against prostate cancer. When the researchers excluded soybeans from the analysis, the protective effects of legumes was just as powerful.[19] A 6-year study of almost 60,000 men living in the Netherlands found that men with the highest intake of legumes had a 29% lower risk of prostate cancer than their peers who consumed the least.[20]

Laboratory studies support the anti-cancer potential of legume-rich diets. Scientists have shown the ability of phytochemicals in legumes (saponins, protease inhibitors, and phytic acid) to block the reproduction of cancer cells and slow the growth of several types of tumours. Isoflavones in soybeans can keep testosterone levels in check, thereby reducing the risk and progression of prostate cancer. (Prostate cancer cells feed off testosterone.) At the time of writing, several studies investigating the possible effects of isoflavones on prostate cancer risk were underway.

SOYBEANS AND BREAST CANCER

Breast cancer rates of women in Asian countries have long been noted to be substantially lower than those among women in North America, a fact that's led researchers to speculate that diet might play a role. Epidemiological studies have linked a high soy intake (soybeans, tofu, miso) among Asian women with a lower risk of breast cancer. But Asians generally have a low-fat diet and eat more fish and vegetables than North Americans do. It's also possible that Asian women are more responsive to the effects of soy. Relatively few studies have measured soy intake and breast cancer risk among North American women.

Despite this, there is some evidence that soy can reduce the risk of breast cancer in non-Asian women. Researchers from Johns Hopkins School of Medicine combined the results of 18 studies that examined soy intake and breast cancer risk. Among all women, high soy intake (tofu and soy foods) was associated with a modest protective effect. Women who consumed the most soy had a 14% lower risk of breast cancer. Soy's protective effect was stronger in premenopausal women than in post-menopausal women. Premenopausal women with high soy intakes were 30% less likely to develop breast cancer compared with premenopausal women who consumed the least.[21]

Isoflavones in soybeans behave like weak forms of the body's own estrogen. That means that isoflavones compete for the same place on breast cells that estrogen does. When isoflavones attach to breast cell receptors, they elbow out estrogen, which can trigger the growth of breast cancer. It's thought that by counteracting the action of estrogen, soybeans and soy foods can reduce a woman's risk of breast cancer.

When it comes to preventing breast cancer, what seems to be most important is when you start consuming it. A study of 3015 women living in China revealed that those who consumed the most soy foods during adolescence (age 13 to 15 years) had only half the breast cancer risk compared with women whose diets contained the least.[22] It's thought that soy isoflavones may confer their protective effects during puberty, when breast cells are maturing and more vulnerable to cancer-causing substances.

If soy isoflavones mimic the action of estrogen in the body, many women worry that eating soy foods could possibly promote the development of breast cancer. The concern is that soy isoflavones could increase a woman's total estrogen levels and encourage the growth of estrogen-dependent breast cancer, especially in women who already have the disease. But it's not that simple. Some studies conducted in animals and test tubes indicate that isoflavones inhibit the development of breast cancer, while others suggest they may increase breast cancer cell growth. It depends on the particular isoflavone studied (soybeans are rich in two types of isoflavones) and the amount used. There's no compelling evidence that soy foods increase breast cancer, but research is ongoing.

That said, I do advise against the use of isoflavone supplements, which offer highly concentrated doses. We just don't have data on the long-term safety of these supplements. Experts also advise women who have had breast cancer to avoid soy supplements and soy protein powders. Although it's believed that eating foods made from soybeans a few times a week is safe, many breast cancer survivors choose to avoid soy altogether. It's clearly a personal decision.

Health concerns about soy

Toxicologists caution that eating large amounts of soy can result in an underactive thyroid gland and goiter (an enlarged thyroid gland) by blocking the production of thyroid hormones. However, this appears to occur only in people who are deficient in iodine, a mineral that's needed for normal thyroid function. In developed countries, salt is fortified with iodine to prevent such a deficiency. It's possible, however, that people who eat soy foods and who don't get enough iodine from their diet could be at risk for goiter.

Critics of soy also warn that soy infant formulas can lead to abnormal sexual development in children. But this finding has never been recognized clinically. American researchers compared 811 adults who were fed either soy or cow's milk formula in infancy and found no differences in growth, maturation, fertility, or other reproductive outcomes. An Italian study of 48 children also concluded soy infant formulas had no hormonal effects.[23]

LEGUMES AND TYPE 2 DIABETES

Several large studies have shown that eating a diet based on low glycemic foods reduces the risk of developing type 2 diabetes.[24] Diets rich in legumes may guard against type 2 diabetes by improving blood sugar control and block decreasing insulin secretion. As well, adding legumes to meals can help prevent weight gain—another risk factor for type 2 diabetes—by delaying the return of hunger after a meal. In fact, a review of the findings from six randomized controlled trials concluded that overweight people on low glycemic diets lost more weight and more body fat than did those who followed high glycemic or other diets.[25] Fending off weight gain and type 2 diabetes are other ways in which a legume-rich diet can help reduce the risk of heart disease.

Enjoying legumes and soy foods

Grocery stores and specialty food stores carry a wide variety of legumes, both dried and canned. Although dried beans have a superior taste and texture to canned beans, they do take longer to prepare. That's why I usually buy canned legumes: All I need to do is open the can, rinse and drain them, and they're ready to add to whatever dish I'm preparing. Some of the less common legumes, however, are available only in their dried form.

Buying

Dried legumes are sold in packages or in bulk food bins. When purchasing from bulk bins, choose firm legumes that are uniform in size. Avoid dried beans that are shrivelled, broken or split. Also, toss any beans that have tiny pinhole markings, which is a sign of insect damage. If buying packaged dried beans, make sure the package is not damaged. When buying canned cooked legumes, avoid cans that are dented, bulged, or rusty. If available, buy brands that are low in sodium.

Storing

Dried legumes can be kept in an airtight container at room temperature for up to 1 year. Keep in mind, though, that older legumes take longer to cook, so don't mix new beans with old legumes in recipes. Cooked legumes stored in a covered container in the refrigerator will stay fresh for up to 4 days.

Cooked legumes freeze well. To freeze legumes so they don't clump together, spread them on a cookie sheet and place in the freezer until frozen. Remove, pack in an airtight container or plastic freezer bag, and return to the freezer. Cooked legumes will keep in the freezer for up to 6 months.

Preparing

The longer preparation time required for dried legumes is often a deterrent for busy people. But as you'll see, cooking dried legumes requires very little effort and can be done while you're attending to other tasks. All dried legumes are prepared in the same way: First they are cleaned and soaked, then they're cooked—ready for your favourite bean dish.

* *Cleaning:* Spread dried legumes in a single layer on paper towel or a light coloured kitchen counter to check for any damaged beans or stones. Place legumes in a colander and rinse thoroughly under lukewarm running water (cold water can cause beans to become tough).

- *Soaking:* The purpose of soaking is to rehydrate the legumes before cooking, which reduces cooking time. Place cleaned legumes in a large pot or bowl and cover with three times the volume of cool water. (Legumes double in size after soaking.) Allow them to soak for 6 to 8 hours at room temperature. During soaking, pour off the water and add fresh water at least once. This helps get rid of some of the indigestible carbohydrates that cause gas. After soaking, drain and rinse the legumes in a colander.

  To save time, use the quick-soak method. Place cleaned legumes in a large pot with three times the volume of cool water. Bring legumes and water to a boil for 2 minutes, then remove from the heat. Cover and let stand for 1 hour. Drain and rinse in a colander.

- *Cooking:* Cooking times vary depending on the type, size, and age of the legume. In general, legumes triple in size after cooking. To cook, add 3 cups (750 ml) of unsalted water for every 1 cup (250 ml) of soaked legumes. The water should be 2 inches (5 cm) above the top of the legumes. Add 1 to 2 tablespoons (15 to 25 ml) of vegetable oil to prevent the water from boiling over. Bring the legumes to a gentle boil, then reduce to a simmer, partially covering the pot. Gently stir legumes occasionally during cooking. Skim off and discard any foam that develops during cooking.

  Small legumes (black beans, pinto beans, navy beans, lentils) may take 30 to 45 minutes to cook; medium-sized legumes (kidney beans, chickpeas, lima beans) can take 1 to 2 hours. Once beans are tender, remove from the heat and allow them to sit in cooking liquid while they cool. This will prevent them from drying out. Once cooked, legumes are ready to be used in recipes.

  Herbs, onion, garlic, celery, or carrots added to the cooking water will enhance the flavour of the beans. Do not add acidic ingredients, such as lemon juice, vinegar, or wine, which will harden the skin of the legumes, preventing them from absorbing water during cooking. Wait until the legumes are almost tender before adding acidic ingredients.

  If you prefer the convenience of canned legumes, you'll only have to open the can, drain the legumes in a colander, and rinse under cool running water. Rinsing canned beans removes unwanted sodium as well as some of the gas-producing carbohydrates.

There are other ways to enjoy the goodness of legumes besides eating cooked beans. A variety of products made from soybeans offer the same nutritional and health benefits. Here's a quick guide.

A guide to soy products

SOYBEANS
These can be bought canned or dried. Add soybeans to soups, casseroles, and curries. Or mash them up and add them to burgers.

MISO
A traditional Asian flavouring, miso is fermented soybean paste made by mixing soybeans with a grain, for example, rice. Use miso as a base for soups or add it to marinades and sauces. For stock, use 1/4 cup (50 ml) of miso for every 4 cups (1 L) of water.

SOY FLOUR
Soy flour is soybeans that have been defatted and finely ground. Because soy flour contains no gluten, the protein that adds structure to wheat-based baked products, it should be mixed with other flours in baking recipes, rather than used alone. Substitute up to half of the all-purpose wheat flour with soy flour in breads, muffins, loaves, cakes, and scones. You'll find soy flour in natural food stores and some grocery stores.

SOY BEVERAGES
There are two types of soy beverages: those made from the juice of ground soybeans and those concocted from soy protein, water, and other ingredients. The flavour varies according to how the product was made, so you may need to try a few brands to find one you like. Buy a brand that is unflavoured (it contains much less added sugar and more protein) or unsweetened (it contains no added sugar) and is fortified with calcium. Use soy beverages as you'd use cow's milk—on cereal and in smoothies, coffee, lattes, and cooking (e.g., soups) and baking.

SOY MEATS
These ready-to-eat or frozen soy foods resemble meat and can be used in place of beef burgers, hot dogs, deli meats, and ground meat. You'll find them in the freezer, deli, or produce section of grocery stores.

Soy nuts

Soy nuts, which are similar in texture and flavour to peanuts, are whole soybeans that have been soaked in water and then baked until crisp and brown. Also called roasted soybeans, soy nuts come in plain, barbecue, and garlic flavours. If you have high blood pressure, choose unsalted soy nuts.

Tempeh

A traditional Indonesian food, tempeh is soybeans that have been fermented using a mould (a tempeh starter), then pressed into a cake form. There are different types of tempeh, including those made with quinoa and kasha. The rich, tender cake has a nutty, yeasty flavour. This may not sound appetizing, but I assure you, tempeh is very tasty. It can be marinated and grilled and added to soups, casseroles, or chili. You can purchase tempeh, refrigerated or frozen, in natural food stores and Asian markets. When selecting tempeh, look for a solid cake with a whitish bloom. Black is also acceptable, but any other colour suggests that the tempeh may have spoiled.

Texturized vegetable protein (TVP)

Made from soy flour that's been defatted and dehydrated, TVP is sold in packages as granules. You can also buy TVP in the bulk section of natural food stores, as flakes or chunks the size of croutons. Rehydrate TVP with an equal amount of water or broth, and then use it to replace ground meat in pasta sauces, lasagna, chili, and tacos.

Tofu

This staple food of traditional Japanese and Chinese cuisine is made from soybeans, water, and a curdling agent. Its relatively bland taste makes it well suited to absorb flavours in spicy curries, stir-fries, and marinades. There are two main kinds of tofu: silken and regular. Both can be found in soft, medium, firm, and extra-firm consistencies. They are made from the same ingredients, but because they are processed slightly differently, they are not interchangeable in a recipe.

Silken tofu, also called soft or Japanese-style tofu, has a softer consistency than regular tofu and will fall apart if not handled carefully. Silken tofu, unlike regular tofu, is often packaged in aseptic boxes that don't require refrigeration. Because of this, silken tofu is sometimes stoked in a different section of the grocery store than regular tofu, which requires refrigeration.

Regular tofu, also called bean curd, is sold in a sealed package or plastic container in the chilled produce section of most grocery stores. Firm or extra-firm regular tofu is best used in stir-fries or any dish in which you will want the tofu to retain its shape. For recipes that call for crumbled or mashed tofu, such as tofu scramble, firm tofu will work just fine, though medium and soft tofu will have a smoother consistency.

TIPS FOR ADDING LEGUMES AND SOY FOODS
TO YOUR MEALS

Substituting protein-rich dried beans, peas, and lentils for meat and poultry is an excellent way to consume less saturated fat and more fibre, folate, magnesium, and phytochemicals. If you're leery of eating more legumes for fear of gas, there's no need to worry. Beans can cause flatulence because they contain oligosaccharides, indigestible carbohydrates that are fermented by bacteria, yeasts, and fungi that reside in the colon. Fortunately, there are ways to minimize this often embarrassing gas production. Some of the oligosaccharides are released when dried beans are soaked—that's why it's important to change the water a few times during soaking.

When adding beans to your diet, start with a small, 1/4 cup (50 ml) portion, and gradually increase your portion size. If you make beans a regular part of your diet, your body will adjust, reducing the gassy effects. Some people, however, are more sensitive to the gas-producing effects of legumes. In these cases, I recommend trying Beano, a digestive enzyme supplement available as tablets or drops in drugstores. If taken with your first bite of the meal, Beano will help the body digest the gas-producing carbohydrates in legumes.

Whether you buy legumes dried or already cooked in cans, there are plenty of tasty ways to incorporate this disease-fighting food into your diet. Below are quick serving suggestions and delicious recipe suggestions for legumes and soybean products, including tofu, tempeh, and soy beverages.

Breakfast
- Add cooked legumes or diced firm tofu to egg dishes—scrambled eggs, frittatas, or omelets.
- Replace bacon with soy-based breakfast meats to reduce saturated fat.
- Enjoy a fruit smoothie made with an unflavoured, calcium-fortified soy beverage for a healthy start to the morning.
- When making muffins, replace up to one-half the all-purpose flour with soy flour.

Lunch and dinner

- Toss cooked legumes into leafy green and pasta salads.
- Add chickpeas to your favourite Greek salad for a boost of protein and fibre.
- Serve soup made from dried beans or peas instead of the usual chicken noodle. Try minestrone, split pea, black bean, or lentil soup.
- Make a three bean salad by mixing red and white kidney beans with black beans. Add chopped parsley, diced onion, and freshly ground black pepper. Toss with a balsamic vinaigrette.
- Add cooked legumes or chopped firm tofu to canned or homemade soups and stews.
- Replace meat or chicken with cubes of firm tofu or tempeh in a stir-fry.
- Spread wrap sandwiches with chickpea purée or hummus (chickpea dip) before filling.
- Add cooked chickpeas to grain dishes, such as couscous or rice pilaf.
- Use a variety of cooked legumes when making chili. Try chickpeas, black beans, and soybeans in addition to kidney beans.
- Add black beans or pinto beans to tacos and burritos. Use half the amount of lean ground meat you normally would and make up the difference with beans.
- Add cooked chickpeas to mashed potatoes or other puréed vegetables, for example, squash.
- Sauté legumes, cubed tofu, or tempeh with chopped spinach and tomatoes and serve over whole-wheat pasta.
- Add white kidney beans to a tomato-based pasta sauce for a Mediterranean-inspired meal.
- Add cooked legumes to sautéed leafy greens such as spinach or Swiss chard for a healthy side dish.

Snacks

- Enjoy hummus (chickpea dip) with baked pita triangles or raw veggies.
- Look for roasted chickpeas or soybeans at your local natural foods store.
- Add cooked lentils to your favourite prepared salsa. Serve with baked tortilla chips.
- Make your own bean dip by puréeing cooked white kidney beans with roasted garlic, cumin, and chili peppers. Serve with raw vegetables.
- Make a Mexican dip by layering black beans, guacamole, chopped fresh tomatoes, low-fat sour cream, diced green onion, and chopped cilantro. Serve with raw vegetables or baked tortilla chips.
- For a twist on bruschetta, mix cooked navy beans with olive oil, chopped sage, and garlic. Serve with toasted whole-grain baguette slices.
- Blend soft tofu with your favourite fruits and honey for a sweet but healthy snack.
- Enjoy edamame (young green soybeans) as a tasty snack. Place frozen edamame (purchased in grocery and natural food stores) in boiling water for 10 minutes. Drain, salt lightly if desired, and enjoy.

RECIPES

★ NUTS AND SEEDS
almonds ★ Brazil nuts ★ cashews ★ hazelnuts
★ macadamia nuts ★ peanuts ★ pecans ★ pine nuts
★ pistachios ★ pumpkin seeds ★ sesame seeds
★ sunflower seeds ★ walnuts

Eat 5 servings per week
1 serving = 1 ounce (30 g) (approx. 1/4 cup/50 ml) shelled nuts *or*
2 tablespoons (25 ml) nut butter *or*
1/4 cup (50 ml) seeds

If you're watching your weight, you might shudder at the idea of adding nuts to your diet. For years, dieters have avoided nuts because of their high fat and calorie content. That's not surprising when you consider that a small handful of mixed nuts—just 1/4 cup (50 ml)—packs in 205 calories and almost 2 tablespoons (25 ml) of oil. But it's their fat content that makes nuts so good for you.

Over the past decade, numerous studies have tied the consumption of nuts with protection from heart attack, high blood pressure, diabetes, even Alzheimer's disease. Eating nuts on a regular basis can also help keep blood cholesterol and blood pressure numbers in check. And believe it or not, it is possible to eat nuts on a regular basis and not gain weight.

Nuts grow on trees and come in many varieties, among them almonds, Brazil nuts, cashews, hazelnuts, macadamia nuts, pecans, pine nuts, pistachios, and walnuts. Peanuts are technically legumes, but their nutrient makeup and health benefits are similar to that of nuts.

Because of their higher protein content, nuts belong in the meat and alternatives food group in Canada's Food Guide. One serving counts as approximately 1/4 cup (50 ml) of shelled nuts or 2 tablespoons (25 ml) of nut butter. Nuts are an important source of protein for vegetarians, many of whom find it challenging to meet their daily protein requirements.

Nutritional benefits of nuts

Nuts are cholesterol-free, but, as you know, they are high in fat. In fact, as much as 90% of the calories in nuts come from fat. The good news is that most of the fat in nuts is the healthy unsaturated kind. Saturated fats, found mainly in animal foods, such as meat and dairy, raise LDL (bad) cholesterol in the bloodstream. (High blood cholesterol can contribute to a buildup of plaque in the arteries, causing them to harden and narrow.) Nuts contain mainly polyunsaturated and monounsaturated fats and only small amounts of saturated fat.

Nuts are high in protein and unusually rich in arginine, an amino acid that may improve blood vessel function. Nuts are also a good source of magnesium, a mineral shown to help maintain a healthy blood pressure. Walnuts are an excellent source of alpha-linolenic acid (ALA), an omega-3 fatty acid that's thought to protect against irregular heart rhythms. Nuts are also a good source of vitamin E, B vitamins (including folate), potassium, and fibre, nutrients demonstrated to have cardio-protective properties.

While nuts are nutritious, they come with a few drawbacks. For starters, they're loaded with calories. A 1 ounce (30 g) serving of nuts delivers between 160 and 200 calories. That's considerably more than 1 ounce (30 g) of chicken or lean meat, which contains roughly 55 calories. One ounce (30 g) of nuts isn't that much—you'll need to count out 8 Brazil nuts, 18 cashews, 14 walnut halves, 24 almonds, or 28 peanuts to make sure you're eating only 1 serving.

Nuts are also easy to overeat. If you eat them by the handful, you're likely to consume plenty of calories that your waistline doesn't need. The best way to eat nuts is portion controlled: pre-portion single servings of nuts in snack-sized Ziploc bags. To prevent weight gain, you will also need to subtract a similar number of calories from your diet. Substitute nuts for less healthy foods, such as cookies, ice cream, candy, soft drinks, chips, and refined starchy foods.

The table below details the serving size and nutrient breakdown of selected nuts.

Serving sizes and nutritional content of nuts

Per 1 ounce (30 g) serving

	How many?	Calories	Noteworthy nutrients
Almonds	24	160	riboflavin, vitamin E, magnesium
Brazil nuts	6–8	190	magnesium, selenium, copper

	How many?	Calories	Noteworthy nutrients
Cashews	18	160	magnesium, copper, plant sterols
Hazelnuts	20	180	vitamin E, copper, manganese
Macadamia nuts	10–12	200	manganese, plant sterols
Peanuts	28	170	niacin, manganese
Pecans	20 halves	200	copper, manganese
Pine nuts	157	190	magnesium, copper, manganese
Pistachios	49	160	vitamin B6, copper, manganese
Walnuts	14 halves	190	copper, maganese, ALA

Nuts and health

NUTS AND HEART HEALTH

More than 40 studies have shown that including nuts in the diet can reduce the risk of heart disease, regardless of the type of nut. Researchers from Harvard Medical School and the Harvard School of Public Heath followed 21,454 healthy men for 17 years and found that over the course of 1 year, men who ate nuts at least twice per week were 47% less likely to die suddenly from heart attack than were men who rarely or never consumed nuts.[26] The ongoing Nurses' Health Study turned up similar results. Among 86,016 women who were tracked for 14 years, those who ate 5 ounces (140 g) of nuts each week were 35% less likely to suffer fatal and non-fatal heart attacks than women who ate less than 1 ounce (30 g) per month. A different report from this study linked regular nut and peanut butter consumption to a lower risk of developing type 2 diabetes.[27]

Even more compelling were the findings of a review of four large studies—including the two studies mentioned above—that examined nut intake and heart disease. When evidence from all four studies was combined, people who ate nuts at least four times per week were 37% less likely to develop heart disease compared with those who seldom or never ate nuts.[28]

The evidence on the cardiovascular benefits of nuts was compelling enough to prompt the U.S. Food and Drug Administration, in 2003, to approve a health claim for seven types of nuts. Packages of almonds, hazelnuts, peanuts, pecans, some pine nuts, pistachios, and walnuts can claim "scientific evidence suggests but does not prove that eating 1 1/2 ounces [45 g] per day of most nuts as part of a diet low in saturated fat and cholesterol may reduce the risk of heart disease." These nuts were approved because they contain less than 4 grams of saturated fat per 1 1/2 ounce (45 g) serving.

Researchers believe it's the type of fat found in nuts that helps keep the heart healthy. When replacing saturated fats, unsaturated fats help lower LDL (bad) blood cholesterol. Studies have consistently shown that adding almonds, peanuts, hazelnuts, macadamia nuts, pecans, pistachios, or walnuts to the diet lowers LDL cholesterol in the bloodstream. One study even found almond butter was effective at lowering blood cholesterol, though not to the same degree as raw almonds.[29] Plant sterols, natural plant chemicals found in nuts, have also been implicated in cholesterol lowering.

Nuts can guard against heart disease in other ways, too. The scientifically tested DASH (Dietary Approaches to Stop Hypertension) diet demonstrated that eating nuts (and legumes) four times per week helped lower elevated blood pressure. Magnesium and arginine (an amino acid) in nuts are thought to help reduce blood pressure. Peanuts also contain resveratrol, an antioxidant also found in red grapes and red wine. Animals studied have demonstrated the ability of this phytochemical to greatly improve blood flow to the brain, thereby reducing the risk of stroke.

NUTS AND TYPE 2 DIABETES

There's also evidence that eating nuts on a regular basis can ward off type 2 diabetes. The ongoing Nurses' Health Study recently found that among 83,818 healthy women who were followed for 16 years, those who ate 1 ounce (30 g) of nuts at least five times per week were 27% less likely to develop type 2 diabetes compared with women who rarely or never consumed nuts. Peanut butter was also protective—women who ate peanut butter five times per week had a 21% lower risk of type 2 diabetes than women who never or almost never ate peanut butter.[30] Researchers suspect that unsaturated fat, fibre, and magnesium in nuts all help protect the body from type 2 diabetes.

What about seeds?

Canada's Food Guide includes seeds in the meat and alternatives food group because they have a similar nutritional profile to nuts. As such, seeds are a heart healthy addition to your diet. You won't hear nutritionists praising their health benefits as often as nuts simply because seeds have not been the focus of scientific studies. But that's no reason to ban them from your diet. One tip for sesame seeds: Because they are so tiny, grind them to a meal before adding them to dishes, for example, salads and stir-fries. Otherwise, they're likely to pass through the intestines undigested.

I tend to count 1 tablespoon (15 ml) of seeds as 1 fat and oil serving, since this is the fat and calorie equivalent to 1 teaspoon (5 ml) of vegetable oil. For more details on healthy fats and oils, see Chapter 7.

What about nut butters?

As you read above, studies have found that eating nut butter can help reduce the risk of type 2 diabetes and lower blood cholesterol. However, the healthy benefits of nut butter are not as powerful as raw nuts. Even so, nut butters are a healthy addition to your diet. (They're certainly a much better choice than highly saturated fat spreads, such as butter and full-fat cream cheese.) Wondering which type of nut butter to use? There are plenty of options besides good old peanut butter.

- *Almond butter* is more nutrient-dense than peanut butter. Per serving, almond butter contains a higher amount of monounsaturated fat, as well as more calcium, magnesium, and potassium, than peanut butter. Many peanut butters have added sugars, for example, icing sugar and corn syrup. Almond butter contains no added ingredients or preservatives—it's simply crushed almonds.
- *Cashew butter* is tasty but contains less protein, fibre, and niacin than peanut and almond butter.
- *Soy butter* is an alternative for people who are allergic to nut butters. It's lower in fat than peanut butter but usually has added sugar to make it palatable.

- *Tahini* (sesame seed butter) is a popular ingredient in Middle Eastern cooking. It can be mixed with ground chickpeas (garbanzo beans) to make hummus or combined with roasted eggplant and spices to make baba ghanoush. I like to mix hummus with roasted garlic for a delicious spread on whole-wheat tortilla wraps.

Enjoying nuts and seeds

Buying

When buying shelled nuts, look for unblanched nuts that are raw or dry-roasted. Roasting nuts does enhance the flavour and reduce spoilage, but it can also alter their essential fatty acid content. Blanched nuts are treated with heat, which may also destroy some nutrients. Oil-roasted nuts contain extra fat that you don't necessarily need. Buy nuts unsalted. Salted nuts contain up to 250 milligrams of sodium per 1 ounce (30 g) or 1/4 cup (50 ml) serving. (Adults should consume no more than 2300 milligrams of sodium per day.)

If buying nuts from a bulk food bin, buy them at a store with a good product turnover to ensure freshness. Choose nuts that are not shrivelled—a sign that they're old. If it is possible to smell the nuts, do so to ensure they smell fresh and not rancid.

When buying unshelled nuts, choose those that feel heavy for their size. The shells of nuts, especially peanuts, should not be cracked, pierced, discoloured, or mouldy. Mouldy peanuts can contain a toxic substance called aflatoxin, a carcinogen produced by a mould that grows naturally on peanuts. You should immediately dispose of any peanuts that appear even a bit mouldy.

When purchasing peanut and other nut butters, read labels. Avoid products that have added sugars and hydrogenated oils. The healthiest nut butters contain nuts, salt, and nothing else.

Most seeds are sold in packages or in bulk food bins. As with nuts, if buying seeds in the bulk food section, buy them from a store that has good turnover, to ensure maximal freshness. If possible, smell the seeds and avoid ones that smell musty or rancid. Avoid unshelled seeds that are broken or shrivelled—a sign the seeds are not fresh.

Storing

Because of their high fat content, nuts can go rancid easily if not stored properly. Store nuts in a tightly sealed container in the refrigerator, where they'll keep for up to 6 months before losing flavour or spoiling. If stored in the freezer, nuts will last for up to 1 year. Nuts still in their shell have the longest shelf life. Unshelled nuts can keep for a few months at room temperature in a cool, dry location.

Natural nut butters have shorter shelf lives than commercially produced peanut butters. Walnut, pecan, and pumpkin seed butters must be refrigerated, even before opening, because of their content of oils that spoil quickly. Cashew butter should be refrigerated after opening. Store other nut butters in a cool, dry cupboard or on a shelf in your pantry. Nut butters are best used within 6 months, when they are freshest.

Store seeds in an airtight container in the refrigerator. Seeds remain edible for several months, but they are best consumed within two months, when they are at maximum freshness.

Preparing

Nuts require little if any preparation. Shelled nuts can be used in recipes whole, chopped, slivered, or ground.

Like nuts, there's little you need to do to make seeds ready to enjoy on their own or in a recipe. Shelled seeds can be used whole, raw or roasted, or ground in many recipes.

TIPS FOR ADDING NUTS AND SEEDS TO YOUR MEALS

Nuts are a good source of protein, contain no cholesterol, and are low in saturated fat. Provided you don't have a nut allergy—and you cut back on something else to balance out the extra calories—nuts are certainly worth adding to your diet. The following tips will help you add a (small) handful of nuts or seeds to your daily diet:

Breakfast

- Top your morning bowl of hot or cold cereal with chopped or whole nuts.
- Add nuts and seeds to your favourite granola.
- Mix slivered or chopped almonds into yogurt.
- Add ground nuts or nut butter to breakfast smoothies.
- Add chopped walnuts or pecans to pancake and waffle batters.
- Add pumpkin seeds to homemade whole-grain muffin batters.

RECIPE

Blueberry Walnut Muesli with Rolled Oats and Flaxseed, page 271

Lunch and dinner

- Toss a handful of peanuts or cashews into an Asian-style stir-fry with vegetables and shrimp or chicken.
- Sauté leafy green vegetables with cashews or pine nuts.
- Sprinkle steamed vegetables with ground sesame seeds.
- Add peanuts or almonds to a spicy curry.
- Mix sliced almonds or pine nuts into chicken salad for a crunchy sandwich filling.
- Toss a handful of toasted nuts and seeds into green salads.
- Add toasted walnuts to whole-grain pasta tossed with extra-virgin olive oil.
- Toss penne or another pasta of your choice with a nut pesto.
- Add nuts to side dishes—hazelnuts to brown rice, pine nuts to couscous, and slivered almonds to green beans.
- Sprinkle casseroles with chopped nuts or seeds after or near the end of cooking time just to brown.
- Add chopped nuts to poultry stuffing.
- Add ground nuts or seeds to burger recipes.

RECIPES
Blueberry and Roasted Walnut Spinach Salad, page 288
Kasha, Walnut, and Apple Salad with Mint, page 300
Spinach Almond Pesto, page 370

Snacks

- Snack on homemade trail mix made with nuts, dried apricots, and raisins.
- Add chopped nuts to muffin and cookie recipes.
- Purée walnuts, cooked lentils, extra-virgin olive oil, and herbs and spices to make a healthy dip for crackers and vegetables.
- Enjoy apple slices dipped in your favourite nut butter.
- Spread nut butter on celery sticks for a tasty midday snack.

RECIPES
Bruce Trail Mix, page 282
Quick Cashew Mango Trail Mix, page 283
Spicy Candied Walnuts, page 284
Tamari Roasted Almonds, page 285
Blueberries topped with Candied Almonds, page 378

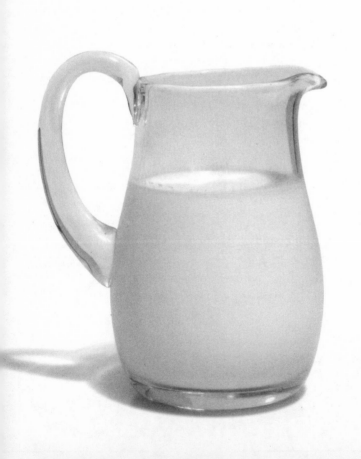

6
Power dairy foods

★ kefir

★ yogurt

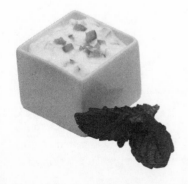

There's no question that dairy products are nutritious. Milk, yogurt, and cheese are most famous for their outstanding calcium content, the mineral needed to help prevent osteoporosis, a bone-thinning disease that leads to fractures. But calcium-rich dairy products do more than maintain strong bones. Research suggests that an adequate intake of the mineral can help guard against colon cancer, kidney stones, and symptoms of premenstrual syndrome. Studies have also shown that low-fat dairy products, as part of a diet rich in fruits and vegetables, help reduce high blood pressure.

Yet there's more to dairy foods than calcium. They're also good sources of protein, vitamin A, riboflavin (vitamin B2), magnesium, zinc, and potassium. Milk (and a few brands of yogurt) is also fortified with vitamin D, a nutrient that's needed to prevent rickets, a disease that causes soft and deformed bones. Vitamin D also plays a vital role in bone health, helping maintain the strength of your bones as you age.

And if you choose low-fat dairy products, you'll get even more nutritional value: all the same nutrients with little or no cholesterol-raising saturated fat. Although all low-fat dairy foods are nutritious, some outshine others when it comes to their disease-fighting components. As you'll read in the pages that follow, a daily serving of fermented milk (i.e., yogurt and kefir) can keep you healthy in ways that plain milk can't.

★ YOGURT AND KEFIR

Eat 1 serving per day
1 serving = 3/4 cup (175 ml or 175 g)

Yogurt and kefir are made by combining milk with bacteria, or "cultures," which go to work fermenting the nutrients in milk while producing substances that curdle and flavour the milk. The end result: a dairy product with a tart flavour and thick, creamy texture that contains live bacteria.

It turns out these live bacteria, called probiotics, do more than simply ferment milk into yogurt or kefir. Studies suggest that regular consumption of foods that contain probiotic organisms can stimulate the immune system, prevent allergies, improve symptoms of lactose intolerance, help treat inflammatory bowel disease (e.g., ulcerative colitis, Crohn's disease), and possibly even lower elevated cholesterol levels. Emerging research also hints that probiotic bacteria may guard against colon cancer.

Probiotics defined

The word *probiotics,* the antonym of *antibiotics,* literally means "for life." Probiotics are live organisms (bacteria and yeast) that, when consumed in certain amounts, exert health benefits. To be called a probiotic, bacteria and other organisms must:

* Grow and be active in the lower intestine. To do this they must survive the acidity of the stomach and pass through to the small intestine.
* Have a health effect that has been demonstrated in clinical trials.
* Improve the balance of bacteria in the gut, so that the activities of so-called good bacteria outweigh those that may be harmful.
* Be properly identified and named strains (i.e., not just a genera, such as lactobacillus, which consists of many strains). These strains must stay alive and remain stable before being consumed.

The two main types of probiotic bacteria in foods and supplements are lactobacillus and bifidobacterium. Within these main types there are dozens of strains, such as *Lactobacillus acidophilus, Lactobacillus GG, Lactobacillus rhamnosus, Bifidobacterium lactis,* and *Bifidobacterium bifidus.*

To make yogurt, manufacturers add two strains of bacteria to milk: *Lactobacillus bulgaricus* and *Streptococcus thermophilus.* These bacteria go to work digesting the nutrients in milk, including lactose, while producing lactic acid (which gives yogurt its sour taste) and folate. Because these bacteria are easily killed by stomach acid, many manufacturers boost the probiotic content of their products with other strains—*Lactobacillus acidophilus,* perhaps, or another bifidus strain. For example, Danone's Activia yogurt contains *Bifidobacterium lactis,* a strain that's been shown to resist stomach acid.

When I refer to yogurt in this chapter, I mean fresh yogurt, not frozen yogurt. Many frozen yogurts contain little if any of the beneficial bacteria because they're made with powdered milk ingredients instead of real yogurt. Even among brands that list fresh yogurt as an ingredient, the numbers of bacteria are most likely too small to exert a health benefit in the intestinal tract. In 2006, the frozen yogurt chain Yogen Früz added probiotic cultures to its non-fat and low-fat frozen yogurts. Whether this product meets the definition of probiotic is tough to say. The company's website does not specify the types or amounts of bacterial strains added.

Kefir is made a little differently in that it contains different cultures from yogurt. In this case, milk is fermented by kefir grains, a combination of Lactobacillus bacteria, yeasts, protein, fat, and sugar. The milk is allowed to ferment for approximately 24 hours, during which time the bacteria and yeast change the texture, taste, and nutrient composition of the milk. Carbon dioxide is also produced, which gives kefir a hint of natural carbonation. Kefir's sparkling mouth feel is why it's often described as the "champagne" of fermented dairy products. Kefir contains unique polysaccharides (long chains of sugar) called kefiran, to which scientists attribute some of kefir's health benefits.

Kefir is best described as a naturally sweet, yet tangy, liquid yogurt. Some people like to drink kefir, while others prefer to eat it with a spoon.

Probiotics and health

The notion that certain bacteria can improve your health is gaining ground among Canadians. Just visit the dairy case at your local grocery store and you'll see rows and rows of colourful cartons of yogurt and kefir in various forms and flavours, and with various fat contents. The live bacterial content of yogurt and kefir makes these foods appealing to scientists and health professionals alike. It seems there isn't a week that goes by without a new report being published linking probiotics and probiotic-containing foods to disease prevention.

Although the health benefits of probiotic foods vary depending on the type and amount of bacteria present, mounting scientific evidence suggests that regular consumption of probiotics is beneficial.

ENHANCED BARRIER AGAINST INFECTION

Probiotic bacteria are normally found in our digestive tract as part of the intestinal flora, a community of hundreds of strains of beneficial bacteria. Here, they help inhibit the growth of unfriendly, disease-causing bacteria by preventing their attachment to the intestinal wall and producing substances that suppress their growth. In the gut, probiotic organisms break down vitamins and digest fibre and carbohydrates that are not absorbed in the small intestine.

Consuming foods that are rich sources of probiotic bacteria is believed to maintain a healthy balance of bacteria in the gut, increasing the number of helpful bacteria and decreasing the number of harmful bacteria. By doing so, probiotic foods can improve the protective barrier of the intestinal tract, one of the body's lines of defence against infection. Numerous animal and laboratory studies have demonstrated the ability of probiotic bacteria in yogurt to increase the production of immune compounds in the gastrointestinal tract.

MAINTAINING REGULARITY

Probiotics appear to do more than build a strong blockade against germs and viruses. The most compelling evidence for their effectiveness is the prevention of diarrhea. A recent analysis of 34 randomized controlled trials concluded that probiotics significantly reduced antibiotic-associated diarrhea by 52%, traveller's diarrhea by 8%, and that of acute diarrhea of different causes by 34%.[1] Acute diarrhea includes rotavirus-induced diarrhea, the leading cause of severe and life-threatening gastroenteritis in children. Traveller's diarrhea is caused by consuming food or water contaminated with disease-causing bacteria.

Children who are treated with antibiotics may benefit from probiotics. Antibiotics disturb the normal intestinal flora, which can result in a range of symptoms, most notably diarrhea. Because antibiotics are prescribed so frequently to children, antibiotic side effects are common. A combined analysis of six studies published in the *Canadian Medical Association Journal* concluded that probiotic bacteria taken along with antibiotics reduced the risk of antibiotic-associated diarrhea in children and teenagers by 57%.[2]

If you suffer from constipation, consuming fermented milk products may help keep you regular. A study conducted among people with chronic constipation showed that drinking milk fermented with *L. bulgaricus* and *S. thermophilus* increased the speed with which waste moved through the intestinal tract and improved bowel function. Drinking the probiotic milk increased the number of bowel movements from three per week to seven per week.[3]

REDUCED LACTOSE INTOLERANCE

Many people with lactose intolerance are able to much better tolerate yogurt and kefir than milk. Lactose intolerance is caused by a shortage of lactase, an enzyme produced in the lining of the small intestine that digests lactose into smaller sugar units (lactose is the naturally occurring sugar in milk). When lactase is deficient, undigested lactose remains in the intestine, causing abdominal cramps, diarrhea, gas, and bloating.

Numerous studies have shown that regularly consuming yogurt and kefir improves the absorption of lactose in children and adults with mild to moderate lactose intolerance. In a study of 15 adults with lactose intolerance, researchers fed participants test meals of milk, yogurt, and kefir. All tests meals contained the same amount of lactose. Compared with milk, the yogurt and kefir meals significantly reduced the severity of digestive complaints, especially flatulence.[4] Another study conducted among 22 people with lactose intolerance found that eating fresh, but not heated, yogurt with live bacterial cultures reduced the severity of gastrointestinal symptoms.[5] Heating yogurt destroys the live bacterial cultures.

Probiotic bacteria found in yogurt and kefir reduce symptoms of lactose intolerance because much of the lactose has been broken down during the fermentation process. That means 1 serving of these foods contains less lactose than 1 serving of cow's milk. Scientists also suspect that certain live cultures in yogurt and kefir actually stimulate the activity of the lactase enzyme in the small intestine.

PROBIOTICS AND CHOLESTEROL LOWERING

More than 25 years ago, researchers reported that Maasai warriors who drank large amounts of fermented milk each day had low blood cholesterol levels. Since then, several animal and human studies have suggested that certain strains of probiotic bacteria have a cholesterol-lowering effect. In one study of 32 men with moderately elevated LDL cholesterol, total and LDL cholesterol levels were reduced in men after consuming about 1/2 cup (125 ml) of yogurt three times per day.[6] A larger study involving 70 otherwise healthy overweight or obese men and women found that a daily intake of almost 2 cups (500 ml) of yogurt fermented with two specific probiotic strains reduced LDL cholesterol by 8.4%.[7]

It's thought that certain types of probiotic bacteria can hamper the absorption of cholesterol from the intestine, thereby reducing the amount in the bloodstream. Studies also suggest that *L. acidophilus* and certain strains of bifidobacteria can inhibit cholesterol production by the liver.

PROBIOTICS AND CANDIDA YEAST INFECTIONS

Research has shown that eating a daily yogurt containing *Lactobacillus acidophilus* helps in the prevention and treatment of vaginal yeast infections caused by *Candida albicans*. Yeast infections are caused by an imbalance of micro-organisms in the vagina. When this balance is disrupted, normally occurring colonies of *Candida albicans* yeast organisms can grow out of control. Symptoms are whitish discharge, burning and/or itching, and a yeasty odour. By restoring a healthy balance of micro-organisms, *L. acidophilus* is believed to crowd out *Candida albicans,* thereby helping treat and prevent yeast infections.

Researchers have shown that eating 1 cup (250 ml) of plain yogurt each day for 6 months can reduce *Candida* growth and infection in women who suffer recurrent vaginal yeast infections.[8] Another study found that eating 2/3 cup (150 ml) of yogurt containing *L. acidophilus* daily increased colonization of the bacteria in the vagina and reduced symptoms.[9]

PROBIOTICS AND INFLAMMATORY BOWEL DISEASE

There are two types of inflammatory bowel disease: Crohn's disease and ulcerative colitis. These disorders cause the intestinal tract to become inflamed, bleed easily, and form sores or scars, causing severe intestinal pain, bloody diarrhea, fever, and fatigue. Mounting evidence suggests that inflammatory bowel disease is triggered by a malfunction in ratio of "bad" to "good" bacteria in the gut. That probiotic bacteria have demonstrated beneficial effects in the gut—increasing the number of "good" bacteria, promoting a barrier to harmful bacteria, and enhancing the immune system—have led researchers to study their effectiveness in treating Crohn's disease and ulcerative colitis.

A recent study published by researchers at the University of Alberta in Edmonton evaluates the effects of 6 weeks of treatment with probiotics in 34 patients with active mild to moderate ulcerative colitis. The researchers found 53% of those treated with probiotics experienced a remission of their disease; 24% had a significant decrease in their symptoms without any significant side effects. The special probiotic mixture used in the study contained eight types of bacteria, including species of lactobacillus, bifidobacteria, and streptococcus.[10]

Although results from preliminary studies are promising, particularly when it comes to ulcerative colitis, scientists are not yet able to recommend probiotic-containing foods or supplements for the management of inflammatory bowel disease. More studies are needed to determine the type of bacteria, the optimal dose, and the duration of therapy required to treat these disorders.

PROBIOTICS AND COLON CANCER PREVENTION

Scientists have long suspected that the intestinal microflora is involved in causing colon cancer. Certain species of bacteria in the colon produce harmful substances laboratory studies have linked to cancer. Probiotic-containing foods may help reduce the risk of colon cancer by preventing the growth of these organisms, boosting the body's immune system, and producing anti-cancer substances. Probiotic bacteria also produce short chain fatty acids, compounds beneficial to colon cells.

Epidemiological studies have found lower rates of colon cancer among populations who consume more fermented milk products, suggesting that these foods might be protective. Studies conducted on human cancer cells in test tubes have demonstrated the ability of probiotics to interfere with the action of carcinogens. And after probiotics are given to laboratory rats, the rats have less damage to DNA in colon cells (an important step in the development of colon cancer) and reduced numbers of tumours in the colon.

The real test, of course, is determining if these effects hold up in human volunteers. At the time of writing, few such studies have been conducted. The EU-sponsored Syncan project found that a combination of probiotics and prebiotics reduced various risk factors for colon cancer. (I discuss prebiotics in the next section.) In the randomized controlled trial, 80 people (43 with colonic polyps and 37 with colon cancer) were assigned to receive either placebo or a special supplement containing a mixture of probiotics Lactobacillus GG and bifidobacteria and prebiotics (chicory inulin) for 12 weeks.[11]

The researchers reported that the beneficial bacterial strains lactobacillus and bifidobacterium increased in all participants. Populations of Clostridium perfringens, a bacterial strain reported to transform dietary substances into cancer-causing compounds, decreased in both groups. In addition, markers of DNA damage were reduced in the supplemented group, compared with the placebo, particularly for the polyp patients.

What are prebiotics?

Prebiotics, found in certain foods and food ingredients, can stimulate the growth and activity of probiotic organisms in the gut. Prebiotics contain non-digestible carbohydrates that reach the large intestine to feed the beneficial bacteria there. A diet high in prebiotics promotes the growth of beneficial bacteria in the colon.

Prebiotics are found naturally in certain foods—allium vegetables (onions, garlic, shallots, leeks), asparagus, chicory root, and Jerusalem artichokes, to name a few. Legumes, flaxseed, barley, and oats contain prebiotics but to a lesser extent. (Now you have one more reason to include these power foods in your diet.) Prebiotic supplements and prebiotic-enriched foods contain inulin, a pure form of the sugar fructose. When probiotics are consumed with prebiotics, as they were in the Syncan study, the combination of both is known as a synbiotic.

Other health benefits of yogurt and kefir

When it comes to maintaining good health, there's more to fermented milk products than probiotic bacteria. The fact that yogurt and kefir (and other dairy products) offer more calcium per serving than other foods makes them important players in disease prevention. Studies show that an adequate intake of calcium guards against high blood pressure, stroke, premenstrual syndrome, kidney stones made from calcium oxalate, and colon cancer.

One of the best-known benefits of consuming calcium-rich foods is the prevention of osteoporosis. Osteoporosis is characterized by low bone mass and deterioration of existing bone, making bones weaker and more vulnerable to fractures. Osteoporosis is not just a woman's issue. Although osteoporosis affects one in four women over the age of 50, one in eight men over 50 have the disease, too. Studies conducted in women and older adults do show that getting adequate calcium can improve bone density and reduce the risk of hip fracture.

That calcium is the most abundant mineral in the body and 99% of it is housed within your bones and teeth underlines its importance to bone health. The remaining 1% of your body's calcium circulates in your bloodstream, where it's used for conducting nerve impulses, contracting muscles, assisting blood clotting, and secreting hormones. If your diet is deficient in calcium, the mineral will be taken from your bones to perform these tasks. Even small reductions in blood calcium can trigger calcium loss from your bones. So when you shortchange your diet, you shortchange your bones, too.

The most effective way to reduce your risk of osteoporosis is to ensure you consume adequate calcium throughout childhood, adolescence, and early adulthood to support bone building. But protecting your bones does not stop when you're young. It's equally important to meet your daily calcium recommendations during adulthood to help maintain bone mass and slow natural age-related bone loss.

Keep in mind, however, that it requires more than an adequate calcium intake to keep your bones healthy. Calcium balance in your body depends on your physical activity level and your intake of other bone-building nutrients—vitamin D, vitamin K, and magnesium. Smoking cigarettes as well as consuming excess animal protein, sodium, and alcohol can cause your body to lose calcium, potentially harming bones. My point: Calcium is definitely important, but it's not the sole factor involved in keeping your bones strong. So consume adequate calcium from foods such as yogurt or kefir and be mindful of other lifestyle factors that increase your chances of developing osteoporosis.

Nutritional benefits of yogurt and kefir

Bacteria aside, it's hard to beat yogurt when it comes to nutrition. A 3/4 cup (175 ml or 175 g) container of plain, low-fat yogurt packs 9 grams of protein and 320 milligrams of calcium, and a fair amount of riboflavin, vitamin B12, zinc, and potassium. All that for only 100 calories. You'll notice from the table below that plain yogurt and kefir contain more protein and calcium than flavoured varieties (adding sugar tends to dilute the nutrient content).

Notable nutrients in yogurt and kefir

Per 3/4 cup (175 ml or 175 g) serving

	Calories	Protein (g)	Riboflavin (mg)	Folate (mcg)	B12 (mcg)
Yogurt, fruit-bottom, 1–2% milk fat (MF)	177	7.0	0.31	20	0.76
Yogurt, flavoured, non-fat	164	7.7	0.31	16	0.8
Yogurt, plain, 1–2% MF	110	9.2	0.37	19	1.0
Yogurt, plain, less than 1% MF	89	8.8	0.35	16	0.92
Yogurt drink, flavoured, non-fat	122	4.4	0.37	21	1.07
Kefir, flavoured, 1% MF	130	10.5	0.30	21	1.0
Kefir, plain, non-fat	87	10.5	0.30	20	1.0

	Calcium (mg)	Magnesium (mg)	Zinc (mg)
Yogurt, fruit-bottom, 1–2% MF	214	22	1.05
Yogurt, flavoured, non-fat	266	26	1.3
Yogurt, plain, 1–2% MF	320	30	1.6
Yogurt, plain, less than 1% MF	294	27	1.2
Yogurt drink, flavoured, non-fat	186	28	0.8
Kefir, flavoured, 1% MF	225	26	0.8
Kefir, plain, non-fat	225	26	0.8

Source: Canadian Nutrient File, 2007.

To help meet your daily recommended intakes for calcium and protein, Canada's Food Guide (2007) advises adults to consume 2 to 3 milk and alternatives servings per day. Teenagers and preteens (age 9 to 13 years) need 3 to 4 servings each day, and younger children require 2 to 3 servings. One serving of milk and alternatives is equivalent to 1 cup (250 ml) of milk, 3/4 cup (175 ml) of yogurt, 3/4 cup (175 ml) of kefir, or 1 1/2 ounces (45 g) of cheese.

Recognizing that not all Canadians drink milk, the food guide now considers fortified soy beverages a member of the milk and alternatives food group (1 serving is equivalent to 1 cup/250 ml). Whichever food you choose, 1 food guide serving supplies roughly 300 milligrams of calcium. What's more, dairy products such as yogurt and kefir contain the most absorbable form of calcium. Even though some vegetables (broccoli, bok choy) supply calcium, natural compounds in plant foods prevent some of this calcium from being absorbed by your body.

As you'll see from the table below, 1 serving of milk and alternatives makes a hefty contribution to your daily calcium requirement.

Recommended daily allowance (RDA) of calcium

Age	RDA (milligrams)
1–3 years	500
4–8 years	800
9–18 years	1300
19–50 years	1000
51+ years	1200
During pregnancy	1000
During breastfeeding	1000
Daily upper limit*	2500

*The daily upper limit is the highest level of calcium intake considered safe for almost all persons.

Source: National Academy of Sciences, Institute of Medicine, Food and Nutrition Board. Dietary Reference Intakes. Calcium, Phosphorus, Magnesium, Vitamin D and Fluoride. The National Academy Press, Washington, DC, 1997.

Although dairy products can go a long way in helping you meet your calcium requirements, by no means do I think that dairy is the only way to get your calcium. Leafy green vegetables, almonds, legumes, canned salmon (with bones), and calcium supplements also supply the mineral. Non-dairy calcium sources are important for people who don't eat dairy products—vegetarians, people who have difficulty digesting the natural sugar in milk (lactose intolerance), and for those who are allergic to the protein in milk.

Enjoying yogurt and kefir

There's no recommended daily intake for probiotics; they are not required for health, yet the emerging scientific data certainly suggest eating probiotic foods such as yogurt and kefir are good for your health. Most experts recommend a daily intake of at least 1 billion active cells (also called CFU or colony forming units) in order to achieve health benefits.

Buying

Read labels when buying yogurt and kefir. Pick a product that contains at least 1 billion active cells per serving. Look for products with well-studied types of bacteria, such as lactobacillus or bifidobacterium. If a label does not state what type or how much bacteria is present, which is the case with many brands, check the company's website or call the manufacturer to ask.

In Canada, all yogurts must contain a standard amount of live (*Lactobacillus bulgaricus* and *Streptococcus thermophilus*) cultures at the time of manufacture. However, not all these organisms survive transit through the acidic stomach to the colon. Brands that contain other acid-resistant bacteria, such as *Lactobacillus acidophilus* and bifidobacteria, include Astro BioBest, President's Choice Too Good to Be True, Liberty Bio, and Danone's Activia.

Added sugars

Extra sugar means more calories, less protein, and less calcium. If you prefer flavoured yogurt over plain, keep in mind that most fruit-bottom or flavoured varieties deliver 4 to 6 teaspoons (20 to 30 ml) of sugar per 3/4 cup (175 ml or 175 g) tub. The grams of sugars listed in the Nutrition Facts box on the packaging include both natural milk sugars and added sugars. Once you account for the naturally occurring sugar, you're usually left with 2 to 4 teaspoons (10 to 20 ml) of added sugars. Ideally, choose a yogurt that has no more than 18 grams of sugar and 2 grams of saturated fat per 3/4 cup (175 ml or 175 g). If you buy smaller containers of yogurt, such as 113 grams, select a yogurt with no more than 10 grams of sugar and 1.5 grams of saturated fat per 113 gram serving.

Calcium

It's not just sugar that squeezes out nutrients. There's also the diminishing size factor. A food guide serving of plain yogurt is 3/4 cup (175 ml). That's how much it takes to get the amount of protein and calcium found in 1 cup (250 ml) of milk. But tubs of yogurt have gotten smaller and smaller. Smaller containers (125 g, 113 g, and 100 g) are great for individuals with small appetites or those counting calories, but if you're looking for a food guide serving of milk, you'll need to eat more than one. A 100 gram container of Yoplait's Source yogurt—that's less than 1/2 cup (125 ml)—may have only 50 calories, but it also contains only 110 milligrams of calcium—roughly one-third of a food guide serving of yogurt.

The percent daily value (% DV) for calcium on nutrition labels is based on the average recommended daily intake for calcium (1100 milligrams); it tells you whether there's a little or a lot of calcium present. To get more nutritional value from yogurt or kefir, choose a brand that supplies at least 20% DV (220 milligrams) for calcium per 3/4 cup (175 ml or 175 g) serving. Smaller tubs of yogurt should supply at least 12% DV for calcium (e.g., 142 milligrams per 113 g container).

Check the best-before or use-by date to make sure the yogurt or kefir is fresh. As fermented milk products sit, their live bacterial counts decline.

Storing

Store yogurt and kefir in the refrigerator in their original containers. If unopened, fermented milk products will stay fresh for 1 week past the best-before date. However, the number of live bacteria will be less than when the product was manufactured.

Preparing

To enjoy the taste and nutrition of yogurt and kefir, there's little you need to do beyond opening up the carton.

TIPS FOR ADDING YOGURT AND KEFIR TO YOUR MEALS

Although fermented milk products are best enjoyed fresh to reap their probiotic benefits, you can add unflavoured yogurt and kefir to muffins, pancakes, and other quick bread recipes to add moistness and a hint of tartness. (Cooking at high temperatures kills probiotic bacteria.) Here are ways to add a serving of fermented milk to your daily diet.

Breakfast

- Stir a large spoonful of plain, low-fat yogurt or kefir into a hot whole-grain cereal, such as oatmeal.
- Alternate layers of yogurt, homemade or low-fat granola, and chopped fresh fruit for a breakfast parfait.
- Toss fresh berries into plain yogurt or kefir and top with a drizzle of honey.
- Top pancakes and waffles with a spoonful of plain yogurt or kefir, toasted walnuts, banana slices, and a drizzle of maple syrup.
- Make a breakfast smoothie with plain or vanilla-flavoured yogurt or kefir, berries, banana, and 1 tablespoon (15 ml) of ground flaxseed. (Grind flaxseed first in a clean coffee grinder before adding to your smoothie. For convenience, you can buy ground flaxseed, called flaxseed meal, at natural food stores.) For a fibre boost, add 1/4 cup (50 ml) of 100% bran cereal to your smoothie.

RECIPES
Blueberry Walnut Muesli with Rolled Oats and Flaxseed, page 271
Blackberry Shake, page 276
Crazy Cranberry Smoothie, page 277

Lunch and dinner

- Toss shredded raw carrots and drained or crushed pineapple with plain low-fat yogurt for a refreshing salad.
- Make a low-fat version of chicken or tuna salad by mixing plain yogurt and Dijon mustard with diced chicken breast or canned light tuna.
- Drop a dollop of plain yogurt or kefir into tomato soup or traditional borscht.
- Spoon plain yogurt or kefir onto sliced fresh tomatoes, cucumbers, and red onions for a tasty side salad.

- Add chopped cucumber, fresh dill, and minced garlic to plain yogurt. Serve as a dip for grilled meats and chicken.
- For tasty grilled salmon, mix plain yogurt or kefir with an equal amount of low-fat mayonnaise. Add 2 to 3 tablespoons (30 to 50 ml) of freshly squeezed lemon juice, freshly ground black pepper, and plenty of chopped fresh dill. Spread on top of salmon fillets before grilling.
- Top a baked potato with plain yogurt or kefir and snipped chives. Or mix plain yogurt with salsa for a Mexican-inspired topping for baked potatoes.
- Make a yogurt- or kefir-based salad dressing by blending yogurt or kefir with water to desired consistency. Add your favourite herbs and salt and pepper to taste.

RECIPES
Creamy Cold Berry Soup, page 304
Creamy Caesar Dressing, page 363
Garlic and Basil Kefir Dressing, page 364
Poppy Seed Dressing, page 369
Tandoori Marinade, page 374

Snacks and desserts

- Swirl vanilla or plain, low-fat yogurt into applesauce or other strained fruits for a nutritious, kid-friendly snack.
- For an afternoon fruit smoothie, blend low-fat yogurt or kefir with your favourite fruit (chopped) and ice.
- Mix yogurt cheese with fresh herbs for a savoury spread for whole-grain crackers.
- Mix yogurt cheese with fruit juice or summer berries for a sweet dip. Serve with fresh fruit pieces for dunking.
- Add a dollop of plain or vanilla low-fat yogurt to desserts—try it on apple crisp and puddings.

RECIPES
Creamy Strawberry Smoothie, page 277
Raspberry Kefir Smoothie, page 281
Yogurt Cheese, page 286
Creamy Dill Dip, page 357
Lemon Ginger Fruit Dip, page 359

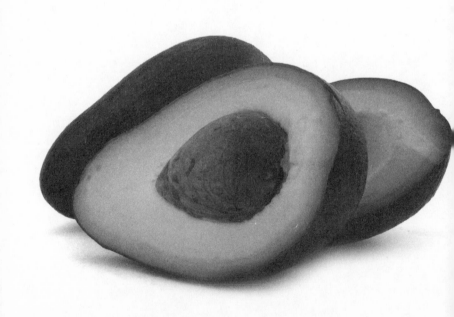

7
Power fats and oils

★ avocado

★ canola oil

★ flaxseed oil

★ olive oil

★ walnut oil

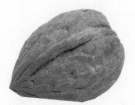

A high-fat diet has been linked to obesity, heart attack, stroke, and breast, colon, and prostate cancers. Since the 1970s, the cornerstone of dietary advice has been to lower our intake of fat, regardless of the type. But conventional wisdom has changed. Dietary fat is not the villain we once thought it to be. Years of research has taught us that not all fats are created equal. When it comes to health, it's now clear that what matters most is the *kind* of fat we eat, rather than how much. A healthy diet can contain as much as 35% of its calories from fat—provided, of course, you choose the right fats. As you'll learn in this chapter, certain types of fat can actually help fight disease.

Unsaturated fats

The so-called "good" fats that you should include in your diet are unsaturated fats—polyunsaturated and monounsaturated fats. In fact, the recently revised Canada's Food Guide (2007) advises we consume 2 to 3 tablespoons (25 to 50 ml) of unsaturated fat each day for optimal health. Polyunsaturated and monounsaturated fats are often referred to as heart healthy fats because they help lower elevated blood cholesterol. In studies in which unsaturated fats were eaten in place of carbohydrates, the fats decreased LDL (bad) cholesterol levels and increased HDL (good) levels.[1] Researchers have also demonstrated that replacing saturated fat (the type that raises blood cholesterol) with polyunsaturated and monounsaturated fats consistently lower total and LDL cholesterol levels.

Vegetable oils, nuts, and seeds are the main source of unsaturated fats in our diet. Dietary fats, including cooking oils, vary in the proportion of monounsaturated (MUFA), polyunsaturated (PUFA), and saturated fatty acids (SFA) they contain but are classified based on which fatty acids are present in the greatest concentration. Safflower oil, sunflower oil, corn oil, walnut oil, and flaxseed oil contain high levels of polyunsaturated fats. Olive oil, canola oil, peanut oil, and avocado contain more monounsaturated fats.

Essential fatty acids

Polyunsaturated fats do more than help keep arteries clear of fatty buildups. They also supply essential fatty acids. As you'll recall from Chapter 1, essential fatty acids—linoleic acid and alpha-linolenic acid—cannot be made by your body and therefore must come from the foods you eat. Essential fatty acids are needed for cell building, hormone production, and the growth and development of infants. When the body lacks essential fatty acids, virtually all organ systems are impaired.

Linoleic acid, an omega-6 fatty acid, is plentiful in sunflower, safflower, corn, and soybean oils. Good sources of alpha-linolenic acid, an omega-3 fatty acid, include flaxseed, walnut, canola, pumpkin seed, and soybean oils. The terms *omega-3* and *omega-6* refer to the chemical structure of fatty acids. A polyunsaturated fat molecule contains two or more carbon double bonds. If the double bond starts after the third carbon, it is classified as an omega-3 fatty acid; if it starts after the sixth carbon, it is an omega-6 fatty acid, and so on. It's important to maintain an appropriate balance of omega-3 and omega-6 fatty acids in the diet, as these two substances work together to promote health.

Once consumed, the body converts some alpha-linolenic acid (ALA) to eiocosapentaenoic acid (EPA) and docosahexaenoic acid (DHA), the omega-3 fatty acids found in oily fish. There's plenty of evidence to suggest getting enough DHA can guard against heart disease, stroke, arthritis, and possibly even Alzheimer's disease. (See Chapter 5, pages 164–166, to learn more about the health benefits of DHA.)

Of the ALA we consume in our diet, only a small amount is converted into DHA. Many factors limit the rate of conversion, including a high intake of linoleic acid. In other words, consuming too much linoleic acid will suppress the body's ability to convert ALA to DHA. Unfortunately, our North American diet contains a high amount of linoleic acid and relatively little alpha-linolenic acid. It's been estimated that the ratio of omega-6 to omega-3 fatty acids in the typical Western diet is almost 10:1 because of our high use of vegetable oils rich in linoleic acid and our declining fish consumption.

ALA AND HEART HEALTH

ALA has other health benefits in addition to being converted to EPA and DHA. Consuming vegetable oils rich in ALA may very well be good for your heart. A study that followed more than 76,000 healthy women for 18 years found that those who consumed the most ALA had a 40% lower risk of fatal heart attack compared with women whose diets provided the least. Interestingly, oil-and-vinegar salad dressing was an important source of ALA. Women who consumed salad dressing at least five times per week were 54% less likely to suddenly die from a heart attack than women who rarely consumed it.[2]

In a 14-year study of 45,722 healthy men, a higher intake of ALA was associated with protection from developing heart disease and dying from a heart attack. In men who ate little or no seafood, each 1 gram per day increase in ALA (about 1 tablespoon/15 ml of canola oil) was associated with a 47% lower risk of heart disease.[3]

ALA is thought to prevent heart disease by reducing the stickiness of blood cells, reducing inflammation, maintaining the integrity of blood vessel walls, and preventing irregular heart beats (arrhythmia). Alpha-linolenic acid has been shown to lower blood cholesterol and triglyceride levels.

Recommended daily allowance (RDA) for alpha-linolenic acid

Age	ALA (grams)
1–3 years	0.7
4–8 years	0.9
Females, 9–13 years	1.0
Females, 14+ years	1.1
Males, 9–13 years	1.2
Males, 14+ years	1.6

OLIVE OIL AND HEART HEALTH

If you've been to Greece or Italy, chances are you brought back a bottle of flavourful, aromatic olive oil to enjoy at home. That people who live in Mediterranean countries use olive oil almost exclusively instead of butter, margarine, or other cooking oils may explain the lower rates of heart disease and cancer observed in these countries. Since mortality statistics first identified that Mediterranean populations were living longer than other

Europeans, scientists have been trying to deduce which components of the Mediterranean diet are responsible for its considerable benefits. And it turns out that olive oil, one of the main components of the Mediterranean diet, is a strong candidate.

A recent study from Italy that followed over 5611 men and women, age 60 and older, for more than 6 years revealed that an "olive oil and salad" pattern of eating lowered the risk of dying by 50%. This eating pattern was characterized by high consumption of olive oil, raw vegetables, salads, soups, and poultry.[4] Another study published in the *New England Journal of Medicine* followed over 22,000 adults living in Greece and reported that adherence to the traditional Mediterranean diet, which is rich in olive oil, improved longevity. The high degree of adherence to this diet was found to significantly reduce the risk of dying from heart disease and cancer.[5]

That olive oil has the highest percentage of monounsaturated fat— 77%—of all the cooking oils may help explain its health benefits. Studies have shown that olive oil can lower LDL cholesterol, raise protective HDL cholesterol, and protect LDL cholesterol particles from becoming oxidized by harmful free radicals. (Oxidized LDL cholesterol is considered more dangerous, since it readily sticks to artery walls.) Researchers from eastern Europe demonstrated that adding 2 tablespoons (25 ml) of olive oil per day for 6 weeks to an otherwise unchanged diet resulted in significant decline in total and LDL cholesterol levels.[6]

The evidence for olive oil's cholesterol-lowering ability was convincing enough for the U.S. Food and Drug Administration to allow a health claim linking olive oil to a reduced risk of heart disease. If you've shopped south of the border since November 2004, you might have seen the following on bottles of olive oil: "Limited and not conclusive scientific evidence suggests that eating about 2 tablespoons [25 ml] of olive oil daily may reduce the risk of coronary heart disease due to the monounsaturated fat in olive oil. To achieve this possible benefit, olive oil is to replace a similar amount of saturated fat and not increase the total number of calories you eat in a day."

By now it's clear that avoiding all types of fat for fear of calories is not good for your health. Monounsaturated and polyunsaturated fats are healthy additions to your diet. That said, as you add these healthy fats to your diet, keep in mind that large portions can lead to weight gain. All dietary fats—olive oil, butter, margarine—deliver 120 calories per tablespoon (15 ml). When it comes to weight control, your waistline doesn't recognize the difference between unsaturated and saturated fats. So drizzle, don't pour, your unsaturated fat.

In addition to being outstanding sources of unsaturated fatty acids, the following power fats contain other disease-fighting compounds, such as alpha-linolenic acid or phytochemicals.

Nutritional benefits of power fats

Eat 2 to 3 servings per day
1 serving = 1 tablespoon (15 ml) *or* 1/3 avocado

★ AVOCADO

Although technically a fruit, avocado is often treated like an added fat because of its relatively high fat content. An avocado derives 84% of its calories from fat, mainly monounsaturated fat. Like olive oil, research has shown that an avocado-rich diet helps lower total and LDL cholesterol and raise HDL cholesterol in people with elevated blood cholesterol.[7]

Avocados are a good source of folate and potassium, two nutrients linked to heart health. In fact, half an avocado provides one-quarter of a day's worth of folate (the recommended daily intake of folate is 400 micrograms). Avocados also contain lutein and zeaxanthin, two phytochemicals associated with a lower risk of cataract and macular degeneration.

Because avocados are high in fat calories, a little goes a long way. Many of my clients are surprised to learn that one whole avocado delivers roughly 330 calories and 30 grams of fat. You need to consider one-eighth of a whole avocado as the equivalent of 1 teaspoon (5 ml) of oil; one-third of an avocado is the equivalent of 1 tablespoon (15 ml) of oil. (Florida avocadoes have a little less fat and calories than those from California, but they're not quite as flavourful.)

★ CANOLA OIL

Once considered a specialty crop of Canada, canola is now a major North American crop. Canola oil comes from canola seeds that are pressed to extract their oil content. If you surf the internet, you might come across negative reports about canola that maintain the oil is toxic and harmful to human health. But there's no need to toss out your bottle of canola: These claims are unfounded. They stem from the fact that, years ago, oil was produced from the rapeseed plant, and rapeseed oil is high in erucic acid, a compound that has been implicated with cancer. In the late 1960s, plant breeders fixed this problem by developing a new plant—canola—that's similar to rapeseed but that contains very low levels of erucic acid. The new, low-erucic-acid oil was called, as you might have guessed, canola oil.

Canola oil is composed of 62% monounsaturated fat and 32% polyunsaturated fat. Of all the commonly used cooking oils, canola has the highest unsaturated fat content (a total of 94%) and lowest saturated fat content (6%). Because of its high unsaturated fat content, the U.S. Food and Drug Administration recently authorized a qualified health claim on bottles of canola oil sold in the United States. The claim states that "limited and not conclusive scientific evidence suggests that eating about 1.5 tablespoons [20 ml] may reduce the risk of coronary heart disease due to the unsaturated fat content in canola oil. To achieve this possible benefit, canola oil is to replace a similar amount of saturated fat and not increase the total number of calories you eat in a day."

Because of its higher polyunsaturated fat content, canola is a very good source of alpha-linolenic acid and linoleic acid. In fact, 1 tablespoon (15 ml) of canola oil supplies 1.3 grams of ALA, a full day's requirement for women.

Canola oil is also a good source of fat-soluble vitamins E and K. One tablespoon (15 ml) of canola oil delivers 20% of the recommended intake for vitamin K, a nutrient that aids in blood clotting and maintaining strong bones. Another bonus: Canola oil contains plant sterols, phytochemicals that can help prevent heart disease by lowering LDL blood cholesterol.

★ FLAXSEED OIL

Flaxseed oil, also called flax oil, is derived from the seeds of the flax plant, which grows mainly in the western Canadian prairies and the northwestern United States. Flaxseed oil has a high proportion of polyunsaturated fat—72% of its fatty acids are polyunsaturated. You'll learn later in this chapter how this nutritional characteristic impacts how you store and use flaxseed oil. When it comes to ALA, flaxseed oil is a nutritional superstar. One tablespoon (15 ml) provides a whopping 7.7 grams, seven times the recommended daily intake for women and almost five times the daily intake for men. Flaxseed oil also contains vitamin E, an antioxidant that protects cell membranes from harmful free radicals.

If you shop for flaxseed oil, you'll notice that some bottles are labelled "lignan-rich." This is flaxseed oil to which manufacturers have added lignans, phytochemicals found in the whole flaxseed. Preliminary studies suggest that lignans have anti-cancer properties and consuming ground flaxseed helps guard against breast and prostate cancers. Lignans are also thought to act like antioxidants and reduce the activity of cell-damaging free radicals. I think you're better off consuming 1 to 2 tablespoons (15 to 25 ml) of ground flaxseed each day if you want to add a good source of lignans to your diet. Not only does it provide an excellent source of lignans, it also offers soluble fibre. Add flaxseed oil to foods for its concentrated source of the essential fatty acid ALA. (See Chapter 4, page 145, for more details on using ground flaxseed.)

★ OLIVE OIL

I told you earlier that olive oil has the highest monounsaturated fat content (77%) of all cooking oils. But there's more to olive oil than monounsaturated fat: Olive oil also contains vitamin K and a hefty dose of antioxidants thanks to its vitamin E and phytochemical content. Olive oil's phytochemicals include chlorophyll, carotenoids, and flavonoids, all of which protect LDL cholesterol particles from free radical damage. Olive oil also contains olecanthal, a phytochemical with anti-inflammatory effects much like Aspirin and ibuprofen. Scientists suspect that olecanthal may be responsible for some of the health benefits associated with the Mediterranean diet.

Researchers believe the nutrients and phytochemicals in olive oil work together to exert their health benefits. As you'll read later, the "virgin" grade of olive oil is the richest source of antioxidants, as it's been processed the least.

★ WALNUT OIL

Its distinctive flavour makes it obvious that this oil is derived from walnut meat. Walnut oil derives almost two-thirds of its fat from heart healthy polyunsaturated oil. It's also an excellent source of ALA—1 tablespoon (15 ml) provides a full day's requirement of this essential fatty acid. Walnut oil also contains some vitamin K.

The table below compares the nutritional characteristics of the fats and oils I've identified as power fats.

Nutritional characteristics of healthy fats

Per 1 tablespoon (15 ml), unless otherwise noted

	Calories (mg)	Vitamin E (mcg)	Vitamin K (g)	ALA (g)	MUFA (%)	PUFA (%)
Avocado, 1/3	107	1.4	14.1	0.08	67	12
Canola oil	125	2	17.3	1.32	62	32
Flaxseed oil	122	2	0.0	7.74	18	72
Olive oil	121	2	8.2	0.11	73	11
Walnut oil	122	0	2.1	1.43	23	63

Source: Canadian Nutrient File, 2007.

Enjoying unsaturated fats

The key to reaping the flavour and nutritional and health benefits of healthy fats and oils is to store and use them properly. All fats, especially unsaturated fats, are sensitive to heat, light, and exposure to oxygen. So if you don't handle them properly, you'll deplete their healthy qualities, not to mention their taste.

Buying

Avoid buying economy-sized bottles of oil unless you plan to share the oil with someone. You may save money, but if you don't use the oil within a certain period, it will go rancid. (Rancid oil has an unpleasant aroma and a pungent or sharp taste. Keep in mind that rancidity can occur long before you can smell or taste it.) It's best to buy small bottles of various types of cooking oils.

Unrefined oils are those that have been cold pressed or expeller pressed to extract the oil from the seed or fruit. This means they were exposed to minimal heat and no chemicals during the extraction process. The method of extraction will be specified on the oil's bottle label. When buying these expensive oils, make sure they have been properly stored or displayed. Heat and bright light cause oils to rapidly deteriorate, so choose oils that are sold in opaque bottles to block light.

Flaxseed oil

Flaxseed oil can be found in the refrigerator section of natural food stores and some large grocery stores. It's packaged in black plastic bottles or dark-brown glass bottles to protect it from light.

Olive oil

Buying olive oil can be a challenge. First, you need to decide whether you want an olive oil extracted from olives grown in Italy, Greece, or California. Then you need to choose a grade of olive oil: extra-virgin, virgin, regular, or light. These grades reflect the degree to which the oil has been processed.

- Extra-virgin. This olive oil comes from the first pressing of the olives. It has the lowest acidity and is judged to have the most superior flavour. Because of its excellent flavour, extra-virgin olive oil is best used as a salad dressing or as a dipping oil. Heating extra-virgin olive oil will cause its flavour to diminish. This is the most expensive type of olive oil.
- *Virgin.* This oil is also derived from the first pressing of the olives, but its acidity can be a little higher than that of extra-virgin olive oil. It's a little less expensive but still flavourful. Keep in mind that the flavour and colour of extra-virgin and virgin olive oils vary considerably, depending on the soil the olives trees are grown in, the time of harvest, the degree of ripeness of the olives, and the extraction process.

  Extra-virgin and virgin olive oils are not refined in any way. Olives are pressed using minimal heat and no chemicals. Because these grades of olive oil are minimally processed, they contain the highest amount of phytochemicals and nutrients.
- *Pure olive oil.* An oil labelled "pure olive oil" or simply "olive oil" is usually refined olive oil with a little extra-virgin or virgin olive oil added to provide flavour, aroma, and colour. Refined olive oil is obtained by treating virgin olive oil that has defects—for example, a relatively high natural acidity, poor flavour, or an unpleasant odour—with heat and/or chemicals to produce a refined oil that's used to make "olive oil" or "pure olive oil." These oils usually contain 85% refined oil and 15% virgin or extra-virgin olive oil.

  Highly refined olive oils can also be labelled as "mild" olive oil or "light" olive oil. These terms refer to the flavour, not calories: These olive oils contain the same amount of fat and calories as any other olive oil. Refined olive oil, which is less expensive, is better suited for sautéing and stir-frying than for salad dressings and dips, where flavour is important.

Avocado

Choose avocadoes according to when you plan to use them. If you're looking for a ripe fruit to eat soon after purchasing, choose one that's slightly soft and free of dark, sunken spots. If you don't intend to eat the avocado for a few days, choose one that's firmer and let it ripen at home at room temperature in a fruit basket or paper bag. Firmer avocadoes are also less likely to have bruises.

Storing

Refined or not, all oils are sensitive to heat, light, and air. Once an oil has turned rancid, not only will it have a unpleasant smell and taste, but its nutritional value will be greatly reduced. It's best to store all oils in the refrigerator or a cool, dry cupboard located away from the oven and out of direct sunlight.

Some oils with a higher monounsaturated fat content, such as olive and canola, may turn semi-solid and cloudy when stored in the fridge. This is not a sign that the oil is past its prime or that the nutritional quality or flavour is reduced. It's simply a chemical reaction that occurs at low temperatures. Once you let the oil sit a room temperature for a while, its fluidity and colour will return.

If stored properly, most unrefined oils (cold or expeller pressed) will keep for 3 to 6 months. Refined oils tend to keep twice as long—at least 6 to 12 months. Polyunsaturated fat is more susceptible to the negative effects of heat and light. That means oils with a high percentage of polyunsaturated fat, such as walnut and flaxseed, have a shorter shelf life than oils with a high monounsaturated fat content.

Here is a guide to storage times of power fats:

Avocado

Once ripe, avocadoes can be stored in the refrigerator for up to 1 week. If you're refrigerating half an avocado, store it in plastic wrap along with its pit to help prevent the browning that occurs when the flesh is exposed to air. Sprinkling avocado flesh with a little lemon or lime juice will also help prevent the oxidation that causes browning.

Canola oil

Canola oil will keep in a cool, dark cupboard for 4 to 6 months or in the refrigerator for up to 9 months.

Flaxseed oil

This oil must be kept refrigerated. It will stay fresh for up to 8 weeks after opening (check the expiry date on the bottle).

Olive oil

If you will not be storing olive oil in its original container, it's best to use storage containers made of either tinted glass (to keep out light) or a non-reactive metal, such as stainless steel. Olive oil can be kept longer than most other oils because of its high monounsaturated fat content. Although it can become rancid, it's less likely to do so than other oils. Make sure the bottle's lid is sealed tightly during storage, otherwise it will spoil more quickly.

The ideal temperature for storing olive oil is 57°F (14°C)—like a fine wine!—though room temperature is okay if it's kept in a dark place. Although olive oil can also be stored in the fridge, I don't recommend refrigerating expensive extra-virgin olive oils. It's possible that condensation can get inside the bottle and affect the oil's flavour.

Olive will keep for 15 months, and if the bottle remains unopened, it will keep for 2 years or more. But for the best flavour, extra-virgin and virgin olive oil should be consumed within a year after pressing. Unlike fine wine, olive oil does not improve with age. As time passes, the oil degrades and its acidity increases.

Walnut oil

Store walnut oil in a cool, dark place for up to 3 months. To prevent rancidity, it's best to keep it refrigerated.

Preparing

How you use a cooking oil should depend on its nutritional characteristics. Oils that are highly polyunsaturated, such as flaxseed and walnut, should not be heated, since high temperatures break down essential fatty acids. Instead, use these oils in salad dressings and dips, or add to hot foods just before serving.

The cooking method will determine which oil is best to use. All oils break down or decompose at a certain temperature, known as the smoke point. When an oil reaches its smoke point, it burns and gives off visible fumes, along with an obnoxious-smelling compound called acreolein. Essential fatty acids are destroyed when the oil reaches its smoke point. Cooking oils with a high smoke point are best suited for high-heat cooking. Unrefined oils have a lower smoke point than refined oils and are not suited for certain high-heat cooking methods; for example, some are fine for sautéing, but none should be used for deep-frying.

Smoke point of commonly used cooking oils

Oil	Smoke point	Best suited to ...
Canola, unrefined	225°F (107°C)	Cold dishes only
Canola, refined	400°F (200°C)	Sauté, pan fry, stir-fry, deep-fry, grill, bake
Corn oil	450°F (230°C)	Sauté, pan fry, stir-fry, deep-fry, grill, bake
Flaxseed oil, unrefined	225°F (107°C)	Cold dishes only
Olive oil, extra-virgin	320°F (160°C)	Sauté, pan fry, stir-fry, grill, bake
Olive oil, virgin	320°F (160°C)	Sauté, pan fry, stir-fry, grill, bake
Olive oil, light	468°F (242°C)	Sauté, pan fry, stir-fry, deep-fry, grill, bake
Peanut oil, refined	450°F (230°C)	Sauté, pan fry, stir-fry, deep-fry, grill, bake
Sesame oil, unrefined	350°F (180°C)	Sauté, pan fry, stir-fry, grill, bake
Sunflower oil, refined	450°F (230°C)	Sauté, pan fry, stir-fry, deep-fry, grill, bake
Walnut oil, unrefined	320°F (160°C)	Sauté, pan fry, stir-fry, grill, bake

Finally, consider taste when deciding which oil to use. Don't waste flavourful oils, such as extra-virgin olive oil, in recipes that mask their flavour. I suggest reserving extra-virgin olive oil for salad dressings, condiments, and baked goods (at temperatures less than 320°F/160°C) and using canola oil instead for cooking and high-heat baking. If you want to use olive oil for sautéing or stir-frying, use either a combination olive oil (one that is a blend of extra-virgin and regular olive oil) or a light olive oil.

TIPS FOR ADDING UNSATURATED FATS TO YOUR MEALS

There are plenty of ways to add flavour and nutrition to your meals with healthy fats and oils. To reap the greatest nutritional benefits, get your 2 to 3 daily servings of unsaturated fat from a variety of power fats. These tips will help you add them to your diet in interesting and tasty ways:

Breakfast

- For a change from peanut butter, spread a slice of whole-grain toast with ripe avocado. Add salt and pepper to taste.
- Garnish an omelet with sliced avocado and tomato salsa.
- Add 1 tablespoon (15 ml) of flaxseed oil to a breakfast smoothie for an ALA boost.
- Mix 1 teaspoon (5 ml) of walnut oil into a bowl of hot oatmeal. Top with chopped walnuts and berries.

Lunch and dinner

- Instead of using butter, margarine, or mayonnaise, add slices of avocado to your next sandwich.
- For a delicious salad, combine slices of avocado, orange, fennel, and red onion. Top with fresh chopped parsley and drizzle with extra-virgin olive oil.
- Add walnut oil's rich nutty flavour to a vinaigrette. Use one part walnut oil to three parts olive or canola oil. Mix with balsamic vinegar, herbs, and spices. Enjoy over an arugula salad.
- Toss whole-grain pasta with a splash of walnut oil, chopped walnuts, and fresh spinach for a flavourful side dish.
- Drizzle a little extra-virgin olive oil over grilled vegetables or brush over cooked meat or fish before serving.

- Drizzle extra-virgin olive oil over crusty bread or an open-faced sandwich.
- Add essential fatty acids to vegetables by sautéing leafy greens or other vegetables in canola oil.
- Add 1 or 2 tablespoons (15 to 25 ml) of flaxseed oil to pasta sauces or soups after cooking.
- Add extra-virgin olive oil or flaxseed oil to mashed potatoes instead of butter. Don't forget the puréed roasted garlic!

RECIPES
Avocado Citrus Salad, page 293
Cilantro-Stuffed Grilled Avocados, page 315
Grapefruit Maple Dressing (olive oil), page 365
Honey Dijon Dressing (olive oil), page 366
Lemon Walnut Dressing (walnut oil), page 367
Pomegranate Maple Dressing (flaxseed oil), page 368
Spinach Almond Pesto (olive oil), page 370
Two Tea Dressing (olive oil), page 371

Desserts and snacks

- Mix chopped avocado, onions, tomatoes, cilantro, and freshly squeezed lime juice for a homemade guacamole. Serve with baked tortilla chips and raw veggie sticks.
- Add 1 tablespoon (15 ml) of flaxseed oil to hummus or yogurt dip.
- Purée extra-virgin olive oil, cooked white kidney beans, roasted garlic, and fresh thyme in the food processor and serve as a dip.
- Mix 1 teaspoon (5 ml) of flaxseed oil into yogurt for a mid-afternoon pick-me-up.
- Replace butter or other oils with regular or light olive oil in bread and dessert recipes. Three tablespoons (50 ml) of olive oil will replace 1/4 cup (50 ml) of butter in baked-good recipes.
- Enhance the flavour of a chocolate dessert by drizzling walnut oil on top.

RECIPE
Jalapeño Guacamole, page 358

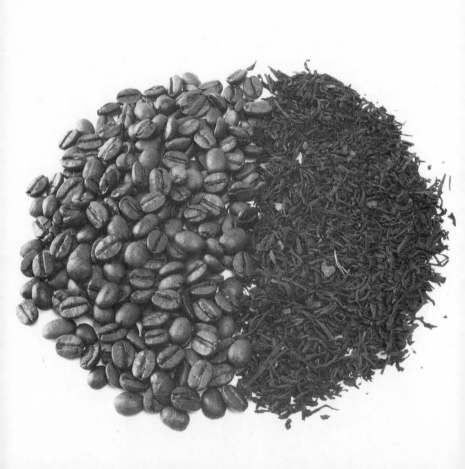

8
Power beverages

★ black tea

★ coffee

★ green tea

★ oolong tea

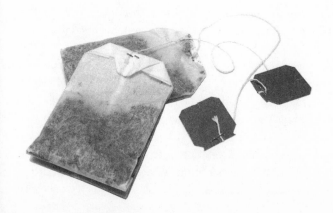

The beverages you drink supply your body with water, an essential nutrient you can't live without. In fact, you can survive longer without food than water. Your body relies on a steady intake of water more than you think. Virtually every chemical reaction in your body takes place in the presence of water. Water also helps transport vitamins, minerals, and phytochemicals to your body's cells. And water acts as a thermostat by regulating your body's internal temperature.

Water can keep you healthy in other ways too. Research suggests that drinking adequate quantities of water can guard against kidney stones, constipation, colon cancer, and bladder cancer. It may even reduce the likelihood of developing heart disease.

You may recall from Chapter 1 that the average woman needs to drink 9 cups (2.2 litres) of water each day and men need 13 cups (3 litres) to replace what the body loses through breathing, sweating, and excreting wastes. Hot, humid weather and physical activity will increase your body's demand for water. (See Chapter 1, pages 24-27, for details on daily water requirements and dehydration symptoms.)

You can meet your daily water requirement by drinking plain water, fruit juice, milk, soy beverages, coffee, tea, herbal tea, clear soups, diet drinks, and—least desirably—sugary soft drinks and fruit drinks. If you're watching your calorie intake, try to get most of your daily water requirement from plain drinking water—it hydrates your body without adding sugar calories, fat calories, or sodium. And keep in mind, too, that alcoholic beverages do *not* count toward your water requirements. I'll tell you why not below.

Perhaps you're wondering why I don't consider plain water a power beverage. Although water is certainly nutritious and supports good health, there are other beverages that go one step farther. Green tea, black tea, and yes, even coffee, hydrate your body with zero calories *and* supply a rich source of phytochemicals. These beverages also offer certain vitamins and minerals, though in much smaller amounts than do fruits and vegetables. As you'll read in the sections below, mounting evidence suggests that drinking tea and coffee can reduce the risk of many diseases. If you're concerned about the caffeine in tea and coffee robbing your body of its much needed water, you'll be relieved by the latest research, which shows that consuming caffeinated beverages on a regular basis does not cause the body to lose water.

Alcohol and health

Alcoholic beverages do not count toward your water requirements because they dehydrate your body. It's well known, however, that a moderate intake of alcohol guards against heart disease. You might even be wondering why I haven't added alcohol—especially red wine—to my list of power beverages. It's true that over 60 studies show that compared with abstainers, people who consume one to two alcoholic drinks per day have a lower risk of heart attack and stroke.

The best-known effect of alcohol is its ability to increase levels of HDL (good) cholesterol. The active ingredient in alcoholic beverages (ethanol) may also help prevent blood clots from forming, providing an effect similar to Aspirin's. The heart benefits of alcohol are not limited to red wine. To date, no one type of alcoholic beverage has been proven to be more protective than the others. (Red wine, made using the skin and seeds of grapes as well as the flesh, contains protective plant chemicals called flavonoids that some experts say offer additional protection. But as you have read in an earlier chapter, you can get plenty of flavonoids by consuming power fruits, vegetables, whole grains, and tea.)

Although a moderate intake of alcohol protects the heart, it also increases the risk of cancer, most notably colon and breast cancers. In September 2007, findings from one of the largest studies to investigate the link between breast cancer and alcohol were reported at a European cancer conference. In the 7-year study of 70,033 women, researchers from California found that moderate drinkers who consumed one or two drinks per day were 10 percent more likely to develop breast cancer than women who had less than one drink a day. A daily intake of three or more drinks increased breast cancer risk by 30 percent—an effect comparable to the risk from smoking one pack of cigarettes per day. What's more, *all* types of alcoholic beverages increased the risk of breast cancer.[1]

When it comes to cancer prevention, experts advise that it is preferable not to drink alcohol. If you do drink, women should limit their intake to one drink per day or seven drinks per week, men one to two drinks per day or nine per week. One drink is defined as 12 ounces (341 ml) of regular beer, 5 ounces (142 ml) of wine, or 1 1/2 ounces (43 ml) of 40% spirits.

★ GREEN, OOLONG, AND BLACK TEAS

Consume 2 to 5 servings per day
1 serving = 1 cup (250 ml)

All teas come from the leaves of an evergreen plant called *Camellia sinensis;* it's how those leaves are processed that determines whether it ends up as green tea, oolong tea, or black tea. (Herbal tea isn't considered a true tea because it's not made from *Camellia sinensis,* but rather, brewed from flowers, grasses, or herbs.) Leaves of *Camellia sinensis* begin to wilt and oxidize if they're not dried quickly after being picked. This process of enzymatic oxidation, called fermentation, can be halted by heating the tea leaves to inactivate the fermentation enzymes.

Green tea is made from mature tea leaves that have not been allowed to oxidize or ferment: The leaves are quickly steamed or heated and then dried. Green tea leaves have a yellow-greenish colour and a flavour that's slightly bitter, similar to the fresh leaf. White tea is produced in a similar manner to green tea except that younger leaves and buds are used.

To make black tea, the leaves are first rolled or broken to release some of the juices necessary for fermentation. The leaves are then allowed to fully ferment before being heated and dried. Fermentation turns the leaves a coppery colour and produces black tea's familiar flavour.

Oolong tea falls in between green and black tea. Leaves that are destined to become oolong tea are partially fermented before they're heated and dried. Oolong tea leaves are greenish-brown in colour, and their flavour is closer to black tea than green tea.

Phytochemicals in tea

Fresh tea leaves are an incredibly rich source of phytochemicals called catechins (a class of flavonoids), which have potent antioxidant properties. In fact, tea is one of the highest sources of antioxidants in the North American diet. I certainly don't mean to imply that drinking tea can replace eating fruits and vegetables, but tea does contain more antioxidants than most types of produce. According to researchers from the United Kingdom, the antioxidant activity in 2 cups (500 ml) of black tea is equal to 1 glass of red wine, 7 glasses of orange juice, and 20 glasses of apple juice.[2] What's more, test tube studies have shown that catechins are more powerful antioxidants than vitamins C and E.

The primary catechin found in tea is epigallocatechin gallate (EGCG), a potent antioxidant that, as you'll learn later in this chapter, appears to lower the risk of heart disease and numerous types of cancer. Because green tea has not been fermented, it contains the highest concentration of catechins—about three times the quantity found in black tea. Steaming the leaves during green tea production inactivates the enzyme that triggers fermentation and the subsequent loss of catechins. White tea is also steamed and so retains high concentrations of antioxidants in the leaves. Black tea, which is fully fermented, contains the least amount of catechins, while oolong tea falls in between green and black tea.

Tea is also a good source of another class of flavonoids, called flavonols, which includes kaempferol, quercitin, and myricitin. Unlike catechins in tea leaves, flavonols are less affected by processing, so they're present in green, black, and oolong tea in similar amounts. (Herbal teas do not contain catechins or flavonols.)

Green tea and health

The vast majority of studies investigating the relationship between tea and health have been on green tea. In studies using animals and cell cultures, green tea has been shown to have several anti-cancer and cardio-protective properties. Among the human studies, many have been conducted in Asia, where green tea consumption is common. Drinking green tea regularly has been linked with lower rates of numerous types of cancers, as well of heart disease. Although the evidence is not as strong, study findings also hint that green tea can prevent arthritis and dental caries (cavities).

The mounting scientific evidence for the many health benefits of tea persuaded Health Canada in May 2007 to approve labelling of three health claims on tea. All types of tea (black, green, and oolong) are recognized as a source of antioxidants for the maintenance of good health. Tea is approved for increasing alertness. And tea is further accredited as helping to maintain and/or support cardiovascular health.

Here are highlights of the hundreds of scientific studies published on the benefits of green tea.

GREEN TEA AND CANCER PREVENTION

Research findings suggest that green tea helps fight against cancer. Observational studies tracking the diets of people over several years have associated regular green tea consumption with a lower risk of cancer of the bladder, colon, stomach, esophagus, and pancreas. Researchers are investigating the therapeutic use of green tea in prostate cancer patients and as a preventative agent against skin cancer.

Breast cancer

Green tea drinkers might be protected from breast cancer. Recently, scientists combined the results from four studies examining the link between green tea and breast cancer—three from Japan and one from Los Angeles—and concluded that green tea is indeed protective. Compared with women who consumed less than 1 cup (250 ml) of green tea per day, those who drank at least 5 cups (1.25 L) daily were 22% less likely to develop breast cancer.[3]

Drinking green tea might also improve a woman's prognosis once diagnosed with breast cancer. Japanese researchers discovered that among women with stage 1 and 2 breast cancer, drinking 5 cups (1.25 L) or more daily lowered the risk of the cancer coming back by 46%. The researchers suspect that phytochemicals in green tea somehow modify breast cancer, making it easier to successfully treat.[4]

Ovarian cancer

Compared with women who seldom or never drink tea, women who regularly drink it—green and black—appear to have a significantly lower risk of developing ovarian cancer. In a 15-year study of 61,057 Swedish women age 40 to 76, drinking at least 2 cups (500 ml) of tea per day, compared with less than 1 cup (250 ml) per month, was associated with a 46% lower risk of ovarian cancer. The findings also suggested that the higher the consumption or the longer the duration of drinking tea, the lower the risk.[5]

Scientists from China think green tea might enhance survival in women with ovarian cancer, too. In their study, conducted among 254 women diagnosed with ovarian cancer, those women who drank at least 1 cup (250 ml) of green tea per day had a 57% lower risk of dying over the 3 years of the study.[6]

Scientists have identified numerous ways in which green tea may help fight cancer. Laboratory studies show antioxidants in green tea powerfully inhibit cancer growth by triggering the death of cancer cells, halting the growth of blood vessels in tumours and arresting the replication of genes in cancer cells. Green tea antioxidants also have anti-inflammatory effects that may play a role in preventing certain types of cancer.

GREEN TEA AND HEART HEALTH

Green tea may ward off heart attacks. In a recent study conducted among Japanese men, those who drank 5 cups (1.25 L) or more of green tea each day were 16% less likely to suffer coronary heart disease.[7] Another study that followed 40,547 healthy Japanese men and women age 40 to 79 for 7 years found that, compared with people who strayed from the traditional Japanese diet, those who adhered closely to the Japanese dietary pattern, which includes daily green tea, had a 23% lower risk of dying from heart disease.[8]

Green tea may protect the heart in several ways. Studies show that drinking green tea daily lowers LDL blood cholesterol, triglycerides (a type of blood fat), and free radicals that damage LDL cholesterol particles. What's more, drinking at least 1/2 cup (125 ml) of green tea each day has been shown to keep blood pressure down. In a study of 1507 men and women living in Taiwan, drinking roughly 1/2 to 2 1/2 cups (125 to 625 ml) of tea per day reduced the risk of developing hypertension by 46%. For those who consumed 2 1/2 cups (625 ml) or more, the risk was reduced by 65%.[9] Lab studies also suggest that green tea catechins can help thin the blood and prevent blood clots from forming.

OTHER HEALTH BENEFITS OF GREEN TEA

Preliminary research suggests that green tea's anti-inflammatory effects might prevent the onset and reduce the severity of painful arthritis in the joints. Research in mice found that green tea antioxidants postponed the beginning and reduced the severity of arthritis.[10] Dentists in Asia have long talked about how drinking green tea can keep your teeth healthy. It turns out, they might be right. Studies in humans and animals have shown green tea to combat oral bacteria that cause cavities. Finally, green tea antioxidants have been demonstrated to protect the liver against certain toxins, including alcohol and cigarette smoke.

Black tea and health

Although the bulk of scientific research has examined green tea's beneficial effects, several studies have revealed black tea's health benefits, especially in the area of cardiovascular health.

BLACK TEA AND HEART HEALTH

In a review of all studies published between 1990 and 2004, researchers found clear evidence that black tea guarded against heart disease. In the report, published in 2007, the authors concluded that drinking at least 3 cups (750 ml) of black tea per day reduced the risk of heart disease.[11] Many studies support this conclusion. The Rotterdam Study, in which 4807 Dutch men and women age 55 years or older were followed for almost 6 years, reported that compared with non–tea drinkers, the risk of heart attack was reduced by 43% in people who drank more than 1 1/2 cups (375 ml) of black tea daily. In the study, black tea offered even greater protection against having a fatal heart attack.[12]

Drinking black tea on a regular basis might also safeguard people with existing heart disease. Researchers from Boston, Massachusetts, found that among 1900 patients hospitalized for heart attack, those who reported being heavy tea drinkers—14 cups (3.5 L) or more per week—had a 44% lower death rate than non–tea drinkers. A moderate tea intake of less than 14 cups (3.5 L) per week was linked with a 28% lower risk of dying from heart disease.[13]

Black tea helps ward off heart disease in the same way green tea does. Catechins in black tea have been shown to lower LDL cholesterol, reduce blood clotting, and prevent the oxidation of LDL cholesterol (oxidized LDL particles are thought to stick more readily to artery walls). It's also hypothesized that the mineral manganese in black tea helps support heart muscle function.

BLACK TEA AND CANCER PREVENTION

The evidence linking black tea to a lower cancer risk is mixed. The large study I mentioned earlier that was conducted in women living in Sweden found that drinking black tea significantly reduced the risk of ovarian cancer. But other studies have not found black tea to lower the risk of breast, colon, stomach, and rectal cancers. Despite this, experiments in animals and human cell cultures have demonstrated the ability of certain flavonols in black tea to suppress the growth of colon cancer cells.

Enjoying green and black tea

Many people think green tea is superior to black tea when it comes to fighting disease. However, both black and green teas have similar and related biochemical effects in the body. One might be more effective than the other in preventing certain diseases, but, overall, both are antioxidant-rich beverages that hydrate the body and promote health. If you don't like the taste of green tea, add a few cups of black tea to your diet. If you're like me and enjoy green and black teas, drink both.

Buying

You can buy tea in two forms: loose leaf or tea bags. Loose leaf teas are usually made up of whole or broken leaves. Tea bags are filled with fannings or dust, the waste product produced from sorting higher quality loose leaf tea. During processing, tea leaves are sorted by passing them over screens with different-sized holes. Tea is then graded, from best (the bud and the first two leaves of the shoot) to worst (fannings).

In my opinion, a cup of brewed loose leaf tea is much better tasting than one brewed with a bag, and it also contains more antioxidants. That's because a whole tea leaf has more surface area for hot water to extract the flavour and the antioxidants from the leaf. Tea bags containing fannings and dust, on the other hand, don't have as much surface area for this extraction.

Although some grocery stores sell packages of loose leaf tea, it's best to buy fresh loose leaf tea from a tea shop or an ethnic market where you can smell and taste the tea. To test for freshness, tightly squeeze a small amount of leaves and smell the aroma—it should smell sweet, flowery, and a little grassy. A high-quality cup of loose leaf tea will be pale green to golden in colour. To ensure your tea stays fresh, buy it in small quantities.

It's not possible to test tea bags for freshness until after you purchase them. To do so, remove the tea fannings from the bag and place the empty bag in a cup. Pour hot water over it and let it steep for 2 to 3 minutes. If the water tastes like hot water, the tea is probably fresh. If the hot water tastes like tea, that means the paper bag has absorbed the tea's flavour and the tea is stale.

A guide to green teas

If you want to experiment with green tea, you'll need to look beyond your grocery store. I've listed below some of the main types of green tea commonly available in tea shops. For added flavour and aroma in your cup of tea, try green teas blended with peppermint, dried fruit, or flowers, also available at many tea shops.

SENCHA   This is the most popular of Japan's green teas. The leaves are slender and long and produce a slightly sweet tea with a fresh, green scent. Bancha is lesser quality sencha tea.

DRAGON WELL   Also called Lung Ching, this is the ultimate Chinese green tea, produced in the Chinese village of Dragon Well. Its leaves are broad and flat and bright green. Its flavour is sweet, delicate, and slightly brisk.

MATCHA   This fine, powdered green tea is famous for its use in the Japanese tea ceremony. When you drink matcha, you consume the powdered leaves, not just the water from steeped tea leaves, as you do with other green teas. As a result, you also consume a higher concentration of phytochemicals. There are two types of matcha: thick, from tea plants older than 30 years, and thin, from plants younger than 30 years. Matcha tea produces a bright green, frothy beverage with a grassy and slightly astringent taste.

GUNPOWDER   This Chinese green tea consists of leaves that are hand rolled into tiny pellets resembling gunpowder. When buying gunpowder tea, look for shiny pellets, an indication of freshness. Gunpowder tea leaves produce brewed tea with a mildly astringent, grassy flavour. Gunpowder tea comes in a few varieties; many have a peppery taste, and some have a hint of smoke.

Storing

Store loose tea or tea bags in a dark, cool, dry cupboard in an air-tight container. With the exception of matcha green tea, refrigeration is not recommended, since tea is susceptible to moisture. Improperly stored tea may lose its flavour and pick up flavours or odours from other foods, or become mouldy.

Black tea can be stored for up to 2 years before being replaced. Green tea loses its freshness faster, usually in less than a year. Matcha can be kept for up to 6 months; check the best-before date on the package.

Preparing

When preparing a cup of antioxidant-rich tea, keep in mind that the antioxidant content increases the longer than tea steeps. Small tea leaves infuse quickly, whereas tightly curled or large leaf teas require a longer infusion time. To extract more antioxidants from tea bags, continuously dunk the bags in the teapot, rather than leaving them to float on top of the water.

Black tea

Warm the teapot before brewing tea by adding a small amount of boiling water to the pot, swirling, and then discarding. (Filtered or spring water make the best-tasting tea.) Steep the loose tea leaves or tea bags in boiling water for not less than 30 seconds and no more than 5 minutes, depending on how strong you like your tea. After 5 minutes, tannins are released, which makes the tea taste bitter. Most experts recommend infusing black tea for 3 to 5 minutes.

Green tea

Water for green tea, according to most experts, should be slightly less than boiling, around 176°F to 185°F (80°C to 85°C); the higher the quality of the leaves, the lower the water temperature should be. Hotter water will burn green tea leaves, producing a bitter taste. It's recommended that the cup or pot you're going to use be warmed first with hot water.

Use approximately 1 teaspoon (5 ml) of green loose tea per 6 to 8 ounce (175 to 250 ml) cup. Once the kettle boils, let the water cool for 1 minute before pouring it over the tea leaves. Green tea should be steeped for 1 to 2 minutes. Although tea leaves will usually sink to the bottom if loose, you may still wish to use a strainer or infuser in your cup or teapot to catch them. Strainers and infusers can be purchased at tea shops and kitchen stores, and often in grocery stores, in the tea or kitchen-utensil section.

Matcha

Add 1/2 to 1 teaspoon (2 to 5 ml) of Matcha to 2 to 3 ounces (60 to 90 ml) of just-below-boiling-temperature water (use filtered spring water). Add more water to desired taste. Stir or whisk until frothy.

TIPS FOR ADDING TEA TO YOUR MEALS

We tend to think of tea as something only to drink, but it's also a versatile ingredient that can be used in many dishes. Tea leaves and brewed tea can be used as ingredients in marinades, sauces, meat tenderizers, and desserts—for example, green tea ice cream. As you experiment drinking a variety of teas, consider also using them to flavour dishes. The following are just a few ideas to help you introduce tea into your diet.

Breakfast

• Kick-start your day with a cup of freshly brewed green or black tea.

Lunch and dinner

• Brew black tea in cold water for 20 minutes and use as a braising liquid or a liquid in marinades, sauces, and gravies.
• For a sophisticated taste, marinate scallops or other shellfish and fish in strong-flavoured tea before cooking.
• Use brewed tea to sauté or stir-fry vegetables.
• Use loose tea leaves in rubs as a coating for meat, fish, and poultry.
• Garnish salads, rice pilafs, casseroles, and stews with dried tea leaves. Add the leaves whole or crush them first.
• When you need liquid to thin a sauce, add brewed green or black tea instead of plain water.
• For a change from water, serve freshly brewed green or black iced tea with lunch or dinner. Garnish with slices of lemon and sweeten to taste. (When making iced tea, double the strength of hot tea, since it will be poured over ice.)
• If you drink soft drinks with meals, replace them with tea.

RECIPES
Lemon Iced Green Tea, page 279
Two Tea Dressing, page 371
Ginger Tea Marinade, page 372

Snacks and desserts

• For a midday break, enjoy a cup of brewed tea with a thin slice each of ginger and lemon.
• For an antioxidant-rich snack, enjoy a green tea latte. Simply brew green tea in hot skim milk or soy beverage and add a dash of cinnamon,

ginger, black pepper, and allspice. Or order one at your local coffee shop—just be sure to ask them to go light on the syrup.
- On a hot summer day, serve homemade popsicles made with a fruit-flavoured green tea.
- For an elegant dessert, serve pears poached in green or black tea with sliced fresh gingerroot. Garnish with fresh mint leaves.
- If you own an ice cream maker, make green tea ice cream. You'll find plenty of recipes online.

★ COFFEE: CAFFEINATED AND DECAFFEINATED

Consume up to 4 servings per day
1 serving = 1 cup (250 ml)

You might be surprised to find coffee on my list of power beverages. It's true that ever since coffee became a major part of the Western diet in the early 16th century, it's been under a cloud of controversy regarding its effect on health. A few hundred years ago, physicians warned that drinking coffee caused sterility, impotence, even paralysis. More recently, coffee has been linked to heart disease, osteoporosis, infertility, and pancreatic cancer.

But the tides have turned. Research now suggests that if you drink enough coffee, you'll lower the risk of a handful of diseases. You'll also feel more alert and work out harder at the gym. It's becoming clear that coffee is more than just a way to consume water. It's a beverage with unique phytochemicals and nutrients that may promote health. So if you drink coffee, there's no reason to feel guilty.

Coffee and health

Mounting evidence suggests that, for most people, drinking coffee does more good than harm. Habitual coffee drinkers appear to be protected from diabetes, liver disease, Parkinson's disease, and gallstones. And as you'll read below, the research does not support the notion that drinking coffee ups the risk of heart disease.

COFFEE AND TYPE 2 DIABETES

The most promising evidence for coffee's health benefits come from studies on diabetes. In a two studies of 41,934 healthy men and 84,276 healthy men, Harvard researchers found that long-term coffee consumption offered significant protection from type 2 diabetes. Among men and women who regularly drank caffeinated coffee, those who drank at least 6 cups (1.5 L) per day were 54% and 30%, respectively, less likely to develop diabetes compared with non–coffee drinkers. Among men, drinking 4 to 5 cups (1 to 1.25 L) per day reduced the risk by 30%. Even decaffeinated coffee offered protection, suggesting there's more than caffeine at work. People who drank at least 4 cups (1 L) of decaf per day had a 26% (men) and 15% (women) reduced risk of type 2 diabetes.[14]

Another study conducted among 28,812 healthy postmenopausal women who were followed for 11 years found that compared with abstainers, women who drank 6 cups (1.5 L) of coffee per day had a 22% lower risk of type 2 diabetes. The researchers noted the effect was largely explained by decaffeinated coffee. When they analyzed the results according to type of coffee, heavy decaf drinkers were 33% less likely to develop diabetes, while regular coffee drinkers had a 21% lower risk.[15]

A report published in the *Journal of the American Medical Association* that combined data from nine large studies concluded that people who drank 4 to 6 cups (1 to 1.5 L) of coffee per day were 28% less likely to develop type 2 diabetes compared with those who drank 2 cups (500 ml) or less daily. Drinking more than 6 cups (1.5 L) each day reduced the risk by 35%.[16]

COFFEE AND HEART DISEASE

Despite earlier concerns that coffee might be bad for your heart, studies haven't found such a connection. In fact, one study conducted among 41,836 healthy women age 55 to 69 found that drinking 1 to 6 cups (250 ml to 1.5 L) of coffee per day—caffeinated or decaffeinated—reduced the risk of dying from heart disease. A daily intake of 4 to 6 cups (1 to 1.5 L) was found to be most protective.[17] Another paper from Harvard University reported no increased risk of fatal or nonfatal heart attack among men and women from drinking 6 cups (1.5 L) or more of coffee each day.[18] What's more, a study published in 2007 that analyzed the results from 23 studies conducted on habitual coffee drinking and coronary heart disease found no association between coffee consumption and heart disease.[19]

COFFEE AND PARKINSON'S DISEASE

Parkinson's disease is a progressive disorder of nerve cells in the part of the brain that helps control muscle movement. The disease usually shows up after the age of 60 and is marked by muscle tremors, rigid muscles, decreased mobility, stooped posture, slow voluntary movements, and a mask-like facial expression.

Several studies have connected habitual coffee consumption with protection from Parkinson's disease. In two studies, Harvard researchers found that men who consumed the most caffeine reduced their risk for Parkinson's disease by 48%. Among women, those who drank 1 to 3 cups (250 to 750 ml) of coffee per day had a 50% reduction in risk.[20] When researchers followed 8004 Japanese-American men for 30 years, they found that compared with men who drank no coffee, those who consumed at least 3 1/2 cups (875 ml) per day were significantly less likely to develop Parkinson's disease. Similar relationships were observed with total caffeine intake, but not with other nutrients in coffee.[21]

COFFEE AND LIVER DISEASE

Coffee seems to protect the liver from the effects of alcohol and toxins. A recent analysis of findings from nine studies conducted in more than 240,000 people with and without a history of liver cirrhosis concluded that the risk of liver cancer was cut by 43% for every 2 cups (500 ml) of coffee consumed per day.[22] (In liver cirrhosis, scar tissue replaces normal, healthy tissue, blocking blood flow and preventing the liver from functioning properly. Chronic alcohol abuse and hepatitis C are the most common causes.)

COFFEE AND PHYSICAL AND MENTAL PERFORMANCE

In terms of performance, studies suggest that as few as 2 cups (500 ml) of coffee can markedly improve endurance performance in activities, such as running, cycling, and cross-country skiing. Coffee also stimulates the brain and enhances mental alertness, particularly if you spread your intake out over the course of the day.

Coffee's bioactive ingredients

Researchers suspect that some of coffee's health benefits are linked to its high phytochemical content. Coffee—both caffeinated and decaffeinated—contains a group of phytochemicals called chlorogenic acids, which in laboratory studies have been shown to have powerful antioxidant activities. Antioxidants in coffee beans may become more potent during roasting. Chlorogenic acids are thought to dampen inflammation in the body and improve how the body uses insulin, the hormone that lowers blood sugar.

If you're a coffee drinker, you probably consume more antioxidants from coffee than you think. In a study from the University of Scranton, in Pennsylvania, coffee was deemed the number one source of antioxidants in the American diet.[23] In other words, Americans get more of their antioxidants from coffee than from any other dietary source. (Black tea came in second place.) Canadians, too, love their coffee: On average, we drink 2.33 cups (575 ml) per day, which means that coffee contributes a considerable amount of antioxidants to our diet.

Caffeine is also thought to play a role in coffee's ability to help fight disease. It's the caffeine in coffee that helps treat asthma symptoms, enhances physical performance, and boosts mental alertness. And coffee's protective effects against gallstones and Parkinson's disease are attributed to caffeine.

Coffee also contains magnesium, a mineral linked to blood sugar regulation, and niacin, a B vitamin necessary for many body processes.

How much caffeine is too much?

Based on a review of the evidence, Health Canada contends that healthy adults are not at risk for adverse effects from caffeine provided daily intake is limited to 450 milligrams. Women are advised to consume no more than 300 milligrams per day during pregnancy, with some experts suggesting a stricter limit of 200 milligrams.

It's important to remember that caffeine is a stimulant drug that's mildly addictive. If you're a habitual coffee drinker and you miss your daily dose, you may experience indigestion, muscle soreness, headache, irritability, even slight depression. Caffeine sensitivity—the amount it takes to elicit an effect—varies from person to person. In general, the smaller the person, the less caffeine it takes to produce side effects. But regardless of body size, the more caffeine you regularly consume, the less sensitive you become to its effects. In other words, it takes more caffeine to feel its jolt.

According to government nutrient databases, a standard cup (8 ounces/250 ml) of coffee is often assumed to provide 100 milligrams of caffeine. However, tests conducted in 2004 for *The Globe and Mail* and CTV News showed that caffeine content of store-bought coffee ranged from 78 to 165 milligrams per cup, depending on the coffee shop. And most coffee shops don't offer 8 ounce (250 ml) cups of coffee—the smallest serving is usually 10 or 12 ounces (300 or 375 ml).

Caffeine content of selected beverages (milligrams)

Coffee, decaffeinated, 8 oz (250 ml)	3
Coffee, brewed, 8 oz (250 ml)	100
Coffee, instant, 8 oz (250 ml)	66
Espresso, 2 oz (60 ml)	54
Starbucks coffee, "venti" size, 20 oz (591 ml)	415
Second Cup coffee, large, 20 oz (591 ml)	391
Timothy's, large, 18 oz (532 ml)	245
Tim Hortons, large, 20 oz (591 ml)	270
Tea, black, 8 oz (250 ml)	45
Tea, green, 8 oz (250 ml)	30
Cola, regular, 12 oz (355 ml)	37
Cola, diet, 12 oz (355 ml)	50
Red Bull energy drink, 8 oz (250 ml)	80
Mountain Dew Energy, 20 oz (591 ml)	91
Snapple iced tea, 16 oz (473 ml)	42
Chocolate milk, 1 cup (250 ml)	8

Keep in mind that the caffeine content of coffee varies greatly depending on the variety of the coffee bean and the brewing equipment used.

Chocolate, too, contains caffeine: 1 ounce (30 g) of dark chocolate contains 20 milligrams. Milk chocolate has considerably less—6 milligrams for the same amount

Should you limit caffeine intake?

Regular coffee isn't for everyone. Despite that epidemiological studies have not found an increased risk of heart disease in coffee drinkers, drinking the beverage could possibly modify risk factors for the disease. Excess caffeine can temporarily boost blood pressure and heart rate, a concern for people with hypertension and heart disease. Research suggests that drinking caffeinated coffee can cause a short-term increase in the stiffening of arterial walls. Coffee has also been shown to increase the level of homocysteine in the bloodstream, a compound linked to heart disease. (Homocysteine is a naturally occurring amino acid produced in the body. In some people it builds up to a high level because of a deficiency in their body's ability to break it down. Elevated homocysteine is thought to damage blood vessel walls.)

Too much caffeine might not be good for your bones, since caffeine increases the amount of calcium the kidneys excrete in the urine. Research has determined that postmenopausal women who don't get enough calcium and consume 450 milligrams of caffeine per day—about three 8 ounce (250 ml) cups of coffee—have lower bone densities. And some studies also suggest that high intakes of caffeine during pregnancy can increase the risk of miscarriage.

So, in my opinion, if you have high blood pressure, existing heart disease, osteoporosis, or suffer from insomnia, it is wise to limit your caffeine intake or switch to decaffeinated coffee. And I agree with those experts who advise pregnant women to limit their caffeine intake to no more than 200 milligrams per day.

For most people, however, coffee in moderation is harmless, and there's no reason to cut back. There is little evidence of health risks and evidence of health benefits from consuming moderate amounts of coffee, 3 to 4 cups (750 ml to 1 L) per day—and up to 450 milligrams of caffeine. Accumulating evidence strongly suggests that coffee's perks extend beyond kick-starting your day.

Enjoying coffee

Unlike the other power foods you learned about in this book, I am not urging you to drink more coffee or start drinking it if you don't already. Earlier in the chapter, I recommended a daily intake of "up to" 4 servings. Although some people can safely drink 3 to 4 servings each day, others are best to consume only 1. And some people don't like the taste of coffee or can't tolerate coffee at all. That's because along with coffee's beneficial antioxidants comes caffeine, a natural compound that can cause side effects in some people. Studies suggest that to obtain the benefits of coffee for type 2 diabetes prevention, you need to drink more than 4 cups (1 L) per day, an intake that translates into at least 400 milligrams of caffeine if you drink regular coffee.

If you're concerned about the caffeine content of coffee, you may want to consider drinking decaf; decaffeinated coffee still retains the antioxidants found in the bean. If you enjoy a cup or more of coffee each day, continue doing so, but monitor your caffeine intake to ensure it isn't negatively affecting you—and make sure you're meeting your daily calcium requirements.

Buying

Coffee is prepared from the roasted seeds—or beans—of the coffee plant. The beans are roasted at a temperature of approximately 400°F (200°C) to a light, medium, or dark brown colour, depending on the desired flavour.

There are two main types of coffee beans: arabica and robusta. Arabica coffee, considered the finest in the world, grows well at high altitudes and has a richer, more refined body and flavour than other species. Arabica coffee is difficult to grow, as it's prone to disease, requires more hand-cultivation, and yields smaller harvests than other varieties. Robusta coffee is a hardier high-yielding plant that's resistant to disease. It grows at lower elevations and produces coffee with a harsher flavour and higher caffeine content.

For the freshest and most flavourful coffee, purchase coffee beans as soon as possible after they've been roasted. (This information will be available at coffee shops that sell coffee beans.) Purchase coffee beans in small amounts—only as much as you can use in a given time. Ideally, buy fresh coffee beans every 2 to 4 weeks.

Storing

The enemies of roasted coffee are moisture, air, light, and heat. Store ground coffee or whole beans in an airtight container in a cool, dark cupboard. Do not store in the refrigerator. Coffee is porous and absorbs odours; make sure you keep it away from onions, garlic, and other strongly aromatic foods.

Once you've opened a bag of coffee, either transfer the coffee to a clean, dry, air-tight container, or simply roll the top of the bag closed, forcing out as much air as possible, and seal the bag with a rubber band. Ground coffee will stay fresh for 2 weeks. Grinding coffee beans releases their oils and exposes the beans to air, which makes the coffee go stale more quickly, no matter how you store it.

If you don't plan on using the ground coffee within 2 weeks, freeze it in a sealable freezer bag. If you know that an unopened bag of coffee—ground or beans—will need to be stored for several weeks or longer, put the unopened bag directly into the freezer. Keep in mind that constant temperature changes can create condensation and affect the quality and flavour of coffee. If you have a lot of coffee to freeze, break it up into smaller packages to prevent having to open the freezer bag numerous times to remove a portion of coffee beans. This increases the chance of moisture in the bag and can affect the quality of the coffee beans.

It's best to buy whole coffee beans and grind them as you need them. Roasted whole coffee beans will stay fresh, in an air-tight container, for up to 1 month. Coffee grinders can be purchased at kitchen stores, coffee shops, and large department stores. You can also buy coffee makers that grind the beans just before brewing—very convenient!

Preparing

The fresher the grind, the more flavourful and aromatic the brewed coffee will be. Ground coffee loses its flavour rapidly, so grind only the beans you need.

The quality of your coffee also depends on the quality of water you use. It's best to use cold, fresh filtered water.

Most coffee experts suggest a 1:1 ratio of coffee to water, meaning 1 tablespoon (15 ml) of freshly ground coffee per 1 cup (250 ml) measure on the coffee maker. For most coffee makers, a 1 cup (250 ml) measure equals 5 ounces (150 ml).

For stronger coffee, increase the ratio of coffee to water. In fact, professional coffee tasters use 2 tablespoons (25 ml) of ground coffee for every 6 ounces (175 ml) of water. If you're using a coffee maker with a built-in grinder, follow the manufacturer's recommendation for coffee bean to water ratio.

To prevent coffee from burning or staling, leave it on the warmer no longer than 20 minutes. If coffee is not to be consumed immediately after brewing, pour it into an insulated thermos or carafe to keep it warm.

Whatever brewing method you choose—drip, percolator, Bodum— keep the equipment clean, inside and out; unclean equipment will affect the flavour.

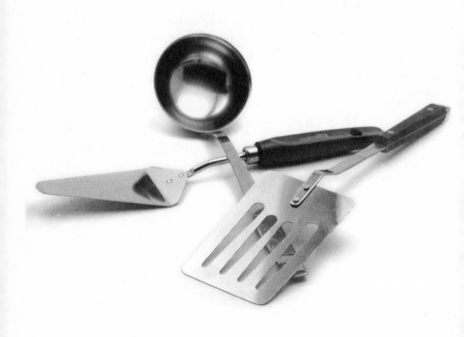

Power recipes that fight disease

Breakfasts

Beverages

Snacks

Salads

Soups

Side dishes

GRAINS

VEGETABLES

Entrees

FISH, MEAT, AND POULTRY

Dips, salad dressings, and marinades

Muffins and quick breads

Desserts

★ RECIPES USING POWER FOODS

Power Vegetables

GARLIC, ONIONS, AND LEEKS

Power fruit

CITRUS

Power grains

OATS

Banana Flax Pancakes	270
Blueberry Walnut Muesli with Rolled Oats and Flaxseed	271
Ginger-Flax Fruit Crisp	381
Hot Apple and Cabbage Salad	289
Whole-Grain Millet Waffles with Orange and Raspberries	275

WHOLE WHEAT

Cranberry Orange Flax Quick Bread	375
Flax Bean Brownies	279
Ginger-Flax Fruit Crisp	381
Low-Fat Lemon Millet Muffins	377
Wheat Berry Salad with Smoked Trout and Gingered Squash	303

FLAXSEED

Banana Flax Pancakes	270
Blueberry Walnut Muesli with Rolled Oats and Flaxseed	271
Cajun Breaded Trout	331
Cinnamon Orange Quinoa Hot Cereal	272
Cranberry Orange Flax Quick Bread	375
Flax Bean Brownies	379
Pomegranate Power Shake	280
Quick Pomegranate Flax Porridge	273

QUINOA

Cinnamon Orange Quinoa Hot Cereal	272
Quinoa-Stuffed Peppers	312

MILLET

Low-Fat Lemon Millet Muffins	377
Whole-Grain Millet Waffles with Orange and Raspberries	275

WHOLE RYE

Blueberry Walnut Muesli with Rolled Oats and Flaxseed   271

BARLEY

Barley Salad   298

Mushroom Barley Casserole   311

KASHA

Kasha Cabbage Rolls   341

Kasha, Walnut, and Apple Salad with Mint   300

BROWN RICE AND WILD RICE

Ginger-Orange Vegetable Stir-fry with Chicken and Brown Rice   339

Hearty Minestrone Soup   307

Wild Rice and Lentil Curry   353

Power dairy foods

YOGURT

Blackberry Shake   276

Blueberry Walnut Muesli with Rolled Oats and Flaxseed   271

Crazy Cranberry Smoothie   277

Creamy Caesar Dressing   363

Creamy Cold Berry Soup   304

Creamy Dill Dip   357

Creamy Strawberry Smoothie   277

Lemon Ginger Fruit Dip   359

Poppy Seed Dressing   369

Tandoori Marinade   374

Yogurt Cheese   286

KEFIR

Garlic and Basil Kefir Dressing   364

Raspberry Kefir Smoothie   281

Power protein foods

FISH

LEGUMES AND SOY

Power fats and oils

Power beverages

Breakfasts

Banana Flax Pancakes

This recipe makes a very thin batter, similar to that of crepes. Gently tilt the pan after pouring in the batter to produce pancakes of uniform thickness. These pancakes freeze well and can be quickly reheated in a skillet or microwave for a fast weekday breakfast.

Tip: If you want, substitute calcium-fortified soy milk for the milk.

1 cup	low-fat (1% MF or less) milk	250 ml
2	medium eggs, lightly beaten	2
1	banana, mashed	1
1/2 tsp	vanilla extract	2 ml
3/4 cup	whole-wheat flour	175 ml
1/2 cup	all-purpose flour	125 ml
1/4 cup	rolled oats	50 ml
2 tbsp	ground flaxseed	25 ml
1/2 tsp	salt	2 ml
2 tsp	baking powder	10 ml
1 tsp	canola oil	5 ml

In a mixing bowl, combine milk, eggs, banana, and vanilla.

In a small bowl, combine flours, oats, flaxseed, salt, and baking powder.

Fold dry ingredients into the wet ingredients. Briskly whisk batter for 10 seconds.

Heat oil in a skillet over medium heat. Add one-quarter of the batter to the hot pan, and tilt pan to spread out the batter as thinly as possible. When bubbles appear on the surface of the batter, flip and continue to cook until golden brown.

Makes 4 large pancakes

Per pancake: 274 cal, 12 g pro, 6 g total fat (1 g saturated fat), 45 g carb, 5 g fibre, 85 mg chol, 518 mg sodium

Excellent source of: vitamin K, magnesium

Good source of: fibre, folate, iron, potassium

Blueberry Walnut Muesli with Rolled Oats and Flaxseed

This hearty muesli is delicious when combined with plain or vanilla yogurt and fresh blueberries. Make the muesli ahead of time and store in an airtight container. For a nuttier flavour, first toast the oats, rye flakes, wheat germ, and walnuts for 5 to 7 minutes at 375°F (190°C) until lightly brown and fragrant.

1 cup	rolled oats	250 ml
1/2 cup	rye flakes	125 ml
1/2 cup	wheat germ	125 ml
1/2 cup	dried cranberries	125 ml
1/4 cup	whole flaxseed	50 ml
1/4 cup	chopped walnuts	50 ml
1 tsp	cinnamon	5 ml
3 cups	low-fat (1% MF or less) plain or vanilla yogurt	750 ml
1 1/2 cups	fresh blueberries	375 ml

In a large bowl, combine rolled oats, rye flakes, wheat germ, cranberries, flaxseed, walnuts, and cinnamon.

When ready to serve, mix with yogurt and fresh blueberries. Serve immediately.

Serves 6

Per 1/2 cup (125 ml) serving of dry muesli: 285 cal, 11 g pro, 9 g total fat (1 g saturated fat), 43 g carb, 9 g fibre, 0 mg chol, 3 mg sodium

Per 1/2 cup (125 ml) serving of muesli with 1/2 cup (125 ml) yogurt and 1/4 cup (50 ml) blueberries: 368 cal, 18 g pro, 9 g total fat (1 g saturated fat), 57 g carb, 10 g fibre, 2 mg chol, 92 mg sodium

With yogurt and blueberries:

Excellent source of: fibre, calcium, magnesium

Good source of: folate, vitamin K, iron, essential fatty acids

Cinnamon Orange Quinoa Hot Cereal

Quinoa is a high-protein grain, making this an ideal breakfast to hold you over until lunchtime. This thick, whole-grain porridge is delicious mixed with fresh fruit.

3/4 cup	orange juice	175 ml
1/2 tsp	cinnamon	2 ml
1/4 tsp	allspice	1 ml
1/4 cup	quinoa	50 ml
1 tbsp	whole flaxseed	15 ml
1 tbsp	dried cranberries	15 ml

In a saucepan, bring orange juice, cinnamon, and allspice to a boil. Add quinoa and flaxseed, stirring to combine. Cover and simmer for 12 to 15 minutes or until most of the liquid is absorbed and the quinoa and flaxseed resemble a thick porridge.

Serve in a bowl, with dried cranberries sprinkled on top.

Serves 1

Per 1/2 cup (125 ml) serving: 329 cal, 9 g pro, 7 g total fat (0 g saturated fat), 60 g carb, 7 g fibre, 0 mg chol, 12 mg sodium

Excellent source of: fibre, vitamin C, iron, magnesium

Good source of: folate, potassium

Quick Pomegranate Flax Porridge

This stick-to-your ribs cereal also tends to stick to your bowl. I recommend that you eat this as soon as it's prepared, and rinse your bowl when you're finished eating. Otherwise you'll need to muster up some elbow grease to get rid of all the dried bits of flaxseed.

1/2 cup	ground flaxseed	125 ml
1/4 cup	pure pomegranate juice, or other 100% fruit juice	50 ml
1/2 tsp	honey	2 ml
	chopped fresh fruit or berries, as garnish	

In a small bowl, combine flaxseed, pomegranate juice, and honey. Stir until the mixture thickens. Top with your choice of fruit or berries.

Serves 2

Per 1/4 cup (50 ml) serving: 174 cal, 5 g pro, 12 g total fat (1 g saturated fat), 15 g carb, 8 g fibre, 0 mg chol, 9 mg sodium

Excellent source of: fibre, magnesium

Good source of: calcium

Tofu Scramble

In this recipe, it is versatile tofu that is scrambled instead of eggs. The result is a high-protein breakfast that's a tasty alternative to eggs.

Tip: For added colour, add freshly chopped chives just before serving.

1 tsp	canola oil	5 ml
1	small onion, chopped	1
2	cloves garlic, chopped	2
1	12 oz/350 g pkg extra-firm tofu	1
1 tsp	turmeric	5 ml
1/2 tsp	chili powder	2 ml
1 tsp	cumin seeds	5 ml
1 tbsp	sodium-reduced soy sauce	15 ml
	freshly ground black pepper to taste	

Heat oil in a skillet over medium heat. Add onion; sauté for 4 to 5 minutes or until golden brown. Add garlic; sauté 1 minute.

With your hands, crumble tofu into 1 inch (2.5 cm) pieces; add to skillet. Stir in turmeric, chili powder, cumin seeds, and soy sauce. Season with black pepper.

Continue to cook over medium heat for 8 to 10 minutes or until most of the moisture from the tofu has evaporated and the tofu begins to brown.

Serves 4

Per 1/2 cup (125 ml) serving: 166 cal, 15 g pro, 9 g total fat (1 g saturated fat), 10 g carb, 2 g fibre, 0 mg chol, 139 mg sodium

Excellent source of: calcium, iron

Good source of: magnesium

Whole-Grain Millet Waffles with Orange and Raspberries

Raspberries add a pale pink hue to these hearty waffles, though you could substitute any fresh berry, including blueberries. You'll find hulled millet in the natural food section of large grocery stores and health food stores. Make extra waffles to freeze, ready for a quick breakfast on a busy morning.

1 cup	hulled millet	250 ml
1 cup	water	250 ml
1 cup	rolled oats	250 ml
3/4 cup	orange juice	175 ml
1/2 cup	raspberries (fresh or frozen)	125 ml
2 tbsp	maple syrup	25 ml
	zest of 1 lemon or orange	
1/2 tsp	cinnamon	2 ml
1/2 tsp	salt	2 ml

Combine millet and water in a large bowl. Stir to combine. Cover and refrigerate for at least 3 hours, or overnight.

Preheat waffle iron.

Drain and rinse millet. Add rolled oats, orange juice, raspberries, maple syrup, lemon or orange zest, cinnamon, and salt. Using a hand blender, mix ingredients to make a thick batter. If batter seems too thin, add up to another 1/4 cup (50 ml) rolled oats, or 2 tbsp (25 ml) ground flaxseed.

Spray waffle iron with cooking spray. Add batter and cook according to manufacturer's directions.

Makes 3 large waffles

Serves 6

Per 1/2 waffle: 264 cal, 8 g pro, 3 g total fat (1 g saturated fat), 51 g carb, 6 g fibre, 0 mg chol, 197 mg sodium

Excellent source of: fibre, vitamin C, magnesium

Good source of: vitamin K, iron

Beverages

Blackberry Shake

You can substitute any 100% unsweetened fruit juice for the orange juice in this recipe. Pomegranate juice works especially well.

1/2 cup	blackberries	125 ml
1/2 cup	low-fat (1% MF or less) plain yogurt	125 ml
1 cup	pure orange juice	250 ml

In a blender, combine blackberries, yogurt, and orange juice. Purée until smooth.

Serve cold.

Serves 1

Per serving: 212 cal, 8 g pro, 1 g total fat (0 g saturated fat), 44 g carb, 4 g fibre, 2 mg chol, 90 mg sodium

Excellent source of: vitamin C, calcium

Good source of: fibre, folate, magnesium, potassium

Blueberry Banana Bonanza Smoothie

Nothing says summer like a basketful of fresh blueberries. If you don't have fresh blueberries on hand, frozen berries work just as well.

1/4 cup	blueberries	50 ml
1	banana	1
1 cup	low-fat (1% MF or less) milk or soy milk	250 ml

In a blender, combine blueberries, banana, and milk. Purée until smooth.

Serve cold.

Serves 1

Per serving: 228 cal, 10 g pro, 3 g total fat (2 g saturated fat), 44 g carb, 3 g fibre, 10 mg chol, 125 mg sodium

Excellent source of: vitamin C, calcium

Good source of: vitamin A, magnesium, potassium

Crazy Cranberry Smoothie

This recipe works just as well with any fresh or frozen berry. For a vitamin C boost, use strawberries.

1 cup	pure cranberry juice	250 ml
3/4 cup	low-fat (1% MF or less) plain yogurt	175 ml
1/4 cup	blueberries	50 ml

In a blender, combine cranberry juice, yogurt, and blueberries. Purée until smooth.

Serve cold.

Serves 1

Per serving: 194 cal, 10 g pro, 0 g total fat (0 g saturated fat), 38 g carb, 1 g fibre, 3 mg chol, 169 mg sodium

Excellent source of: calcium

Good source of: vitamin C

Creamy Strawberry Smoothie

If you prefer your smoothies on the thick side, add a few more strawberries, or increase the proportion of yogurt to milk.

1/2 cup	sliced strawberries	125 ml
1/2 cup	low-fat (1% MF or less) plain yogurt	125 ml
1 cup	skim or 1% milk or soy milk	250 ml

In a blender, combine strawberries, yogurt, and milk. Purée until smooth.

Serve cold.

Serves 1

Per serving: 173 cal, 15 g pro, 1 g total fat (0 g saturated fat), 27 g carb, 2 g fibre, 7 mg chol, 215 mg sodium

Excellent source of: vitamin C, calcium

Good source of: vitamin A, vitamin D, magnesium, potassium

Lemon Ginger Infusion

This soothing drink is ideal when you're feeling under the weather or just wanting a caffeine-free alternative to tea or coffee. This beverage can be served warm or cold. For a spicier version, double the amount of ginger.

2 cups	water	500 ml
3 tbsp	freshly squeezed lemon juice	50 ml
1 tbsp	chopped gingerroot (large chunks)	15 ml

In a small saucepan, combine water, lemon juice, and gingerroot. Bring to a boil, cover, and simmer for 3 to 5 minutes. Remove from heat and scoop out the pieces of ginger. Serve warm.

Serves 2

Per serving: 8 cal, 0 g pro, 0 g total fat (0 g saturated fat), 3 g carb, 0 g fibre, 0 mg chol, 8 mg sodium

Excellent source of: vitamin C

Lemon Iced Green Tea

This refreshing iced tea has very little sugar, making it a much healthier alternative to store-bought versions. For variety, use different types of green or black teas, including tea leaves blended with dried fruit or flowers.

6 cups	boiling water	1.5 L
6	green tea bags	6
1/4 cup	lemon juice	50 ml
2 tbsp	honey	25 ml
	fresh mint leaves, as garnish	

Pour boiling water over tea bags in a large pitcher. Steep for 5 to 10 minutes, depending on desired strength.

Remove tea bags. Stir in lemon juice and honey. Allow the tea to cool before pouring into 6 large ice-filled glasses. Garnish with fresh mint leaves. Serve immediately.

Serves 6

Per 1 cup (250 ml) serving: 30 cal, 0 g pro, 0 g total fat (0 g saturated fat), 8 g carb, 0 g fibre, 0 mg chol, 3 mg sodium

Pomegranate Power Shake

Ground flaxseed adds a boost of fibre to this antioxidant-rich smoothie. If you prefer your smoothies thin, add 1/4 cup (50 ml) skim milk or low-fat soy milk.

1 cup	pure pomegranate juice	250 ml
1/2 cup	whole strawberries	125 ml
1	banana	1
1 tbsp	ground flaxseed	15 ml

In a blender, combine pomegranate juice, strawberries, banana, and flaxseed. Purée until smooth.

Serve cold.

Serves 1

Per serving: 313 cal, 3 g pro, 4 g total fat (1 g saturated fat), 71 g carb, 5 g fibre, 0 mg chol, 13 mg sodium

Excellent source of: vitamin C

Good source of: fibre, magnesium, potassium

Raspberry Kefir Smoothie

This recipe works well with any berry, not just raspberries. Try blueberries, strawberries, or blackberries. You'll find kefir, a fermented milk product, in the dairy section of most grocery stores and natural food stores.

1 cup	plain kefir	250 ml
1/2 cup	fresh or frozen raspberries	125 ml
1	banana	1

In a blender, combine kefir, raspberries, and banana. Purée until smooth.

Serve cold.

Serves 1

Per serving: 257 cal, 10 g pro, 6 g total fat (3 g saturated fat), 45 g carb, 5 g fibre, 14 mg chol, 123 mg sodium

Excellent source of: vitamin C, calcium, potassium

Good source of: fibre, magnesium

Snacks

Bruce Trail Mix

Whether it's for the West Coast Trail, Cabot Trail, or Bruce Trail, this trail mix is the perfect snack to keep you energized while hiking.

1/2 cup	slivered almonds	125 ml
1/4 cup	walnuts halves	50 ml
2 tbsp	dried cranberries	25 ml
2 tbsp	dark chocolate chips	25 ml
1/2 cup	rolled oats	125 ml

In a bowl, combine almonds, walnuts, cranberries, chocolate chips, and rolled oats. Store in an airtight container.

Serves 6

Per 1/4 cup (50 ml) serving: 159 cal, 5 g pro, 11 g total fat (2 g saturated fat), 12 g carb, 3 g fibre, 0 mg chol, 4 mg sodium

Good source of: magnesium

Quick Cashew Mango Trail Mix

Keep this tasty snack on hand for those days when you need a mid-afternoon energy boost.

1/2 cup	unsalted cashews	125 ml
1/4 cup	shelled unsalted sunflower seeds	50 ml
1/4 cup	shredded unsweetened coconut	50 ml
2	strips dried mango, cut into chunks	2
1/3 cup	dried banana chips	75 ml

In a small bowl, combine cashews, sunflower seeds, coconut, dried mango, and banana chips. Store in an airtight container.

Serves 4

Per 1/3 cup (75 ml) serving: 222 cal, 5 g pro, 17 g total fat (6 g saturated fat), 17 g carb, 3 g fibre, 0 mg chol, 16 mg sodium

Excellent source of: magnesium

Good source of: iron

Spicy Candied Walnuts

Sweet, salty, and spicy—these walnuts have it all! Although this recipe makes an addictive cocktail snack all year round, it's also a special treat for holiday parties.

1 1/2 cups	walnuts halves	375 ml
1/4 cup	shredded unsweetened coconut	50 ml
2 tbsp	honey	25 ml
1/8 tsp	cayenne pepper, or to taste	0.5 ml
pinch	salt, or to taste	pinch
1/3 cup	dried cranberries	75 ml

Preheat oven to 350°F (180°C).

In a medium bowl, combine walnuts, coconut, honey, cayenne pepper, and salt.

Spread walnut mixture onto a baking sheet and bake, turning once, for 8 to 10 minutes or until brown and slightly crispy.

Transfer walnut mixture to a bowl to cool. Toss with cranberries. Store in an airtight container.

Serves 6

Per 1/4 cup (50 ml) serving: 251 cal, 8 g pro, 19 g total fat (2 g saturated fat), 18 g carb, 2 g fibre, 0 mg chol, 59 mg sodium

Excellent source of: essential fatty acids, especially alpha-linolenic acid

Good source of: magnesium

Tamari Roasted Almonds

These almonds take only minutes to prepare and are a tasty variation on regular toasted almonds. Add lemon zest for extra flavour.

1 1/2 cups	raw unsalted almonds	375 ml
2 tbsp	tamari or sodium-reduced soy sauce	25 ml
2 tbsp	freshly squeezed lemon juice	25 ml

Heat a skillet over medium heat. Add almonds and heat for 3 to 5 minutes, or until nuts become fragrant, stirring frequently.

Drizzle tamari and lemon juice over almonds and as soon as pan begins to dry out, remove from heat.

Serve warm, or transfer almonds to a bowl to cool and then store in an airtight container.

Serves 6

Per 1/4 cup (50 ml) serving: 214 cal, 8 g pro, 18 g total fat (1 g saturated fat), 8 g carb, 4 g fibre, 0 mg chol, 171 mg sodium

Excellent source of: magnesium

Good source of: fibre

Tofu "Yogurt"

This dairy-free alternative to yogurt is great paired with granola and fresh fruit. Silken tofu is available in different flavours, including plain or almond; either works well in this recipe.

1 1/2 cups	frozen mixed berries	375 ml
1	10 1/2 oz (300 g) package soft silken tofu	1
1 tbsp	honey	15 ml

In a blender, combine berries, tofu, and honey. Purée until smooth.

Serves 4

Per 1/2 cup (125 ml) serving: 87 cal, 4 g pro, 2 g total fat (0 g saturated fat), 14 g carb, 2 g fibre, 0 mg chol, 6 mg sodium

Excellent source of: vitamin C

Yogurt Cheese

When the excess liquid is drained from yogurt, the yogurt takes on the consistency of soft cheese. It can then be served as a fat-free spread with whole-grain crackers or as a topping for baked potatoes, or used to replace mayonnaise and butter on sandwiches.

1 cup	low-fat (1% MF or less) Balkan-style plain yogurt	250 ml

Secure 4 layers of cheesecloth over a bowl. Place yogurt in cheesecloth, ensuring it remains suspended over the bowl; refrigerate for 6 to 8 hours, allowing the liquid to drain from the yogurt.

Makes 1/2 to 3/4 cup (125 to 175 ml)

Per 2 tbsp (25 ml) serving: 31 cal, 3 g pro, 0 g total fat (0 g saturated fat), 4 g carb, 0 g fibre, 1 mg chol, 44 mg sodium

Zesty Edamame

Edamame, or green soybeans in pods, are a popular appetizer served at Japanese restaurants. You'll find bags of edamame in the freezer section of grocery stores and health food stores. And they're a quick snack to prepare—they need only be boiled for a few minutes and they're ready to enjoy.

1	1 lb/450 g bag frozen edamame	1
	zest of 1 lemon	
1/2 tsp	coarse sea salt	2 ml
1/8 tsp	red pepper flakes	0.5 ml

Fill a saucepan with water and bring to a boil. Add edamame and bring water back to a boil. When edamame rises to the surface (about 3 to 4 minutes), remove from heat and drain.

Place edamame in a serving bowl and toss with lemon zest, salt, and red pepper flakes. Serve warm.

Serves 4

Per 1 cup (250 ml) serving: 127 cal, 12 g pro, 5 g total fat (0 g saturated fat), 10 g carb, 6 g fibre, 0 mg chol, 296 mg sodium

Excellent source of: fibre, folate

Good source of: vitamin C, iron, magnesium

Salads

Vegetables

Blueberry and Roasted Walnut Spinach Salad

This power salad tastes as good as it sounds—and looks. If you have other types of berries on hand, such as raspberries or strawberries, feel free to add them for extra flavour and colour. Drizzle the salad with dressing just before serving, otherwise the spinach will wilt. This salad goes especially well with the Lemon Walnut Dressing (page 367).

1/4 cup	walnut halves	50 ml
8 cups	spinach (about 1 lb/450 g)	2 L
1 cup	fresh blueberries	250 ml
1/4 cup	dried cranberries	50 ml
	zest of 1 lemon	

Preheat oven to 375°F (190°C).

Bake nuts on a baking sheet for 5 to 7 minutes, or until nuts are slightly brown and fragrant. Remove from oven and set aside to cool.

In a large bowl, toss spinach with blueberries, cranberries, and toasted walnuts.

Drizzle with salad dressing of your choice and transfer to individual plates. Garnish each with lemon zest.

Serves 4

Per 2 cup (500 ml) serving of undressed salad: 117 cal, 5 g pro, 5 g total fat (0 g saturated fat), 16 g carb, 5 g fibre, 0 mg chol, 91 mg sodium

Per 2 cup (500 ml) serving of salad with 2 tbsp (25 ml) Lemon Walnut Dressing: 255 cal, 5 g pro, 19 g total fat (1 g saturated fat), 20 g carb, 5 g fibre, 0 mg chol, 134 mg sodium

Excellent source of: vitamin A, folate, vitamin C, vitamin K, iron, magnesium

Good source of: fibre

Hot Apple and Cabbage Salad

This colourful cruciferous salad makes for a hearty meal all by itself. And it's very low in fat and sodium: only 1 gram of fat and 12 milligrams of sodium per serving.

1 cup	water	250 ml
1/2	medium red cabbage, shredded	1/2
2	apples, peeled, cored, and grated	2
1/4 cup	rolled oats	50 ml
2 tbsp	brown sugar	25 ml
1 tbsp	apple cider vinegar	15 ml
1/4 tsp	ground cloves	1 ml

In a large saucepan, combine water, cabbage, apples, oats, sugar, vinegar, and cloves, and bring to a boil. Reduce heat and simmer for 40 to 45 minutes or until cabbage is tender.

Serve hot or cold.

Serves 6

Per 3/4 cup (175 ml) serving: 79 cal, 2 g pro, 1 g total fat (0 g saturated fat), 18 g carb, 3 g fibre, 0 mg chol, 12 mg sodium

Excellent source of: vitamin C

Pomegranate Garden Salad

I suggest serving this colourful salad with Pomegranate Maple Dressing (page 368). If you don't have cherry tomatoes on hand, diced tomatoes will work equally well.

4 cups	mixed baby greens, such as mesculin mix	1 L
1 cup	halved cherry tomatoes	250 ml
1/2 cup	shredded carrot	125 ml
1/2 cup	pomegranate seeds	125 ml
2 tbsp	sunflower seeds	25 ml

In a large bowl, combine greens, tomatoes, carrot, pomegranate seeds, and sunflower seeds.

Toss with Pomegranate Maple Dressing or dressing of your choice just before serving.

Serves 4

Per 1 1/2 cup (375 ml) serving of undressed salad: 83 cal, 3 g pro, 3 g total fat (0 g saturated fat), 15 g carb, 3 g fibre, 0 mg chol, 40 mg sodium

Per 1 1/2 cup (375 ml) serving of salad with 2 tbsp (25 ml) Pomegranate Maple Dressing: 161 cal, 3 g pro, 10 g total fat (1 g saturated fat), 19 g carb, 3 g fibre, 0 mg chol, 69 mg sodium

Excellent source of: vitamin A, folate, vitamin C, vitamin K

Sesame Coleslaw

The sesame oil and rice vinegar in this recipe turn regular coleslaw into a flavourful, Asian-inspired salad.

Tip: This salad tastes better the longer it is allowed to sit, so make it a few hours or up to a day before you plan to serve it.

6 cups	shredded Savoy cabbage (about 1/2 head)	1.5 L
1 1/2 cups	shredded carrot	375 ml
2	green onions, thinly sliced	2
1/4 cup	seasoned rice wine vinegar	50 ml
2 tbsp	dark sesame oil	25 ml
1 tsp	granulated sugar	5 ml
1 tsp	mustard seeds	5 ml

In a large bowl, combine cabbage, carrot, and green onion.

In a small bowl, whisk together rice vinegar, sesame oil, sugar, and mustard seeds. Drizzle over cabbage mixture. Toss to mix thoroughly.

Cover and refrigerate for at least 3 hours before serving.

Serves 6

Per 1 1/4 cup (300 ml) serving: 89 cal, 2 g pro, 5 g total fat (1 g saturated fat), 11 g carb, 4 g fibre, 0 mg chol, 39 mg sodium

Excellent source of: vitamin A, vitamin C

Good source of: fibre

Spinach and Grapefruit Salad

This is a refreshing combination of three power foods: spinach, grapefruit, and walnuts. For added colour, toss in a handful of fresh berries. Or serve this salad warm by sautéing the mushrooms with onions in balsamic vinegar before tossing with spinach. Serve with Grapefruit Maple Dressing (page 365).

1/4 cup	walnuts halves	50 ml
4 cups	spinach	1 L
1	grapefruit, peeled and sectioned	1
1	small red onion, thinly sliced	1
1 cup	sliced mushrooms	250 ml
1/2 cup	low-fat goat cheese	125 ml

Preheat oven to 375°F (190°C).

Bake walnuts on a baking sheet for 5 to 7 minutes, until lightly brown and fragrant. Remove from oven; set aside to cool.

In a large bowl, toss spinach with grapefruit, onion, mushrooms, toasted walnuts, and goat cheese.

Drizzle salad with Grapefruit Maple Dressing just before serving.

Serves 4

Per 1 3/4 cup (425 ml) serving of undressed salad: 156 cal, 8 g pro, 10 g total fat (0 g saturated fat), 11 g carb, 3 g fibre, 0 mg chol, 146 mg sodium

Per 1 3/4 cup (425 ml) serving of salad with 2 tbsp (25 ml) Grapefruit Maple Dressing: 208 cal, 8 g pro, 14 g total fat (1 g saturated fat), 16 g carb, 3 g fibre, 0 mg chol, 168 mg sodium

Excellent source of: vitamin A, folate, vitamin C, vitamin K

Good source of: iron, magnesium

Fruit

Avocado Citrus Salad

Avocado goes well with both grapefruit and strawberries. If you have a fairly firm avocado, consider tossing the slices with the fruit. If the avocado is medium firm or soft, I suggest you serve it with the slices fanned on the side.

2	pink grapefruit, peeled and sectioned	2
1 cup	sliced strawberries	250 ml
2 tbsp	maple syrup	25 ml
2 tbsp	freshly squeezed lime juice	25 ml
1	medium-firm avocado, pitted, peeled, and sliced	1
	fresh mint leaves, as garnish	

In a medium-sized bowl, combine grapefruit and strawberries.

In a small bowl, whisk together maple syrup and lime juice.

Drizzle dressing over fruit, cover, and refrigerate for at least 2 hours before serving to allow flavours to blend.

Garnish with avocado slices and fresh mint.

Serves 4

Per 1 cup (250 ml) serving: 154 cal, 2 g pro, 8 g total fat (1 g saturated fat), 23 g carb, 1 g fibre, 0 mg chol, 7 mg sodium

Excellent source of: vitamin C, vitamin E

Balsamic Strawberries and Oranges

The key to this dish is letting it sit for a couple of hours to allow the sweet juice from the strawberries to meld its flavour with that of the balsamic vinegar.

2 tbsp	brown sugar	25 ml
2 tbsp	balsamic vinegar	25 ml
2	oranges, peeled and sectioned	2
2 cups	sliced strawberries	500 ml
	fresh mint sprigs, as garnish	

In a large bowl, whisk together sugar and balsamic vinegar.

Gently toss oranges and strawberries with vinegar mixture.

Cover and refrigerate for at least 2 hours to allow flavours to blend.

Serve chilled, garnished with sprigs of fresh mint.

Serves 4

Per 1 cup (250 ml) serving: 86 cal, 1 g pro, 1 g total fat (0 g saturated fat), 22 g carb, 4 g fibre, 0 mg chol, 4 mg sodium

Excellent source of: vitamin C

Mixed Berry Fruit Salad with Candied Lemon Zest

Candied lemon zest turns ordinary fruit into extraordinary. This simple yet elegant dish makes a light and delicious dessert to serve at a special dinner party, with a square of bittersweet dark chocolate.

Salad:

2 cups	mixed berries (such as strawberries, blackberries, raspberries, and blueberries)	500 ml
2 tbsp	chopped fresh mint	25 ml

Candied lemon zest:

	zest of 1 lemon	
1 tbsp	granulated sugar	15 ml

In a large bowl, gently toss berries with mint.

To prepare candied lemon zest, combine lemon zest and sugar in a small bowl. Set aside for 30 minutes, until zest and sugar begin to crystallize.

Just before serving, top berries with crystallized zest. Serve cold.

Serves 4

Per 1/2 cup (125 ml) serving: 45 cal, 1 g pro, 0 g total fat (0 g saturated fat), 11 g carb, 2 g fibre, 0 mg chol, 3 mg sodium

Excellent source of: vitamin C

Pomegranate and Blueberry Fruit Salad with Fresh Ginger

This simple but colourful salad combines some of my favourite fruits—
fresh blueberries and mangoes—with shiny pomegranate seeds.

1 1/2 cups	pomegranate seeds (about 2 pomegranates)	375 ml
1 cup	fresh blueberries, washed and trimmed	250 ml
1	mango, peeled and diced	1
2 tbsp	pure pomegranate juice	25 ml
1 tbsp	minced gingerroot	15 ml

In a large bowl, combine pomegranate seeds with blueberries and mango.
In a small bowl, whisk together pomegranate juice and gingerroot. Drizzle
over the fruit just before serving.

Serves 4

Per 1 cup (250 ml) serving: 113 cal, 1 g pro, 1 g total fat (0 g saturated fat), 29 g
carb, 3 g fibre, 0 mg chol, 6 mg sodium

Excellent source of: vitamin A, vitamin C, beta carotene

Strawberry and Kiwi Salad

This eye-catching salad combines bright red strawberries with vibrant green kiwi. I suggest finely chopping the mint and mixing it in with the fruit. But if you prefer instead, use whole mint leaves as a garnish. This salad pairs nicely with Poppy Seed Dressing (page 369).

2 cups	sliced strawberries	500 ml
2	kiwi, peeled and sliced	2
2 tbsp	finely chopped fresh mint	25 ml

In a bowl, combine strawberries, kiwi, and mint. Cover and refrigerate until ready to serve.

Toss with Poppy Seed Dressing just before serving.

Serves 4

Per 3/4 cup (175 ml) serving of undressed salad: 53 cal, 1 g pro, 1 g total fat (0 g saturated fat), 13 g carb, 3 g fibre, 0 mg chol, 3 mg sodium

Per 3/4 cup (175 ml) serving of salad with 1/4 cup (50 ml) Poppy Seed Dressing: 95 cal, 4 g pro, 1 g total fat (0 g saturated fat), 19 g carb, 3 g fibre, 1 mg chol, 47 mg sodium

Excellent source of: vitamin C

Grains and Legumes

Barley Salad

If you don't have a bottle of wine open, you can easily substitute the same amount of orange juice for a vitamin C boost.

2 1/2 cups	water	625 ml
1/2 cup	dry white wine	125 ml
1 cup	pot barley	250 ml
2 tbsp	extra-virgin olive oil	25 ml
2 tbsp	white wine vinegar	25 ml
1 tbsp	freshly squeezed lemon juice	15 ml
1 tsp	Dijon mustard	5 ml
1/2 tsp	coarse sea salt	2 ml
2	carrots, shredded	2
1/4 cup	sliced pitted black olives	50 ml
2 tbsp	capers	25 ml
2	green onions, finely sliced	2

In a medium saucepan, bring water and wine to a boil. Add barley; cover and simmer for 1 hour or until barley is tender. Remove from heat, drain any excess liquid, and set aside to cool.

In a small bowl, whisk together olive oil, vinegar, lemon juice, mustard, and salt.

Combine barley with carrots, olives, capers, and onions. Drizzle with the vinaigrette, tossing to combine. Cover and refrigerate for 2 hours before serving.

Serve cold or at room temperature.

Serves 6

Per 3/4 cup (175 ml) serving: 192 cal, 4 g pro, 6 g total fat (1 g saturated fat), 30 g carb, 4 g fibre, 0 mg chol, 444 mg sodium

Excellent source of: vitamin A

Easy Lentil Salad

This is an easy salad to make, and it's loaded with flavour. It's a perfect dish for picnics and barbecues. The salad is best if made a day ahead, to allow the lentils to marinate.

1/3 cup	red wine vinegar	75 ml
2 tbsp	extra-virgin olive oil	25 ml
2 tsp	Dijon mustard	10 ml
2	19 oz/540 ml cans lentils, drained and rinsed	2
1	red bell pepper, seeded and diced	1
1/2	cucumber, diced	1/2
1	green onion, chopped	1

In a small bowl, whisk together vinegar, olive oil, and mustard.

In a large serving bowl, combine lentils, bell pepper, cucumber, and green onion. Drizzle with vinaigrette, tossing to coat.

Cover and refrigerate for at least 2 hours before serving. Serve cold.

Serves 8

Per 3/4 cup (175 ml) serving: 172 cal, 11 g pro, 4 g total fat (1 g saturated fat), 25 g carb, 5 g fibre, 0 mg chol, 18 mg sodium

Excellent source of: folate, vitamin C, iron

Good source of: fibre, vitamin A, magnesium

Kasha, Walnut, and Apple Salad with Fresh Mint

This flavourful and colourful whole-grain salad is as nice to look at as it is to eat. Ideally, make this salad a day or two in advance of serving to allow the flavours to blend. If you don't have seasoned rice vinegar, apple cider vinegar makes for a tasty alternative.

2	cups water	500 ml
1 cup	kasha	250 ml
1	apple, diced	1
1	carrot, shredded	1
1/4 cup	dried cranberries	50 ml
1/4 cup	walnuts, chopped	50 ml
1/4 cup	finely chopped fresh mint	50 ml
2	green onions, chopped	2
2 tbsp	seasoned rice vinegar	25 ml
2 tbsp	freshly squeezed lemon juice	25 ml
1 tbsp	Dijon mustard	15 ml
1 tbsp	extra-virgin olive oil	15 ml
1 tsp	honey	5 ml

In a large saucepan, heat water to a boil. Add kasha; cover and simmer for 10 to 12 minutes or until most of the liquid has been absorbed. Rinse kasha with cold water and set aside to cool.

Meanwhile, in large bowl, combine apple, carrot, cranberries, walnuts, mint, and green onions.

In a small bowl, whisk together rice vinegar, lemon juice, mustard, olive oil, and honey.

Toss kasha with apple mixture. Drizzle with dressing. Cover and refrigerate until ready to serve.

Serves 6

Per 3/4 cup (175 ml) serving: 190 cal, 5 g pro, 6 g total fat (1 g saturated fat), 32 g carb, 4 g fibre, 0 mg chol, 39 mg sodium

Excellent source of: vitamin A, magnesium

Good source of: fibre

Spicy Black Bean and Pepper Salad with Chili Dressing

Consider doubling this recipe—not only is it a hit at picnics and barbecues, but also its flavour gets even better after sitting in the refrigerator for a few days. If you like your food spicy, retain the jalapeño seeds.

1	19 oz/540 ml can black beans, drained and rinsed	1
1	red bell pepper, seeded and diced	1
1	green bell pepper, seeded and diced	1
1	small jalapeño, seeded and diced	1
1/2	red onion, chopped	1/2
2	fresh tomatoes, diced	2
1/2 cup	chopped cilantro	125 ml
1/4 cup	freshly squeezed lemon juice	50 ml
1 tbsp	extra-virgin olive oil	15 ml
3	cloves garlic, chopped	3
	freshly ground black pepper to taste	

In a large bowl, combine beans, bell peppers, jalapeño, onion, tomatoes, and cilantro.

In a small bowl, whisk together lemon juice, olive oil, garlic, and black pepper.

Toss bean mixture with dressing. Cover and refrigerate for at least 1 hour before serving, stirring occasionally. Serve cold.

Serves 4

Per 1 1/4 cup (300 ml) serving: 214 cal, 11 g pro, 4 g total fat (1 g saturated fat), 36 g carb, 10 g fibre, 0 mg chol, 13 mg sodium

Excellent source of: fibre, vitamin A, folate, vitamin C, magnesium

Good source of: vitamin K, iron, potassium

Wheat Berry Salad with Smoked Trout and Gingered Squash

Smoked trout paired with gingered squash makes for an incredible flavour combination. Serve this salad on its own cold, or heat, bundled in Swiss chard leaves.

Miso is a thick paste made from fermented soybeans. It adds a unique flavour to salad dressings, marinades, baked tofu, and vegetable dishes. You'll find miso in the refrigerator section of Asian grocery stores and natural food stores.

3 1/2 cups	water	875 ml
1/2 tsp	salt	2 ml
1 cup	wheat berries	250 ml
4 oz	smoked trout	120 g
1	carrot, shredded	1
2 cups	Roasted Gingered Squash (p. 326)	500 ml
1	green onion, chopped	1
2 tsp	minced gingerroot	10 ml
2 tsp	frozen orange juice concentrate	10 ml
1 tsp	miso	5 ml

In a large pot, bring salted water to a boil. Add wheat berries; cover and simmer for 60 to 70 minutes or until wheat berries are tender and slightly chewy. Drain and rinse berries under cold water.

When wheat berries are cool, transfer to a large bowl. Toss with trout, carrot, squash, and green onion.

In a small bowl, whisk together gingerroot, orange juice concentrate, and miso. Drizzle over wheat berry mixture.

Serve cold, or wrap 1/4 cup (50 ml) of the salad in a Swiss chard leaf, making a small bundle; bake at 350°F (180°C) until heated through.

Serves 6

Per 1 cup (250 ml) serving: 214 cal, 11 g pro, 4 g total fat (1 g saturated fat), 37 g carb, 5 g fibre, 14 mg chol, 246 mg sodium

Excellent source of: vitamin A

Good source of: fibre, vitamin C, iron, magnesium

Soups

Creamy Cold Berry Soup

This anthocyanin-rich soup is a colourful addition to any meal—as a starter or a dessert. Or eat it as a snack, or even breakfast. Just about any type of berry can be substituted for the strawberries or blueberries.

2 cups	fresh strawberries, washed and trimmed	500 ml
1	pear, peeled and cored	1
1/2 cup	blueberries	125 ml
1/2 cup	pure pomegranate juice	125 ml
1 1/2 cups	low-fat (1% MF or less) plain yogurt	375 ml
	fresh mint sprigs, as garnish	

In batches, blend strawberries, pear, blueberries, pomegranate juice, and yogurt. Combine blended ingredients in a large bowl. Refrigerate until ready to serve.

Garnish with sprigs of fresh mint.

Serve cold.

Serves 4

Per 1 cup (250 ml) serving: 127 cal, 5 g pro, 1 g total fat (0 g saturated fat), 26 g carb, 4 g fibre, 2 mg chol, 69 mg sodium

Excellent source of: vitamin C

Good source of: fibre, calcium

Curried Pumpkin Soup

The combination of orange juice, pumpkin, and curry powder gives this soup a creamy consistency and rich flavour. But the best part is that it's low in sodium: Per serving, this soup contains about one-third of the sodium as most commercial soups.

Using less broth—or in this, case fewer bouillon cubes—and more spices results in a soup that has plenty of flavour without the added sodium.

Tip: This recipe calls for soy milk, which can be substituted with 1% or skim milk. Add the milk at the end of cooking to prevent it from curdling. This soup also freezes well, handy to have on hand for brown-bag lunches or a warm meal when you're in a hurry.

1 tsp	canola oil	5 ml
1	onion, finely chopped	1
8 cups	water	2 L
2	1/2 oz/11 g vegetable bouillon cubes	2
1	28 oz/796 ml can pure pumpkin purée	1
1 cup	orange juice	250 ml
1 tbsp	curry powder	15 ml
1 tsp	cumin	5 ml
1 tsp	coriander	5 ml
1 cup	unflavoured soy milk	250 ml
	freshly ground black pepper to taste	
	fresh cilantro sprigs, as garnish	

In a large pan, heat oil over medium heat. Add onion; sauté for 5 to 6 minutes or until onion is golden yellow.

Add water, bouillon cubes, pumpkin purée, orange juice, curry powder, cumin, and coriander. Cover and simmer for 10 minutes. Remove from heat and stir in soy milk.

Season with black pepper. Garnish with fresh cilantro and serve.

Serves 8

Per 1 1/2 cup (375 ml) serving: 84 cal, 3 g pro, 2 g total fat (0 g saturated fat), 16 g carb, 4 g fibre, 0 mg chol, 488 mg sodium

Excellent source of: vitamin A, vitamin C

Good source of: fibre, vitamin K, iron, magnesium

French Onion Soup

With only 153 calories and 369 milligrams of sodium per serving, this version of French onion soup is much healthier than most traditional recipes. Another bonus: This soup is a breeze to make and freezes well. Serve with whole-grain crusty bread.

2 tbsp	canola oil	25 ml
3 lbs	onions (about 6 large), sliced	1.4 kg
3	cloves garlic, chopped	3
6 cups	water	1.5 L
4	4.5 g reduced-sodium beef bouillon sachets	4
1/2 cup	dry red wine	125 ml
	freshly ground black pepper to taste	

Heat oil in a large saucepan over medium heat. Add onions; sauté for 10 minutes or until golden yellow. Add garlic; sauté for another 1 to 2 minutes.

Add water, bouillon cubes, red wine, and black pepper; bring to a boil. Cover and simmer for 10 minutes.

Serves 6

Per 1 1/2 cup (375 ml) serving: 153 cal, 3 g pro, 5 g total fat (0 g saturated fat), 22 g carb, 4 g fibre, 0 mg chol, 369 mg sodium

Excellent source of: vitamin K

Good source of: fibre, vitamin C

Hearty Minestrone Soup

This hearty bean and whole-grain soup is truly a meal in a bowl. The combination of wild rice, beans, and veggies results in a tasty soup that's low in fat and high in fibre. This soup freezes extremely well—I suggest freezing it in individual portions, ready to grab to take to work or school for lunch.

1 tbsp	canola oil	15 ml
1	onion, chopped	1
3	cloves garlic, chopped	3
8 cups	water	2 L
1 tbsp	tomato paste	15 ml
1	carrot, chopped	1
1/4 cup	uncooked wild rice	50 ml
1	28 oz/796 ml can diced tomatoes	1
1	19 oz/540 ml can chickpeas, drained and rinsed	1
1	19 oz/540 ml can kidney beans, drained and rinsed	1
6	Brussels sprouts, trimmed and halved	6
1/2	zucchini, sliced	1/2
3 tbsp	sodium-reduced soy sauce	50 ml
2 cups	sliced bok choy	500 ml
2 tbsp	chopped fresh basil	25 ml
	freshly ground black pepper, to taste	

In a large saucepan, heat oil over medium heat. Add onions; sauté for 4 to 5 minutes or until golden brown. Add garlic; sauté for 1 minute.

Add water, tomato paste, carrot, wild rice, tomatoes, chickpeas, kidney beans, Brussels sprouts, zucchini, and soy sauce. Cover and simmer for 55 minutes or until rice is tender.

Add bok choy and basil. Season with black pepper. Simmer for 5 minutes.

Serves 8

Per 1 1/2 cup (375 ml) serving: 235 cal, 12 g pro, 3 g total fat (0 g saturated fat), 43 g carb, 7 g fibre, 0 mg chol, 817 mg sodium

Excellent source of: fibre, vitamin A, folate, vitamin C, iron, magnesium

Good source of: vitamin K, calcium, potassium

Moroccan Lentil Soup

The secret to making this soup is puréeing it to the right consistency; the cooked lentils will give it a rich, creamy texture. Adjust cayenne pepper to taste, keeping in mind that this soup tends to get slightly spicer after being refrigerated.

1 tbsp	canola oil	15 ml
1	onion, chopped	1
2	cloves garlic, chopped	2
1 tbsp	chopped gingerroot	15 ml
8 cups	water	2 L
1 cup	dried brown lentils, rinsed and picked over	250 ml
1 cup	chopped carrots	250 ml
1	28 oz/796 ml can plum tomatoes	1
3 tbsp	freshly squeezed lemon juice	50 ml
1 tsp	salt	5 ml
1 tsp	turmeric	5 ml
1/8 tsp	cayenne pepper, or to taste	0.5 ml
1/8 tsp	cinnamon	0.5 ml
	freshly ground black pepper to taste	

Heat oil in a large saucepan over medium heat. Add onion; sauté until softened and lightly brown, about 4 to 5 minutes. Add garlic and gingerroot; sauté 1 minute. Add water, lentils, carrots, tomatoes, lemon juice, turmeric, cayenne pepper, cinnamon, and salt. Stir to combine. Season with black pepper.

Cover and simmer for 60 minutes. Remove from heat. Purée using a hand blender until carrots and lentils are a uniform creamy consistency.

Serves 8

Per 1 1/2 cup (375 ml) serving: 141 cal, 8 g pro, 2 g total fat (0 g saturated fat), 24 g carb, 5 g fibre, 0 mg chol, 458 mg sodium

Excellent source of: vitamin A, folate, vitamin C, vitamin K, iron

Good source of: fibre, magnesium

Mushroom Leek Soup

This soup uses low-sodium soy sauce in place of vegetable broth. As a result, it's low in sodium—fewer than 300 milligrams per serving. That's hard to beat for soup! Although I usually use white button mushrooms for this recipe, other varieties would also work well—try cremini, portobello, or shiitake.

Tip: The longer you cook the mushrooms and leeks, the more flavourful the soup will be. Make this recipe a few days in advance, as it always tastes better after sitting in the refrigerator for at least one day.

1 tbsp	canola oil	15 ml
2	leeks	2
8 cups	sliced mushrooms	2 L
2 tbsp	all-purpose flour	25 ml
1/8 tsp	cayenne pepper, or to taste	0.5 ml
4 cups	water	1 L
2 cups	skim milk or non-flavoured soy milk	500 ml
2 tbsp	sodium-reduced soy sauce	25 ml

Heat oil in a large saucepan over medium heat. Wash the leeks well to remove sand, trim ends, and slice. Add leeks and mushrooms to pan; sauté until tender, about 10 minutes.

Add flour and cayenne pepper, stir to blend. Gradually pour in water, stirring frequently until the mixture begins to thicken.

Cover and simmer for 30 minutes. Remove from heat and stir in milk and soy sauce. Using a hand blender, purée until smooth.

Serves 6

Per 1 1/2 cup (375 ml) serving: 115 cal, 7 g pro, 4 g total fat (1 g saturated fat), 16 g carb, 2 g fibre, 3 mg chol, 219 mg sodium

Excellent source of: vitamin K

Good source of: iron

Side Dishes

Grains

Mushroom Barley Casserole

Some liquid may be left on the bottom of the pan after cooking this casserole, but don't worry—the barley will quickly absorb it.

2 tbsp	canola oil	25 ml
1	large onion, chopped	1
4 cups	sliced mushrooms of your choice	1 L
1 tbsp	balsamic vinegar	15 ml
1 cup	pot barley	250 ml
2 1/2 cups	water	625 ml
1 tsp	thyme	5 ml
	freshly ground black pepper to taste	

Preheat oven to 375°F (190°C).

Heat 1 tbsp (15 ml) of the oil in a skillet over medium heat. Add onion and mushrooms; sauté until onions are brown and mushrooms begin to dry out. Transfer mushroom mixture to a glass baking dish.

Add the vineger to the skillet, then scrape the bottom to lift up any onion and mushroom bits. Pour vinegar mixture into the baking dish.

Heat the remaining 1 tbsp (15 ml) of oil in skillet over medium heat. Add barley; sauté until lightly brown. Add toasted barley to mushroom mixture. Add water to baking dish; season with thyme and black pepper. Cover and bake for 60 to 65 minutes or until barley is soft.

Serve warm or cold.

Serves 6

Per 1 cup (250 ml) serving: 184 cal, 5 g pro, 5 g total fat (0 g saturated fat), 31 g carb, 4 g fibre, 0 mg chol, 10 mg sodium

Excellent source of: vitamin K

Good source of: fibre

Quinoa-Stuffed Peppers

Pale yellow quinoa is the most widely available variety of this high-protein whole grain, though some natural food stores carry a dark reddish-brown variety. Both are prepared the same way. If you want a more colourful dish, use equal parts yellow and red quinoa.

6	small red bell peppers	6
2 cups	cooked quinoa	500 ml
1/2 cup	chopped onion	125 ml
3	cloves garlic, chopped	3
1	carrot, shredded	1
2 tbsp	chopped chives	25 ml
1 tbsp	chopped fresh basil	15 ml
1 tbsp	freshly squeezed lemon juice	15 ml

Preheat oven to 375°F (190°C).

Cut off and reserve the tops of the bell peppers. Scoop out and discard the seeds.

In a large bowl, combine quinoa, onion, garlic, carrot, chives, basil, and lemon juice. Stuff each pepper with the quinoa mixture, evenly distributing the mixture among the peppers. Place a reserved top on each of the peppers.

Gently place the peppers in a glass baking dish. Bake for 30 minutes. If the peppers begin to burn on the bottom, add about 2 tbsp (25 ml) water to the baking dish.

Serves 6

Per stuffed pepper: 276 cal, 10 g pro, 4 g total fat (0 g saturated fat), 54 g carb, 7 g fibre, 0 mg chol, 21 mg sodium

Excellent source of: fibre, vitamin A, vitamin C, iron, magnesium

Good source of: potassium

Vegetables

Balsamic Swiss Chard

Swiss chard with pale green stems is the most common kind available in grocery stores. You can also find rainbow and ruby chard—with brightly coloured red and yellow stems respectively—at most farmers' markets during the summer.

If you grow Swiss chard in your garden, you probably know that it often grows faster than you can eat it. If this is the case, double or triple this recipe and freeze the leftovers so you can enjoy the bounty of your garden throughout the winter months.

1 tsp	canola oil	5 ml
2	cloves garlic, minced	2
1	large bunch of chard (Swiss, rainbow, or ruby), washed and trimmed (about 6 cups/1.5 L)	1
1 tbsp	balsamic vinegar	15 ml
	freshly ground black pepper to taste	

Heat oil in a skillet over medium heat. Add garlic; sauté for 1 minute. Add Swiss chard; cover and steam for 4 to 5 minutes, until chard begins to wilt. Remove from heat, sprinkle with vinegar. Season with black pepper.

Serves 4

Per 1/2 cup (125 ml) serving: 23 cal, 1 g pro, 1 g total fat (0 g saturated fat), 3 g carb, 1 g fibre, 0 mg chol, 116 mg sodium

Good source of: vitamin C, magnesium

Broccoli with Sesame Thai Dressing

The combination of rice wine vinegar, sesame oil, gingerroot, and sesame seeds is a perfect match for broccoli. When sautéing the broccoli, be careful not to overcook it—it should be slightly crunchy. Overcooked broccoli will become soggy once dressed.

1 tsp	canola oil	5 ml
3	cloves garlic, chopped	3
3 cups	broccoli, cut into bite-sized pieces	750 ml
1 tbsp	seasoned rice wine vinegar	15 ml
1 tbsp	dark sesame oil	15 ml
1 tsp	chopped gingerroot	5 ml
1 tbsp	sesame seeds	15 ml

Heat oil in a skillet over medium heat. Add garlic and broccoli; sauté until garlic is fragrant and broccoli is tender, about 4 to 5 minutes.

Transfer broccoli to a large bowl; set aside to cool.

Meanwhile, in a small bowl, whisk together rice wine vinegar, sesame oil, and gingerroot. Drizzle over broccoli. Sprinkle sesame seeds on top. Serve warm or cold.

Serves 6

Per 1/2 cup (125 ml) serving: 127 cal, 10 g pro, 5 g total fat (1 g saturated fat), 18 g carb, 8 g fibre, 0 mg chol, 86 mg sodium

Excellent source of: fibre, vitamin A, folate, vitamin C, vitamin K, iron, magnesium

Good source of: potassium

Cilantro-Stuffed Grilled Avocados

This attractive dish pairs well with grilled chicken, white fish, or steak. Although avocado is technically a fruit, this side dish can be served in lieu of a vegetable. Use medium-firm avocados for best results.

Avocado:

3	avocados	3
2 tbsp	freshly squeezed lime juice	25 ml
1/2 tsp	light olive oil	2 ml

Tomato filling:

1	tomato, diced	1
2	cloves garlic, minced	2
1/4 cup	finely chopped cilantro	50 ml
1/4 tsp	red pepper flakes	1 ml

Preheat grill to medium.

Halve and pit the avocadoes, but keep the skin on.

In a small bowl, whisk together lime juice and oil; rub on each avocado half.

Gently place avocados face down on grill. Grill for 2 to 3 minutes or until lightly brown. Remove from heat; set aside to cool.

Meanwhile, in a small bowl, combine tomato, garlic, cilantro, and red pepper flakes. Fill each avocado half with tomato mixture.

Serve chilled or at room temperature.

Serves 6

Per 1/2 stuffed avocado: 173 cal, 2 g pro, 16 g total fat (3 g saturated fat), 9 g carb, 5 g fibre, 0 mg chol, 13 mg sodium

Good source of: fibre, folate, vitamin C, vitamin E, magnesium

Cinnamon Sweet Potato Bake with Toasted Pecan Topping

Warm sweet potatoes mixed with cinnamon and pecans probably conjure up images of Thanksgiving and cool autumn weather. But I assure you this antioxidant-rich dish is a treat all year round. This dish can be assembled ahead of time, frozen, and then baked (no need to thaw first) whenever you want.

2	medium sweet potatoes, peeled	2
1/4 cup	pecans	50 ml
2 tbsp	orange juice	25 ml
1 tsp	cinnamon	5 ml
1/2 tsp	allspice	2 ml
2 tbsp	ground flaxseed	25 ml

Preheat oven to 375°F (190°C).

Cut each sweet potato into 6 to 8 pieces. Place in a large pot and cover with water. Bring water to boil over high heat; reduce heat and simmer for 20 minutes or until sweet potatoes are tender. Drain potatoes and transfer to a mixing bowl.

Spread pecans on a baking sheet; bake 5 to 7 minutes or until lightly brown and fragrant.

While the pecans are toasting, mash the sweet potatoes with the orange juice, cinnamon, and allspice, until thoroughly combined. Spread potato mixture into a 4.5 x 8.5 inch (1.5 L) glass loaf pan.

Let toasted pecans cool, then coarsely grind in a food processor. Combine pecans with flaxseed. Spread pecan mixture on top of potatoes.

Bake for 30 minutes or until the casserole lightly browns on top.

Serves 4

Per 1 cup (250 ml) serving: 128 cal, 2 g pro, 7 g total fat (1 g saturated fat), 17 g carb, 4 g fibre, 0 mg chol, 38mg sodium

Excellent source of: beta carotene

Good source of: fibre

Garlic Roasted Brussels Sprouts

If members of your family turn up their noses at Brussels sprouts, this recipe is sure to change their opinion. Roasting these humble sprouts mellows their earthy flavour—they taste almost like an entirely different vegetable.

Cooking time depends largely on the size of the sprouts, so keep an eye on them. They're done when they can be easily pierced with a fork.

2 cups	Brussels sprouts, ends trimmed	500 ml
2 tsp	light olive oil	10 ml
2	cloves garlic, chopped	2
	freshly ground black pepper to taste	

Preheat oven to 400°F (20°C).

In a bowl, toss Brussels sprouts with oil and garlic. Season with black pepper. Transfer to a baking sheet. Bake for 25 minutes or until Brussels sprouts are tender when pricked with a fork.

Serves 4

Per 1/2 cup (125 ml) serving: 66 cal, 4 g pro, 3 g total fat (0 g saturated fat), 10 g carb, 4 g fibre, 0 mg chol, 26 mg sodium

Excellent source of: vitamin C

Good source of: fibre, folate, vitamin K

Garlic Sautéed Spinach

Although 8 cups (2 L) of spinach may sound like a lot, it wilts and quickly reduces in volume when cooked. If you have other leafy greens on hand, such as Swiss chard or kale, substitute for a portion of the spinach, if you like. Keep in mind, however, that kale and chard take a little longer to cook than spinach, so add them to the pan a minute or two before the spinach.

1 tsp	light olive oil	5 ml
2	cloves garlic, minced	2
8 cups	spinach (about 1 lb/450 g)	2 L
	freshly ground black pepper to taste	

Heat oil in a skillet over medium heat. Add garlic; sauté for 1 minute. Add spinach; cover and steam for 3 to 4 minutes or until spinach begins to wilt.

Remove from heat. Season with black pepper.

Serves 4

Per 1/4 cup (50 ml) serving: 37 cal, 3 g pro, 2 g total fat (0 g saturated fat), 4 g carb, 3 g fibre, 0 mg chol, 89 mg sodium

Excellent source of: vitamin A, folate, vitamin C, vitamin K, iron, magnesium

Honey Dijon Carrots

This quick beta carotene–rich side dish feeds a crowd. If you're a mustard fan, try making this recipe with different variations of mustard, such as whole grain or honey Dijon.

4 cups	sliced carrots	1 L
1 tbsp	honey	15 ml
1 tsp	Dijon mustard	5 ml
	freshly ground black pepper to taste	

Fill a medium saucepan with water. Add carrots and bring to a boil. Reduce heat; simmer until carrots are tender, about 8 to 10 minutes.

Drain carrots. Stir in honey and mustard. Season with black pepper.

Serves 8

Per 1/2 cup (125 ml) serving: 55 cal, 1 g pro, 0 g total fat (0 g saturated fat), 13 g carb, 3 g fibre, 0 mg chol, 44 mg sodium

Excellent source of: beta carotene

Good source of: vitamin K

Maple Mashed Sweet Potatoes

I'm convinced orange zest and sweet potatoes were meant to be paired together, and I think you'll agree after tasting this dish. For a lower sugar version, substitute the maple syrup with orange juice.

2	large sweet potatoes, peeled and quartered	2
1 tsp	canola oil	5 ml
2 tbsp	maple syrup	25 ml
	zest of 1/2 orange	

Preheat oven to 375°F (190°C).

In a bowl, toss sweet potatoes with oil to coat. Transfer to a baking sheet. Bake for 45 minutes or until tender.

Transfer potatoes to a large bowl. Add maple syrup and orange zest. With a potato masher, mash potatoes to a smooth consistency.

Serves 4

Per 1 cup (250 ml) serving: 92 cal, 1 g pro, 1 g total fat (0 g saturated fat), 20 g carb, 2 g fibre, 0 mg chol, 37 mg sodium

Excellent source of: vitamin A

Oven-Roasted Root Vegetables

This is a basic recipe for roasted vegetables—feel free to substitute or add any other root vegetables you have on hand. Before serving, add lemon zest for a burst of flavour and phytochemicals. (Remember those limonoids you read about earlier in the book?)

4	carrots	4
2	parsnips	2
1	sweet potato	1
1/2	turnip	1/2
2	stalks celery	2
12	scrubbed baby red potatoes	12
2	small onions, quartered	2
1 tsp	peppercorns	5 ml
5	cloves garlic	5
2	bay leaves	2
2 tbsp	light olive oil	25 ml
2 tbsp	chopped fresh rosemary	25 ml
	freshly ground black pepper to taste	

Preheat oven to 375°F (190°C).

Peel the carrots, parsnips, sweet potato, and turnip. Cut, along with the celery, into 1 inch (2.5 cm) pieces.

In a 13 x 9 (3.5 L) glass baking dish, toss red potatoes and onion with the carrots, parsnips, sweet potato, turnip, celery, peppercorns, garlic, and bay leaves. Sprinkle oil and rosemary on top and toss vegetables again to coat. Season with black pepper.

Bake uncovered for 50 to 55 minutes or until vegetables are tender when pricked with a fork. If the baking dish begins to dry out during cooking, add a little water.

Serves 6

Per approximately 1 cup (250 ml) serving: 190 cal, 4 g pro, 5 g total fat (1 g saturated fat), 35 g carb, 6 g fibre, 0 mg chol, 81 mg sodium

Excellent source of: fibre, vitamin A, vitamin C

Good source of: magnesium, potassium

Oven-Roasted Tomatoes with Feta Cheese

This attractive side dish is easy to prepare and very flavourful. Although regular beefsteak or other common-variety tomatoes work well in this recipe, you can also substitute heirloom tomatoes, which come in a variety of colours—pink, yellow, purple, green, and orange. For a twist, drizzle lemon-infused olive oil over the tomatoes just before serving.

2	large tomatoes	2
	freshly ground black pepper to taste	
1/4 cup	low-fat feta cheese	50 ml
	few sprigs fresh basil leaves, finely chopped	

Preheat oven to 375°F (190°C).

Slice tomatoes in half lengthwise. Place, cut side up, in a glass baking dish. Season with black pepper.

In a small bowl, combine feta cheese and basil. Top each tomato with one-quarter of the feta mixture.

Cover with a foil tent; bake for 20 to 30 minutes.

Serves 4

Per serving: 55 cal, 3 g pro, 4 g total fat (2 g saturated fat), 4 g carb, 1 g fibre, 14 mg chol, 183 mg sodium

Pepper and Rapini Sauté

Rapini, also called broccoli raab, is a leafy green with a slightly nutty and bitter flavour. This recipe combines deep green rapini with bright red and yellow peppers for a burst of colour and taste. Green onions can be used in place of the chives.

4 cups	rapini, trimmed and cut into 1 inch/2.5 cm pieces	1 L
1 tsp	canola oil	5 ml
2	cloves garlic, minced	2
1	red bell pepper, seeded and chopped	1
1	yellow bell pepper, seeded and chopped	1
2 tbsp	chopped chives	25 ml
	freshly ground black pepper to taste	

Bring a large pot of water to a boil.

Add rapini to pot and boil until tender but still brightly coloured, about 5 minutes. Remove from heat and drain.

Heat oil in a skillet over medium heat. Add garlic; sauté for 1 to 2 minutes.

Add bell peppers and rapini; sauté for 5 to 6 minutes or until tender. Remove from heat. Toss with the chives. Season with black pepper.

Serves 4

Per 3/4 cup (175 ml) serving: 46 cal, 3 g pro, 2 g total fat (0 g saturated fat), 8 g carb, 2 g fibre, 0 mg chol, 17 mg sodium

Excellent source of: vitamin A, vitamin C, vitamin K

Good source of: folate

Raspberry Grilled Kale

Here, the peppery taste of kale complements the sweet fresh raspberries. The contrast between the deep green leaves and bright red berries make for an attractive dish. Although the recipe calls for the kale to be placed directly on the grill, you can also use a grilling basket. Either way, be sure to keep an eye on the kale to ensure it doesn't burn.

12	large kale leaves, washed and patted dry	12
6 tbsp	raspberry-flavoured vinegar	100 ml
2 tbsp	canola oil	25 ml
4	cloves garlic, chopped	4
	freshly ground black pepper to taste	
1/2 cup	fresh raspberries	125 ml

Preheat grill to medium.

Place kale in a large bowl, and toss with vinegar, oil, garlic, and black pepper.

Place kale directly on grill. Turn once every minute until kale is slightly wilted and brown around the edges, about 5 to 7 minutes, being careful not to let it burn. Remove from heat.

When kale leaves are cool, roughly shred leaves into bite-sized pieces, discarding the tough stem.

Toss kale with fresh raspberries. Serve warm or cold.

Alternatively, shred kale after washing and rinsing. Place leaves in a grilling basket and drizzle with vinegar, oil, and garlic. Season with black pepper. Grill kale until it is slightly wilted. Remove from heat and toss with the raspberries.

Serves 4

Per 1/2 cup (125 ml) serving: 131 cal, 4 g pro, 8 g total fat (1 g saturated fat), 15 g carb, 4 g fibre, 0 mg chol, 49 mg sodium

Excellent source of: vitamin A, vitamin C, vitamin E, vitamin K

Good source of: fibre, calcium, iron, magnesium

Roasted Cauliflower with Red Pepper

If you're looking for a new way to cook cauliflower, look no farther. Roasting the cauliflower produces an appealing light brown colour and nutty flavour. If you're not a fan of red bell peppers, you can just as easily leave them out, though they do add a splash of colour and make this recipe an excellent source of vitamin C.

1	head cauliflower, cut into florets	1
1	red bell pepper, cut into strips	1
2 tsp	canola oil	10 ml
1	clove garlic, chopped	1
	freshly ground black pepper to taste	

Preheat oven to 375°F (190°C).

In a large bowl, toss cauliflower, bell pepper, oil, and garlic. Season with black pepper. Spread mixture on a baking sheet. Bake for 30 to 40 minutes or until cauliflower begins to brown and is tender when pierced with a fork.

Serves 6

Per 1 cup (250 ml) serving: 46 cal, 2 g pro, 2 g total fat (0 g saturated fat), 7 g carb, 2 g fibre, 0 mg chol, 31 mg sodium

Excellent source of: vitamin A, vitamin C

Good source of: folate

Roasted Gingered Squash

Roasting the squash with gingerroot and orange zest adds plenty of mouth-watering flavour. This squash tastes wonderful in the Wheat Berry Salad with Smoked Trout and Gingered Squash (page 303).

2 cups	butternut squash, diced (about 1 squash)	500 ml
2 tbsp	finely sliced gingerroot	25 ml
2 tbsp	honey	25 ml
1 tbsp	orange zest	15 ml
1 tsp	light olive oil	5 ml

Preheat oven to 375°F (190°C).

Cut squash into 1 inch (2.5 cm) cubes. In a large bowl, toss squash with gingerroot, honey, orange zest, and oil.

Spread squash on a baking sheet and bake for 30 to 40 minutes, until tender.

Serve immediately, or cool and use in Wheat Berry Salad with Smoked Trout and Gingered Squash (page 303).

Serves 4

Per 1/2 cup (125 ml) serving: 83 cal, 1 g pro, 1 g total fat (0 g saturated fat), 19 g carb, 1 g fibre, 0 mg chol, 4 mg sodium

Excellent source of: beta carotene

Good source of: vitamin C

Spicy Sautéed Collard Greens

This recipe is an easy way to use collard greens, a leafy green that's rich in calcium, folate, vitamin K, and the phytochemical lutein. If you don't have fresh lemons on hand, substitute an acidic liquid, such as balsamic vinegar or apple cider vinegar.

1 tbsp	canola oil	15 ml
2	cloves garlic, minced	2
1 lb	collard greens (about 2 bunches), chopped	450 g
2 tbsp	freshly squeezed lemon juice	25 ml
1/4 tsp	red pepper flakes	1 ml
1/8 tsp	coarse sea salt	0.5 ml
	freshly ground black pepper to taste	

Heat oil in a skillet over medium heat. Add garlic; sauté for 1 minute. Add collard greens, sautéing for 4 to 5 minutes or until greens are wilting and tender. If pan begins to dry out, add 2 tbsp (25 ml) water.

When greens are wilted, season with lemon juice, red pepper flakes, sea salt, and black pepper.

Serves 4

Per 1/2 cup (125 ml) serving: 69 cal, 3 g pro, 4 g total fat (0 g saturated fat), 8 g carb, 4 g fibre, 0 mg chol, 98 mg sodium

Excellent source of: vitamin A, folate, vitamin C, vitamin K

Good source of: fibre, calcium

Spicy Sweet Potato Wedges

This is one of those easy-to-make recipes that guests of all ages will love. Turn the potatoes once or twice while baking to prevent them from burning. Try them dipped in Jalapeño Guacamole (page 358).

2	medium sweet potatoes, peeled	2
2 tsp	canola oil	10 ml
2 tsp	cumin seeds	10 ml
1/8 tsp	cayenne pepper, or to taste	0.5 ml
1/8 tsp	coarse sea salt	0.5 ml
	freshly ground black pepper to taste	

Preheat oven to 375°F (190°C).

Cut each sweet potato into 8 wedges. In a bowl, toss sweet potato wedges with oil to coat. Add cumin seeds, cayenne pepper, and sea salt. Season with black pepper. Toss to mix.

Spread potato wedges on a baking sheet. Bake for 35 to 45 minutes, turning once or twice, until potatoes are slightly crispy and tender.

Serves 4

Per 4 wedges (1/2 sweet potato): 89 cal, 1 g pro, 3 g total fat (3 g saturated fat), 14 g carb, 2 g fibre, 0 mg chol, 113 mg sodium

Excellent source of: beta carotene

Good source of: vitamin K

Spinach with Spicy Peanut Sauce

The peanut sauce in this recipe tastes wonderful on spinach, but it can also be used on grilled vegetables or chicken breast. Or try it as a dipping sauce for Tempeh Vegetable Rolls (page 349).

1 tsp	canola oil	5 ml
2	cloves garlic, chopped	2
1 tbsp	minced gingerroot	15 ml
8 cups	spinach (about 1 lb/450 g)	2 L
2 tbsp	peanut butter	25 ml
2 tbsp	freshly squeezed lime juice	25 ml
1 tsp	sodium-reduced soy sauce	5 ml
pinch	cayenne pepper, or to taste	pinch

Heat oil in a skillet over medium heat. Add garlic and gingerroot; sauté for 1 minute. Add spinach, cover pan, and let steam for 2 to 3 minutes until wilted.

Meanwhile, in a small bowl, whisk together peanut butter, lime juice, soy sauce, and cayenne pepper.

When spinach is just wilted, pour peanut sauce into pan; heat for 30 seconds. Serve immediately.

Serves 4

Per 1/4 cup (50 ml) serving: 88 cal, 5 g pro, 6 g total fat (1 g saturated fat), 7 g carb, 4 g fibre, 0 mg chol, 168 mg sodium

Excellent source of: vitamin A, folate, vitamin C, vitamin K, iron, magnesium

Good source of: fibre, potassium

Tarragon Sautéed Cherry Tomatoes

This side dish is ready in 10 minutes or less and can be enjoyed warm or cold. You can substitute just about any fresh herbs—basil, thyme, oregano, even chives—for the tarragon; use whichever you have on hand.

1 tsp	light olive oil	5 ml
2	cloves garlic, chopped	2
4 cups	cherry tomatoes	1 L
2 tbsp	chopped fresh tarragon	25 ml
	freshly ground black pepper to taste	

Heat oil in a skillet over medium heat. Add garlic; sauté for 1 minute. Add tomatoes and tarragon; sauté for 3 to 4 minutes.

Remove from heat. Season with black pepper. Serve warm or cold.

Serves 4

Per 1/2 cup (125 ml) serving: 59 cal, 2 g pro, 2 g total fat (0 g saturated fat), 11 g carb, 3 g fibre, 0 mg chol, 20 mg sodium

Excellent source of: vitamin C, vitamin K

Good source of: vitamin A

Entrees

Fish, Meat, and Poultry

Cajun Breaded Trout

In this recipe, Cajun rub is paired with trout, but it works well with just about any type of fish, including salmon, tilapia, and sole. If you enjoy spicy food, increase the cayenne pepper to 1/4 teaspoon (1 ml).

4	4 oz/120 g trout fillets	4
1 tsp	canola oil	5 ml
1/4 cup	whole-wheat breadcrumbs	50 ml
2 tbsp	ground flaxseed	25 ml
1 tsp	chili powder	5 ml
1/2 tsp	garlic powder	2 ml
1/2 tsp	black pepper	2 ml
1/8 tsp	cayenne pepper	0.5 ml

Preheat oven to 375°F (190°C).

Lightly coat fillets with oil.

In a small bowl, combine breadcrumbs, flaxseed, chili powder, garlic powder, black pepper, and cayenne pepper. Pat the breadcrumb mixture onto the fillets.

Place fillets on a baking sheet lightly coated with cooking spray. Bake for 8 to 10 minutes or until fish flakes easily when tested with a fork.

Serves 4

Per fillet: 175 cal, 24 g pro, 7 g total fat (1 g saturated fat), 4 g carb, 1 g fibre, 65 mg chol, 39 mg sodium

Good source of: iron, magnesium

Coconut Curry Tilapia

This thick and creamy curry sauce is delicious with mild-flavoured tilapia. It also works well with chicken, chickpeas, and tofu.

1 tsp	canola oil	5 ml
1/2 tsp	cumin seeds	2 ml
2	cloves garlic, chopped	2
1 tsp	finely chopped gingerroot	5 ml
1 cup	crushed tomatoes	250 ml
1/2 cup	light coconut milk	125 ml
1/2 tsp	cumin	2 ml
1/2 tsp	turmeric	2 ml
1/8 tsp	chili powder	0.5 ml
4	4 oz/120 g tilapia fillets	4
1/4 cup	chopped cilantro	50 ml

Heat oil in a skillet over medium heat. Add cumin seeds; fry until they start to pop. Add garlic and gingerroot; sauté for 1 minute.

Add tomatoes, coconut milk, cumin, turmeric, and chili powder; stir to combine. Gently place fillets in sauce and cook for 8 to 10 minutes or until fish flakes easily when tested with a fork.

Sprinkle with cilantro and serve immediately.

Serves 4

Per fillet: 198 cal, 24 g pro, 9 g total fat (6 g saturated fat), 6 g carb, 1 g fibre, 57 mg chol, 148 mg sodium

Good source of: iron, magnesium

Easy Baked Pesto Salmon

This colourful dish is rich in heart-healthy omega-3 fats and requires next to no time to prepare. For the pesto, I suggest using Spinach Almond Pesto (page 370), but if you're pressed for time, a store-bought pesto will do just fine.

4	4 oz/120 g salmon fillets	4
2 tbsp	Spinach Almond Pesto (p. 370), or store-bought variety	25 ml
4	lemon wedges	4

Preheat oven to 375°F (190°C).

Place fillets in a baking dish and spread 1/2 tbsp (7 ml) pesto on each fillet. Bake for 8 to 10 minutes or until fish flakes easily when tested with a fork.

Serve each fillet with a lemon wedge.

Serves 4

Per fillet: 198 cal, 24 g pro, 11 g total fat (2 g saturated fat), 1 g carb, 1 g fibre, 63 mg chol, 50 mg sodium

Hoisin Chili Halibut

In this recipe, the hoisin and chili sauces are spread on the fish after it is cooked, to prevent them from burning. Hoisin sauce can be found in the ethnic food section of your grocery store. It's a staple item in my kitchen. The hoisin-chili combination also makes a great dipping sauce for Tempeh Vegetable Rolls (page 349).

4	4 oz/120 g halibut fillets	4
2 tbsp	hoisin sauce	25 ml
2 tbsp	sweet chili sauce	25 ml
1	green onion, thinly sliced	1

Preheat oven to 375°F (190°C).

Place fillets on a baking sheet lightly coated with cooking spray. Bake for 8 to 10 minutes or until fish flakes easily when tested with a fork.

Meanwhile, in a small bowl combine hoisin sauce, chili sauce, and green onions.

Evenly spread hoisin-chili mixture onto cooked fillets and serve.

Serves 4

Per fillet: 144 cal, 24 g pro, 3 g total fat (0 g saturated fat), 4 g carb, 0 g fibre, 37 mg chol, 191 mg sodium

Excellent source of: magnesium

Good source of: vitamin A

Lemon Dill Salmon

This simple yet elegant dish combines the flavours of dill and lemon with heart-healthy salmon. If you don't have fresh dill, substitute 2 teaspoons (10 ml) of dried dill. For added flavour, garnish each fillet with freshly grated lemon zest before serving.

4	4 oz/120 g salmon fillets	4
2	cloves garlic, chopped	2
2 tbsp	finely chopped fresh dill	25 ml
	freshly ground black pepper to taste	
4	lemon slices	4
	zest of 1/2 lemon to garnish, optional	

Preheat oven to 375°F (190°C).

Place fillets on a baking sheet lightly coated with cooking spray. Evenly sprinkle the fillets with the garlic and dill. Season with black pepper. Place a lemon slice on top of each fillet.

Bake for 8 to 10 minutes or until fish flakes easily when tested with a fork.

Garnish with lemon zest if desired.

Serves 4

Per fillet: 165 cal, 23 g pro, 7 g total fat (1 g saturated fat), 1 g carb, 0 g fibre, 63 mg chol, 51 mg sodium

Miso-Glazed Trout

Trout, a rich source of omega-3 fatty acids, is a great alternative to salmon. If you don't want the hassle of peeling and chopping fresh gingerroot, use puréed ginger (sold in jars)—it works especially well in this recipe, giving the sauce a thick consistency and creamy texture.

Tip: The miso sauce can double as a salad dressing.

4	4 oz/120 g trout fillets	4
4 tsp	chopped gingerroot	20 ml
4 tsp	frozen orange juice concentrate	20 ml
2 tsp	miso	10 ml
1 tbsp	chopped fresh chives	15 ml

Preheat oven to 375°F (190°C).

Place fillets on a baking sheet lightly coated with cooking spray and bake for 10 to 12 minutes or until fish flakes easily when tested with a fork.

Meanwhile, in a small bowl, whisk together gingerroot, orange juice concentrate, and miso. Pour sauce over cooked fillets; sprinkle with chives.

Serves 4

Per fillet: 151 cal, 24 g pro, 4 g total fat (1 g saturated fat), 3 g carb, 0 g fibre, 65 mg chol, 135 mg sodium

Good source of: vitamin C, iron

Spicy Sesame Salmon

The flavours of spicy chili sauce and tart lime juice go incredibly well with salmon. For extra flavour and a little unsaturated fat, sprinkle the cooked salmon with sesame seeds just before serving.

1 tsp	sesame oil	5 ml
2	cloves garlic, chopped	2
1 tbsp	chili garlic sauce	15 ml
1 tbsp	freshly squeezed lime juice	15 ml
4	4 oz/120 g salmon fillets	4
	sprigs fresh cilantro to garnish, optional	
	sesame seeds to garnish, optional	

In a small bowl, whisk together sesame oil, garlic, chili sauce, and lime juice.

Pour sesame-chili mixture over fillets and marinate for 20 minutes.

Heat a skillet over medium heat. Add salmon and sesame-chili marinade. Cook for 4 to 5 minutes per side or until fish flakes easily when tested with a fork.

Sprinkle with fresh cilantro and sesame seeds, if desired, and serve immediately.

Serves 4

Per fillet: 175 cal, 23 g pro, 8 g total fat (1 g saturated fat), 1 g carb, 0 g fibre, 63 mg chol, 51 mg sodium

Pork Tenderloin with Blackberry Dijon Sauce

This recipe combines the flavours of antioxidant-rich pomegranate, and blackberries, and a hint of clove with pork. The cayenne pepper lends a touch of heat. After adding the blackberries to the pan, you can either leave them whole or crush them with the back of a spoon to make the sauce slightly thicker.

1 tbsp	canola oil	15 ml
1 lb	pork tenderloin	450 g
3/4 cup	pure pomegranate juice	175 ml
2 tbsp	apple cider vinegar	25 ml
1 tbsp	maple syrup	15 ml
1 tsp	Dijon mustard	5 ml
1/8 tsp	cayenne pepper	0.5 ml
1/8 tsp	ground cloves	0.5 ml
2	green onions, chopped	2
2	cloves garlic, minced	2
1 cup	blackberries	250 ml

Heat oil in a skillet over medium-high heat. Add pork and, turning to brown well on all sides, cook through, about 18 to 22 minutes, depending on the shape of the tenderloin.

Meanwhile, in a small bowl whisk together pomegranate juice, vinegar, maple syrup, mustard, cayenne pepper, and cloves.

Transfer the cooked pork to a plate, cover, and set aside.

Reduce the heat under the pan to medium. Add the green onions and garlic to pan; cook for 1 to 2 minutes, until softened. Add the pomegranate juice mixture to the pan, scraping the bottom of the pan with a spatula to lift up all the browned bits of pork. Simmer for 3 to 4 minutes until liquid reduces and is slightly thickened.

Add blackberries and continue to simmer for 1 to 2 minutes.

Arrange pork on a serving dish. Drizzle with pomegranate-blackberry glaze. Serve immediately.

Serves 4

Per 1/4 lb (125 g) pork tenderloin and approximately 1/2 cup (125 ml) sauce: 238 cal, 28 g pro, 7 g total fat (1 g saturated fat), 17 g carb, 2 g fibre, 67 mg chol, 74 mg sodium

Excellent source of: vitamin K

Ginger-Orange Vegetable Stir-Fry with Chicken and Brown Rice

This tasty stir-fry combines ginger-infused whole-grain rice with a medley of power vegetables: bright orange, cruciferous, allium. The red pepper adds a hit of vitamin C. It's sure to please parents and kids alike.

1 1/2 cups	water	375 ml
2 tsp	chopped gingerroot	10 ml
3/4 cup	uncooked long-grain brown rice	175 ml
12 oz	chicken breast, boneless and skinless	340 g
1 tsp	sesame oil	5 ml
1	clove garlic, chopped	1
2 cups	roughly chopped bok choy	500 ml
1 cup	broccoli florets	250 ml
2	carrots, shredded	2
1	red bell pepper, chopped	1
2 tbsp	frozen orange juice concentrate	25 ml
1 tbsp	sodium-reduced soy sauce	15 ml

Bring water and 1 teaspoon (5 ml) of the gingerroot to a boil in a large saucepan. Add rice, cover, and simmer for 40 minutes or until most of the liquid is absorbed and rice is tender.

Meanwhile, preheat grill to medium. Grill chicken until cooked through (cooking time will depend on the thickness of the chicken breast).

Once both the rice and chicken are cooked, heat sesame oil in a large wok or skillet over medium heat. Add the remaining 1 teaspoon (5 ml) of the gingerroot and the garlic; sauté for 1 minute. Add bok choy, broccoli, carrots, and bell pepper; cook for 4 to 5 minutes, until vegetables are warmed through and bok choy is wilted.

Add orange juice concentrate and soy sauce, stirring until heated through, about 30 seconds.

Transfer rice, chicken, and vegetables to a large serving dish. Toss to combine.

Serves 4

Per 1/2 cup (125 ml) rice and 1/4 of the chicken and vegetables: 329 cal, 29 g pro, 4 g total fat (1 g saturated fat), 47 g carb, 8 g fibre, 49 mg chol, 254 mg sodium

Excellent source of: fibre, vitamin A, folate, vitamin C, vitamin K, iron, magnesium, potassium

Good source of: calcium

Kasha Cabbage Rolls

This recipe is a new take on a classic. The nutty-flavoured kasha (roasted buckwheat groats) means that these tasty cabbage rolls are high in fibre (13 grams per serving) The cabbage lends the disease-fighting phytochemicals of cruciferous vegetables.

These cabbage rolls freeze well after they've been baked—they're ideal to have on hand for quick, stress-free dinners and brown bag lunches.

12	medium cabbage leaves	12
1 lb	ground chicken, turkey, or soy ground round	450 g
2 cups	cooked, cooled kasha	500 ml
2 cups	chopped onion	500 ml
1/4 cup	ground flaxseed	50 ml
1 tbsp	basil	15 ml
1 tsp	red pepper flakes	5 ml
1 tsp	salt	5 ml
3	cloves garlic, chopped	3
2	eggs	2
2	28 oz/796 ml cans diced tomatoes	2
	freshly ground pepper to taste	

Preheat oven to 375°F (190°C).

Blanch cabbage leaves by plunging them into a pot of boiling water; remove them once they're slightly softened and wilted. Shake off any water.

In a large bowl, combine ground poultry, kasha, onion, flaxseed, basil, red pepper flakes, salt, garlic, and eggs.

Cover the bottom of a large Dutch oven with half of the tomatoes.

Scoop 1/2 cup (125 ml) of the kasha mixture onto one end of a cabbage leaf and roll up, firmly folding the ends under. Place roll in the Dutch oven. Continue making the rolls in this way until all the cabbage and kasha mixture is used up, arranging the rolls in the bottom of the pot in a snug single layer.

Pour remaining tomatoes over rolls. Season with black pepper.

Cover and bake for 2 to 2 1/2 hours or until tomato mixture in bubbling and meat is cooked through.

Makes 12 rolls

Serves 6

Per 2 cabbage rolls: 377 cal, 26 g pro, 6 g total fat (1 g saturated fat), 63 g carb, 13 g fibre, 56 mg chol, 826 mg sodium

Excellent source of: fibre, vitamin A, folate, vitamin C, iron, magnesium, potassium

Good source of: calcium

Legumes

Black Bean Burritos

This hearty Mexican-inspired dish is easy to make and sure to be a crowd-pleaser. At 12 grams of fibre each thanks to the beans and whole-wheat tortilla, these burritos are an outstanding source of fibre.

Tip: After wrapping the burritos, warm them on a hot grill for 2 to 3 minutes.

1 tsp	canola oil	5 ml
1	red bell pepper, seeded and diced	1
2 tsp	cumin	10 ml
2	cloves garlic, chopped	2
2 tbsp	freshly squeezed lime juice	25 ml
1/4 tsp	red pepper flakes	1 ml
1	19 oz/540 ml can black beans, drained and rinsed	1
1	fresh tomato, chopped	1
6	10 inch/25 cm whole-wheat tortillas	6
2 cups	spinach leaves, washed and dried	500 ml
1/2 cup	store-bought salsa	125 ml
1/2 cup	chopped cilantro	125 ml
1	avocado, pitted, peeled, and diced	1

Heat oil in a skillet over medium heat. Add bell pepper; sauté until softened, about 4 minutes. Stir in cumin and garlic; sauté for 1 minute.

Stir in lime juice, red pepper flakes, black beans, and tomato; reduce heat to medium-low. Continue to cook, stirring occasionally, until thickened, about 10 minutes. If mixture begins to dry out, add a little water.

Meanwhile, warm tortillas one at a time in a skillet over medium heat (about 1 minute each).

Divide bean mixture, spinach, salsa, cilantro, and avocado among the tortillas. Fold each tortilla over to create a wrap. Serve warm.

Serves 6

Per burrito: 365 cal, 13 g pro, 12 g total fat (2 g saturated fat), 55 g carb, 12 g fibre, 0 mg chol, 588 mg sodium

Excellent source of: fibre, vitamin A, folate, vitamin C, vitamin K, iron, magnesium

Good source of: potassium

Chickpea Curry

Here, the curry sauce is paired with chickpeas, but if you want, substitute another protein-rich food, such as lentils, chicken breast, or white fish, for the chickpeas.

1 tsp	canola oil	5 ml
6	black peppercorns	6
6	cloves	6
1	onion, chopped	1
1 tbsp	chopped gingerroot	15 ml
3	cloves garlic, chopped	3
2	19 oz/540 ml cans chickpeas, drained and rinsed	2
1 cup	crushed tomatoes	250 ml
1 cup	water	250 ml
2 tsp	coriander	10 ml
2 tsp	cumin	10 ml
1/2 tsp	each chili powder and turmeric	2 ml
1/4 cup	chopped cilantro	50 ml

Heat oil in a medium saucepan over medium heat. Add peppercorns and cloves; allow to sizzle. Add onion; sauté until golden brown, about 4 minutes. Add gingerroot and garlic; sauté for 1 minute.

Add chickpeas, tomatoes, water, coriander, cumin, chili powder, and turmeric. Stir to combine. Cover and simmer for 20 minutes.

Transfer to a serving plate and sprinkle with cilantro.

Serves 6

Per 1 cup (250 ml) serving: 259 cal, 10 g pro, 3 g total fat (0 g saturated fat), 49 g carb, 9 g fibre, 0 mg chol, 648 mg sodium

Excellent source of: fibre, folate, iron

Good source of: vitamin C, magnesium

Mushroom Lentil Patties

These patties are tasty on their own or served on a whole-grain bun with horseradish, fresh spinach leaves, sliced avocado, and tomato slices. Although I usually use white button mushrooms, crimini or shiitake mushrooms also work well in this recipe.

1 tbsp	canola oil	15 ml
1	small onion, chopped	1
4 cups	thinly sliced mushrooms	1 L
2 tbsp	balsamic vinegar	25 ml
2 cups	shredded carrot	500 ml
1 1/2 cups	cooked or canned (drained and rinsed) brown lentils	375 ml
1/2 cup	whole wheat breadcrumbs	125 ml
1/2 cup	rolled oats	125 ml
1/4 cup	ground flaxseed	50 ml
1/4 cup	slivered almonds, coarsely chopped	50 ml
2	eggs, beaten	2
1 tbsp	Dijon mustard	15 ml
1/2 tsp	coarse sea salt	2 ml
1/8 tsp	cayenne pepper, or to taste	0.5 ml
	freshly ground black pepper to taste	

Heat oil in a skillet over medium heat. Sauté onion for 4 to 5 minutes, until lightly brown. Add mushrooms; sauté for 8 to 10 minutes or until all the moisture from the mushrooms has evaporated. Transfer mushrooms and onions to a large mixing bowl.

Deglaze the skillet by pouring in the balsamic vinegar and scraping the bottom to lift up any onion or mushroom bits. Pour the vinegar mixture over the mushrooms.

Preheat oven to 350°F (180°C).

Add the carrot, lentils, breadcrumbs, oats, flaxseed, almonds, eggs, mustard, sea salt, and cayenne pepper to the bowl. Stir until well combined with the mushrooms and onions. Season with black pepper.

Spray a baking sheet with cooking spray. With your hands, form mushroom and lentil mixture into 8 patties. Place on baking sheet; bake for 20 to 25 minutes.

Serves 4

Per 2 patties: 206 cal, 10 g pro, 8 g total fat (1 g saturated fat), 27 g carb, 6 g fibre, 37 mg chol, 260 mg sodium

Excellent source of: fibre, vitamin A, folate, vitamin K, iron

Good source of: magnesium

Sesame-Crusted Tofu

Although the tofu in this recipe needs marinating for only 1 hour, it's even more flavourful when marinated overnight. Enjoy these tofu cutlets on their own, in a burrito, or as a sandwich filling.

1	12 oz/350 g pkg extra-firm tofu	1
2 tbsp	sodium-reduced soy sauce	25 ml
2 tbsp	freshly squeezed lime juice	25 ml
1 tbsp	sesame oil	15 ml
3	cloves garlic, chopped	3
1/4 cup	sesame seeds	50 ml
1 tbsp	canola oil	15 ml

Cut tofu widthwise into 1/4 inch (5 mm) thick strips—about 20 strips. Place in a glass baking dish.

In a small bowl, whisk together soy sauce, lime juice, sesame oil, and garlic.

Pour soy sauce mixture over tofu and let marinate for at least 1 hour (or cover and refrigerate overnight).

Spread sesame seeds onto a plate. Remove tofu from marinade one piece at a time and dredge in sesame seeds.

Heat oil in a skillet over medium heat. Add tofu and fry for 2 to 3 minutes per side or until slightly crispy.

Serves 4

Per 5 slices: 248 cal, 16 g pro, 19 g total fat (3 g saturated fat), 8 g carb, 2 g fibre, 0 mg chol, 256 mg sodium

Excellent source of: vitamin K, calcium, iron, magnesium

Tempeh Vegetable Rolls

Like tofu, tempeh is extremely versatile, taking on the flavour of whatever it is cooked with. There are different types of tempeh, including those made from quinoa and kasha. Any type can be used in this recipe. If you have Swiss chard in your vegetable crisper, consider substituting it for the spinach. Fresh mint leaves add a refreshing flavour when added to these rolls.

These tempeh rolls are perfect for dipping—try them with peanut sauce, the directions for which you'll find as part of the Spinach with Spicy Peanut Sauce recipe (page 329)—just leave out the spinach—or with hoisin chili sauce, the directions for which you'll find as part of the Hoisin Chili Halibut recipe (page 334).

1	8 1/2 oz/240 g block tempeh	1
1/2	8 3/4 ounce/250 g package vermicelli noodles	1/2
1 tsp	canola oil	5 ml
2	cloves garlic, chopped	2
1 tbsp	minced gingerroot	15 ml
1 tbsp	sodium-reduced soy sauce	15 ml
2 cups	whole spinach leaves	500 ml
1 cup	shredded carrot	250 ml
1 cup	chopped cilantro	250 ml
1	red bell pepper, cut into thin strips	1
12	9 inch/23 cm pieces rice paper	12

Cut tempeh into 1/4 inch (5 mm) thick strips; set aside.

Fill a large saucepan with water and bring to a boil. When water begins to boil, remove from heat. Soak noodles in the water for 2 to 3 minutes, until noodles become soft; drain.

Meanwhile, heat oil in a skillet over medium heat. Add garlic and ginger-root; sauté for 1 minute. Add tempeh and soy sauce; cook until tempeh is slightly crispy. Remove from heat.

Arrange the spinach, carrot, cilantro, and bell pepper within easy reach.

Fill a large bowl with lukewarm water. Add one piece of rice paper and gently move it around with your fingers until the paper is soft and flexible (about 30 seconds); remove from water, gently shaking off any excess moisture. Lay the rice paper on a plate.

In the middle of the rice paper, add a small handful (about 1/4 cup/50 ml) of noodles, a couple of strips of tempeh, a few spinach leaves, some shredded carrots, cilantro, and red peppers strips. Gently fold the top and bottom of the paper over the filling. Gently roll the remaining sides to make an enclosed pocket. Seal any seams with a dab of water.

Serve cold.

Serves 6

Per 2 rolls: 275 cal, 10 g pro, 5 g total fat (1 g saturated fat), 48 g carb, 5 g fibre, 1 mg chol, 393 mg sodium

Excellent source of: vitamin A, vitamin C, vitamin K

Good source of: fibre

Three Bean Garden Chili

This hearty meal is packed with fibre-rich legumes, providing 16 grams of fibre per serving. Cocoa and cinnamon give the chili a unique, subtle flavour that will leave your guests guessing at the secret ingredient that makes it tastes so good. This chili is a breeze to make and freezes well.

1 tbsp	canola oil	15 ml
1	large onion, chopped	1
3	cloves garlic, chopped	3
1	red bell pepper, seeded and diced	1
1	green bell pepper, seeded and diced	1
2	28 oz/796 ml cans diced tomatoes	2
1	19 oz/540 ml can kidney beans, drained and rinsed	1
1	19 oz/540 ml can black beans, drained and rinsed	1
1	19 oz/540 ml can chickpeas, drained and rinsed	1
1/2 cup	canned whole-kernel corn	125 ml
2–3 tbsp	chili powder	25–50 ml
2 tbsp	unsweetened cocoa	25 ml
1/2 tsp	cinnamon	2 ml
1/4 tsp	cayenne pepper	1 ml
1	carrot, chopped	1
2 tbsp	tomato paste	25 ml
	freshly ground black pepper to taste	

Heat oil in a large saucepan over medium heat. Add onion; sauté for 4 to 5 minutes or until golden brown. Add garlic and bell peppers; sauté for 2 to 3 minutes.

Add tomatoes, kidney beans, black beans, chickpeas, corn, chili powder, cocoa, cinnamon, cayenne pepper, carrot, and tomato paste. Stir to combine. Season with black pepper. Cover and simmer for 35 minutes.

Serves 8

Per 1 1/2 cup (375 ml) serving: 318 cal, 16 g pro, 4 g total fat (1 g saturated fat), 60 g carb, 16 g fibre, 0 mg chol, 789 mg sodium

Excellent source of: fibre, vitamin A, folate, vitamin C, iron, magnesium, potassium

Good source of: vitamin K, calcium

Wild Rice and Lentil Curry

This hearty curry casserole may take a while to cook, but you'll enjoy the aroma. Feel free to substitute long-grain brown rice for the wild rice, or white wine for the lemon juice.

1/2 cup	uncooked wild rice	125 ml
1/2 cup	dried brown lentils, rinsed and picked over	125 ml
4	cloves garlic, minced	4
1 tbsp	chopped gingerroot	15 ml
1	1 inch/2.5 cm cinnamon stick	1
1 tbsp	curry powder	15 ml
1/2 tsp	cumin	2 ml
2 cups	water	500 ml
1/2 cup	crushed canned tomatoes	125 ml
1/4 cup	freshly squeezed lemon juice	50 ml
1/2 tsp	coarse sea salt	2 ml
	freshly ground black pepper to taste	

Preheat oven to 350°F (180°C).

In an 8 x 8 inch (2 L) casserole dish, combine rice, lentils, garlic, ginger-root, cinnamon, curry powder, and cumin. Pour in the water, then add the tomatoes, lemon juice, and salt. Season with black pepper.

Cover and bake for 70 to 75 minutes, stirring 2 or 3 times.

Serves 4

Per 1 1/4 cup (300 ml) serving: 178 cal, 11 g pro, 1 g total fat (0 g saturated fat), 35 g carb, 5 g fibre, 0 mg chol, 369 mg sodium

Excellent source of: folate, vitamin K, iron

Good source of: fibre, vitamin C, magnesium

Pasta

Garden Vegetable Lasagna

This lycopene-rich and whole-grain lasagna incorporates plenty of vegetables, including spinach and beta carotene–rich carrots. Slices of zucchini and eggplant serve as an additional layer of "noodles."

Tip: This lasagna can be made so it's dairy-free—just omit the cheese and add an extra 1/2 cup (125 ml) water.

12	whole-wheat lasagna noodles	12
1	24 oz/700 ml jar low-fat pasta sauce	1
6	cloves garlic, minced	6
1 cup	low-fat ricotta cheese	250 ml
2	eggs	2
2 cups	fresh spinach leaves	500 ml
2 cups	sliced mushrooms	500 ml
1	eggplant, cut into long strips lengthwise	1
1	large zucchini, cut into long strips lengthwise	1
1	red bell pepper, diced	1
1 1/2 cups	shredded carrot	375 ml
1	bunch fresh basil, chopped	1
1/2 cup	low-fat grated Parmesan cheese	125 ml
1 cup	water	250 ml
	freshly ground black pepper to taste	

Cook lasagna noodles according to package directions.

Preheat oven to 375°F (190°C).

Combine pasta sauce and garlic.

In a small bowl, whisk together ricotta cheese and eggs.

Spread 1/4 cup (50 ml) pasta sauce on the bottom of a 15 x 10 inch (3.75 L) baking dish.

Arrange 4 noodles on the bottom of the dish, followed by one-third of the remaining sauce, and half of all the vegetables, basil, and cheese-and-egg mixture. Repeat layering with 4 more noodles, one-third of the sauce, and the remaining vegetables, basil, and cheese-and-egg mixture. Finish by laying 4 noodles, the remaining sauce, and Parmesan cheese on top. Sprinkle lasagna with freshly ground black pepper. Pour 1 cup (250 ml) water into the baking dish at the edge.

Cover and bake for 70 minutes. Uncover and continue to bake for 5 minutes, until cheese begins to bubble.

Serves 12

Per 3 3/4 x 3 1/3 inch (6 cm x 13 cm) piece: 285 cal, 18 g pro, 10 g total fat (5 g saturated fat), 31 g carb, 8 g fibre, 53 mg chol, 553 mg sodium

Excellent source of: fibre, vitamin A, vitamin C, vitamin K, calcium

Good source of: folate, magnesium

Spaghetti with Olive and Rosemary Sauce

This spaghetti sauce is chock-full of flavourful ingredients—garlic, olives, capers, and sun-dried tomatoes. Although a little goes a long way, it never hurts to double the recipe when making it and stores the extra in the freezer for no-fuss dinners later.

For an especially quick dinner, freeze individual portions of cooked whole-grain pasta. When you're ready to eat, just take the amount of pasta you need out of the freezer, pour boiling water over it, and let sit until heated through. Toss with sauce, and you're ready to go.

Feel free to substitute a whole-grain pasta of your choice for the spaghetti.

1 tbsp	canola oil	15 ml
1	small onion, chopped	1
3	cloves garlic, chopped	3
1	28 oz/796 ml can plum tomatoes	1
1/4 cup	chopped pitted black olives	50 ml
1 tbsp	capers	15 ml
1/4 cup	dry white wine	50 ml
1 tbsp	chopped sun-dried tomatoes	15 ml
	freshly ground black pepper to taste	
2 tbsp	chopped fresh rosemary	25 ml
2 tbsp	chopped fresh basil	25 ml

Heat oil in a saucepan over medium heat. Add onion; sauté for 4 to 5 minutes or until golden yellow. Add garlic; sauté 1 minute.

Stir in tomatoes, olives, capers, wine, and sun-dried tomatoes. Break up tomatoes with the back of a spoon; stir to combine with other ingredients. Season with black pepper. Cover and simmer for 30 minutes. Just before serving, stir in rosemary and basil.

Serve over whole-wheat spaghetti.

Serves 6

Per 2/3 cup (150 ml) sauce (not including pasta): 85 cal, 2 g pro, 3 g total fat (1 g saturated fat), 12 g carb, 2 g fibre, 0 mg chol, 515 mg sodium

Excellent source of: vitamin C

Dips, Salad Dressings, and Marinades

Dips

Creamy Dill Dip

This creamy dip is great with sliced fresh vegetables, or it can be used as a salad dressing or as a condiment for grilled salmon.

1 cup	low-fat (1% MF or less) plain yogurt	250 ml
2 tbsp	chopped fresh dill	25 ml
1 tbsp	freshly squeezed lemon juice	15 ml
1	clove garlic, minced	1

In a small bowl, combine yogurt, dill, lemon juice, and garlic. Cover and refrigerate until ready to serve.

Makes 1 cup (250 ml)

Serves 4

Per 1/4 cup (50 ml) serving: 33 cal, 3 g pro, 0 g total fat (0 g saturated fat), 5 g carb, 0 g fibre, 1 mg chol, 44 mg sodium

Jalapeño Guacamole

If you have ripe avocados on hand, this recipe makes for a great last-minute appetizer or mid-afternoon snack with baked tortilla chips. If you have avocados that aren't quite ripe, you can quicken the ripening process by storing them in a paper bag with a tomato. They should be ready to use within a day or two. Note that most of the heat in the jalapeño comes from the seeds. If you're a fan of spicy food, you can leave the seeds in, otherwise carefully discard them.

3	avocados, mashed	3
2	cloves garlic, minced	2
3 tbsp	freshly squeezed lime juice	50 ml
1	small jalapeño, finely chopped	1
1/8 tsp	coarse sea salt	0.5 ml

In a small bowl, combine avocado, garlic, lime juice, jalapeño, and salt. Mash to desired consistency.

Makes about 3 cups

Serves 6

Per 1/2 cup (125 ml) serving: 165 cal, 2 g pro, 15 g total fat (2 g saturated fat), 9 g carb, 5 g fibre, 0 mg chol, 60 mg sodium

Good source of: fibre, folate, vitamin C

Lemon Ginger Fruit Dip

This dip is an excellent accompaniment to Roasted Fruit Kebabs (page 382), or to slices of your favourite fresh fruit.

1 1/2 cups	low-fat (1% MF or less) vanilla yogurt	375 ml
2 tbsp	honey	25 ml
1 tsp	minced gingerroot	5 ml
	zest of 1/2 lemon	

In a bowl, combine yogurt, honey, gingerroot, and lemon zest. Cover and refrigerate until ready to serve.

Makes 1 1/2 cups (375 ml)

Serves 6

Per 1/4 cup (50 ml) serving: 57 cal, 3 g pro, 0 g total fat (0 g saturated fat), 11 g carb, 0 g fibre, 1 mg chol, 44 mg sodium

Lemon Hummus

This basic hummus is delicious just the way it is. If you're feeling adventurous, add fresh herbs, such as dill or lemon thyme. Or spice things up by adding chopped fresh jalapeño (it's up to you whether you include the seeds—just remember that they contain most of the heat found in the pepper). Tahini (ground sesame seed paste) is available in supermarkets, often in the ethnic foods section, and in natural food stores.

1/4 cup	tahini	50 ml
1/4 cup	freshly squeezed lemon juice	50 ml
1 tbsp	extra-virgin olive oil	15 ml
1	19 oz/540 ml can chickpeas, drained and rinsed	1
2	cloves garlic, minced	2

In a food processor, process tahini, lemon juice, olive oil, and chickpeas, and garlic to a smooth consistency. If hummus is too thick, add 1 tbsp (15 ml) water.

Makes 1 1/2 cups (375 ml)

Serves 6

Per 1/4 cup (50 ml) serving: 190 cal, 6 g pro, 8 g total fat (1 g saturated fat), 25 g carb, 5 g fibre, 0 mg chol, 281 mg sodium

Good source of: fibre, folate

Roasted Garlic

Roasted garlic is a rich-tasting low-fat spread for crusty whole-grain bread, as well as a flavourful addition to dips, salad dressings, and pasta sauce. I often add roasted garlic to Lemon Hummus (page 360).

4	heads garlic	4
1 tsp	extra-virgin olive oil	5 ml
	freshly ground black pepper to taste	

Preheat oven to 375°F (190°C).

Cut off the top eighth of each head of garlic and remove any loose outer skin. Sprinkle each head with olive oil and freshly ground black pepper. Wrap each head individually in foil or place in a clay garlic roaster.

Bake for 40 to 45 minutes. Remove from heat and let cool, then unwrap each head. Gently squeeze the pulp from the cloves. Store the roasted garlic pulp in an airtight container in the refrigerator.

Makes about 1 cup (250 ml)

Serves 4

Per 1/4 cup (50 ml) serving: 46 cal, 2 g pro, 1 g total fat (0 g saturated fat), 8 g carb, 1 g fibre, 0 mg chol, 4 mg sodium

Roasted Squash and Garlic Dip

This dip may take longer to prepare than others, but it's well worth the effort. It's an incredibly versatile dip that pairs well with raw vegetables and crackers. It's also a great low-fat alternative to butter, margarine, or mayonnaise on sandwiches. This dip can be made in advance and refrigerated for up to 5 days.

1	acorn squash	1
1/2 cup	water	125 ml
1	apple, peeled, cored, and halved	1
2 tbsp	orange juice	25 ml
2	heads garlic	2
1 tsp	extra-virgin olive oil	5 ml
	freshly ground black pepper to taste	

Preheat oven to 375°F (190°C).

Cut squash in half lengthwise, removing seeds. Place squash cut side up in a shallow casserole dish. Pour water into the bottom of the dish.

Place an apple half into the hollow of each squash half. Drizzle 1 tbsp (15 ml) of the orange juice onto each squash half. Cover casserole dish with foil and set aside.

Cut off the top eighth of each head of garlic and remove any loose skin. Drizzle with olive oil. Wrap each garlic head in foil or place in a clay garlic roaster.

Place squash and garlic in the oven and bake for 55 to 60 minutes or until the squash is tender when pricked with a fork.

Remove squash and garlic from oven and cool slightly.

Gently scoop out squash flesh and apple; place in a mixing bowl. Unwrap garlic heads and gently squeeze the garlic pulp from the cloves and into the mixing bowl. Mash squash, apple, and garlic with a fork until smooth and combined. Season with black pepper.

Makes about 2 cups (500 ml)

Serves 8

Per 1/4 cup (50 ml) serving: 49 cal, 1 g pro, 1 g total fat (0 g saturated fat), 12 g carb, 2 g fibre, 0 mg chol, 3 mg sodium

Good source of: vitamin C, beta carotene

Dressings

Creamy Caesar Dressing
The only thing missing from this recipe is the fat. This dressing has just as much flavour as any full-fat recipe, but with zero grams of fat per serving. You'll find anchovy paste in packaged tubes in the refrigerator section (usually by the seafood counter) of most grocery stores.

1 cup	low-fat (1% MF or less) plain yogurt	250 ml
2 tbsp	freshly squeezed lemon juice	25 ml
1 tbsp	anchovy paste	15 ml
1 tsp	Dijon mustard	5 ml
1 tsp	Worcestershire sauce	5 ml
2	cloves garlic, minced	2

In a small bowl, whisk together yogurt, lemon juice, anchovy paste, mustard, Worcestershire sauce, and garlic. Cover and refrigerate until ready to use.

Makes 1 1/4 cups (300 ml)

Serves 10

Per 2 tbsp (25 ml) serving: 18 cal, 2 g pro, 0 g total fat (0 g saturated fat), 2 g carb, 0 g fibre, 2 mg chol, 123 mg sodium

Garlic and Basil Kefir Dressing

With only 1 gram per serving, this dressing may be low in fat, but I promise you it's big on taste.

Tip: If you don't have fresh basil on hand, substitute 1/4 tsp (1 ml) dried basil.

1/2 cup	unflavoured kefir	125 ml
1 tsp	minced gingerroot	5 ml
1 tsp	chopped fresh basil	5 ml
1	clove garlic, minced	1

In a small bowl, whisk together kefir, gingerroot, basil, and garlic. Cover and refrigerate until ready to use.

Makes 1/2 cup (125 ml)

Serves 4

Per 2 tbsp (25 ml) serving: 17 cal, 1 g pro, 1 g total fat (0 g saturated fat), 2 g carb, 0 g fibre, 2 mg chol, 15 mg sodium

Grapefruit Maple Dressing

As with the Pomegranate Maple Dressing (page 368), this dressing contains very little oil and as a result has a thin consistency. It can be made up to 5 days in advance and kept covered in the refrigerator until ready to use. I suggest pairing it with the Spinach and Grapefruit Salad (page 292).

1/4 cup	freshly squeezed grapefruit juice	50 ml
1 tbsp	freshly squeezed lemon juice	15 ml
1 tbsp	maple syrup	15 ml
1 tbsp	extra-virgin olive oil	15 ml
1/2 tbsp	Dijon mustard	7 ml
1/2 tsp	minced gingerroot	2 ml
1	clove garlic, minced	1

In a small bowl, whisk together grapefruit juice, lemon juice, maple syrup, olive oil, mustard, gingerroot, and garlic. Cover and refrigerate until ready to use.

Makes 1/2 cup (125 ml)

Serves 4

Per 2 tbsp (25 ml) serving: 52 cal, 0 g pro, 4 g total fat (1 g saturated fat), 5 g carb, 0 g fibre, 0 mg chol, 22 mg sodium

Honey Dijon Dressing

This salad dressing doubles as a marinade for fish, poultry, meat, or veggies.

1/4 cup	extra-virgin olive oil	50 ml
2 tbsp	balsamic vinegar	25 ml
1 tbsp	Dijon mustard	15 ml
2 tsp	honey	10 ml
1	clove garlic, minced	1

In a small bowl, whisk together olive oil, vinegar, mustard, honey, and garlic.

Makes 1/2 cup (125 ml)

Serves 4

Per 2 tbsp (25 ml) serving: 137 cal, 0 g pro, 14 g total fat (2 g saturated fat), 4 g carb, 0 g fibre, 0 mg chol, 44 mg sodium

Lemon Walnut Dressing

Use unrefined walnut oil in this recipe. Not only does it have more flavour than refined walnut oil, but unrefined walnut oil also tends to be higher in essential fatty acids, since it's been processed to a lesser extent. Unrefined oils are more prone to the effects of heat, light, and air, so be sure to store your walnut oil in the refrigerator. Drizzle this dressing over a mixed green salad.

1/4 cup	walnut oil	50 ml
2 tbsp	freshly squeezed lemon juice	25 ml
1 tbsp	Dijon mustard	15 ml
2 tsp	honey	10 ml
	zest of 1 lemon	

In a small bowl, whisk together walnut oil, lemon juice, mustard, honey, and lemon zest until consistency is thick and creamy. Cover and refrigerate until ready to serve.

Makes 1/2 cup (125 ml)

Serves 4

Per 2 tbsp (25 ml) serving: 138 cal, 0 g pro, 14 g total fat (1 g saturated fat), 4 g carb, 0 g fibre, 0 mg chol, 43 mg sodium

Pomegranate Maple Dressing

This is an attractive salad dressing with a deep red colour (from the pomegranate juice) and a lovely nutty flavour (from the flaxseed oil). This dressing contains very little oil, so it has a very thin consistency; I suggest you make it in a jar with a lid, so you can shake it well before serving. Serve this dressing, rich in alpha-linolenic acid, with Pomegranate Garden Salad (page 290).

1/4 cup	pure pomegranate juice	50 ml
2 tbsp	apple cider vinegar	25 ml
2 tbsp	flaxseed oil	25 ml
2 tsp	Dijon mustard	10 ml
2 tsp	freshly squeezed lemon juice	10 ml
1 tsp	maple syrup	5 ml

In a small bowl, whisk together pomegranate juice, vinegar, flaxseed oil, mustard, lemon juice, and maple syrup. Cover and refrigerate until ready to serve.

Makes 1/2 cup (125 ml)

Serves 4

Per 2 tbsp (25 ml) serving: 78 cal, 0 g pro, 7 g total fat (1 g saturated fat), 4 g carb, 0 g fibre, 0 mg chol, 29 mg sodium

Poppy Seed Dressing

Serve this zesty dressing with Strawberry and Kiwi Salad (page 297).

1 cup	low-fat (1% MF or less) plain yogurt	250 ml
1 tbsp	frozen orange juice concentrate	15 ml
1 tsp	poppy seeds	5 ml

In a small bowl, combine yogurt, orange juice, and poppy seeds. Cover and refrigerate until ready to use.

Makes 1 cup (250 ml)

Serves 4

Per 1/4 cup (50 ml) serving: 42 cal, 3 g pro, 0 g total fat (0 g saturated fat), 6 g carb, 0 g fibre, 1 mg chol, 44 mg sodium

Spinach Almond Pesto

Two ingredients—spinach and almonds—that aren't commonly found in pesto are what make this version so interesting. This recipe also omits the usually called-for Parmesan cheese. The result is an incredibly flavourful pesto that's lower in fat and calories than most store-bought varieties. You can substitute the almonds with any nut or seed, including cashews, walnuts, and pumpkin seeds. If you have leftover pesto, freeze individual portions in an ice cube tray.

2 cups	fresh basil leaves, loosely packed	500 ml
2 cups	fresh spinach leaves, loosely packed	500 ml
3 tbsp	extra-virgin olive oil	50 ml
2 tbsp	slivered almonds	25 ml
2 tbsp	pine nuts	25 ml
1/2 tsp	sea salt	2 ml
4	cloves garlic, minced	4

In a blender, purée basil, spinach, olive oil, almonds, pine nuts, sea salt, and garlic to a smooth consistency.

Makes 3/4 cup (175 ml)

Serves 4

Per 3 tbsp (50 ml) serving: 161 cal, 4 g pro, 15 g total fat (2 g saturated fat), 4 g carb, 3 g fibre, 0 mg chol, 313 mg sodium

Excellent source of: vitamin A, vitamin K

Good source of: folate

Two Tea Dressing

Ideally, make this catechin-rich dressing 2 to 8 hours in advance to allow the tea's full flavour to infuse the dressing.

1/4 cup	extra-virgin olive oil	50 ml
1/4 cup	apple cider vinegar	50 ml
1 tsp	Dijon mustard	5 ml
1 tsp	honey	5 ml
	zest of 1 lemon	
1	Earl Grey tea bag	1
1	peppermint tea bag	1

In a small bowl, whisk together oil, vinegar, mustard, honey, and lemon zest. Add Earl Grey and peppermint tea bags and let sit for at least 2 hours. Remove tea bags before serving.

Makes 1/2 cup (125 ml)

Serves 4

Per 2 tbsp (25 ml) serving: 129 cal, 0 g pro, 14 g total fat (2 g saturated fat), 3 g carb, 0 g fibre, 0 mg chol, 15 mg sodium

Marinades

Ginger Tea Marinade

This marinade has an intriguing taste that pairs well with chicken, white fish, or scallops. Use whatever type of tea suits your taste, from fragrant Earl Grey to grassy Chinese green tea to sweet and slightly nutty rooibos tea.

Tip: If using loose tea, brew 1 tsp (5 ml) in 3/4 cup (175 ml) water. Use an infuser or strain the tea from the leaves after brewing.

3/4 cup	boiling water	175 ml
2	tea bags of your choice	2
2 tbsp	sodium-reduced soy sauce	25 ml
1 tbsp	minced gingerroot	15 ml
1 tbsp	freshly squeezed lime juice	15 ml

In a heat-proof measuring cup, pour boiling water over tea bags; let steep for 10 minutes. Remove tea bags.

Stir in soy sauce, gingerroot, and lime juice.

Makes 1 cup (250 ml)

Per 1/4 cup (50 ml): 6 cal, 0 g pro, 0 g total fat (0 g saturated fat), 1 g carb, 0 g fibre, 0 mg chol, 243 mg sodium

Spicy Pomegranate Glaze

This spicy glaze adds both colour and flavour to grilled and roasted meats, especially pork, as well as to fish, poultry, even vegetables. Just brush on at the end of cooking. To turn down the spice factor, add fewer red pepper flakes.

1 cup	pure pomegranate juice	250 ml
1/4 cup	honey	50 ml
1/4 tsp	red pepper flakes	1 ml
	freshly ground black pepper to taste	

In a medium saucepan, combine pomegranate juice, honey, red pepper flakes, and black pepper. Bring to a hard boil; boil for 5 minutes. Remove from heat.

Makes 1 1/4 cups (300 ml)

Per 2 tbsp (25 ml): 58 cal, 0 g pro, 0 g total fat (0 g saturated fat), 15 g carb, 0 g fibre, 0 mg chol, 2 mg sodium

Tandoori Marinade

This Indian-inspired marinade is fantastic with chicken, mild fish, or vegetables. Garam masala is a blend of spices commonly used in Indian cuisine. If you can't find it at your local grocery store, look for it in ethnic food markets. This recipe makes enough to marinate 6 chicken breasts or fish fillets.

1 tsp	canola oil	5 ml
1/2	onion, chopped	1/2
2	cloves garlic, minced	2
1 tbsp	minced gingerroot	15 ml
1 tsp	cumin	5 ml
1 tsp	coriander	5 ml
1 tsp	garam masala	5 ml
1 cup	low-fat (1% MF or less) plain yogurt	250 ml

Heat oil in a skillet over medium heat. Add onion; sauté for 4 to 5 minutes or until light brown. Add garlic, gingerroot, cumin, coriander, and garam masala; sauté for 1 minute. Remove from heat.

In a medium bowl, combine onion mixture with yogurt.

Makes 1 cup (250 ml)

Per 1/6 cup (38 ml): 39 cal, 2 g pro, 1 g total fat (0 g saturated fat), 5 g carb, 1 g fibre, 1 mg chol, 31 mg sodium

Muffins and Quick Breads

Cranberry Orange Flax Quick Bread

It's hard to believe that this low-fat bread—only 4 grams per slice—is so moist. The ground flaxseed sprinkled on top resembles brown sugar but adds a nutty flavour.

3/4 cup	whole-wheat flour	175 ml
1/2 cup	all-purpose flour	125 ml
1/2 cup	granulated sugar	125 ml
1/2 cup	dried cranberries	125 ml
1 tbsp	whole flaxseed	15 ml
1/2 tbsp	baking powder	7 ml
1/2 tsp	baking soda	2 ml
1/2 cup	low-fat (1% MF or less) plain yogurt	125 ml
1/4 cup	light ricotta cheese	50 ml
1	large egg	1
2 tbsp	frozen orange juice concentrate	25 ml
1 tbsp	canola oil	15 ml
1 tsp	vanilla extract	5 ml
1/2 tbsp	ground flaxseed	7 ml

Preheat oven to 400°F (200°C).

Grease and flour a 9 x 5 inch (2 L) loaf pan.

In a large bowl, combine whole-wheat and all-purpose flours, sugar, cranberries, flaxseed, baking powder, and baking soda.

In a small bowl, combine yogurt, ricotta cheese, egg, orange juice concentrate, oil, and vanilla extract.

Add wet ingredients to dry ingredients, mixing just enough to combine. Pour batter into loaf pan. Sprinkle ground flaxseed on top.

Bake for 35 minutes or until cooked through (when a knife inserted in the centre comes out clean).

Serves 9

Per 1 inch (2.5 cm) slice: 178 cal, 5 g pro, 4 g total fat (1 g saturated fat), 33 g carb, 2 g fibre, 23 mg chol, 152 mg sodium

Good source of: vitamin K

Low-Fat Lemon Millet Muffins

These healthy muffins have only 2 grams of fat per muffin, whereas store-bought muffins can have up to 20 grams of fat per muffin. Not to worry, the fact that they're low in fat does not compromise their taste.

3/4 cup	all-purpose flour	175 ml
3/4 cup	whole-wheat flour	175 ml
1/2 cup	soy flour	125 ml
1/2 cup	granulated sugar	125 ml
2 tbsp	hulled millet	25 ml
1 tsp	baking powder	5 ml
1 tsp	baking soda	5 ml
1/4 tsp	salt	1 ml
1 cup	low-fat (1% MF or less) plain yogurt	250 ml
1	egg	1
3 tbsp	freshly squeezed lemon juice	50 ml
2 tbsp	poppy seeds	25 ml
1 tsp	freshly grated lemon zest	5 ml

Preheat oven to 375°F (190°C).

In a large bowl, combine all-purpose, whole-wheat, and soy flours, sugar, millet, baking powder, baking soda, and salt.

In a small bowl, combine yogurt, egg, lemon juice, poppy seeds, and lemon zest.

Add wet ingredients to dry ingredients, mixing just enough to combine. Pour batter into 12-cup lined muffin tin.

Bake for 30 to 35 minutes.

Serves 12

Per muffin: 133 cal, 6 g pro, 2 g total fat (0 g saturated fat), 25 g carb, 2 g fibre, 14 mg chol, 202 mg sodium

Desserts

Blueberries Topped with Candied Almonds

You'll be lucky if these candied almonds last until dessert—they're so good, you can't help but nibble on them. The almonds can be made up to 1 week in advance and stored in an airtight container in the refrigerator. You'll find shaved almonds in the baking section of most grocery stores— look for them in 3 1/2 ounce (100 g) packages.

1	egg white	1
1 1/2 tbsp	granulated sugar	20 ml
3/4 cup	shaved almonds	175 ml
1 tsp	almond extract	5 ml
2 cups	fresh blueberries	500 ml
	lemon zest or sprigs fresh mint, as garnish	

Preheat oven to 350°F (180°C).

In a small bowl, whisk egg white until frothy. Add sugar, continuing to whisk until egg white is light and airy. Add almonds and almond extract. Stir to coat almonds with egg white.

Spread almond mixture onto a baking sheet lined with waxed paper. Bake for 10 to 12 minutes or until almond mixture begins to harden and brown. Remove from heat; set aside to cool.

When almonds are cool, break up into small pieces.

Divide blueberries into 4 bowls, sprinkle with almond mixture, and garnish with lemon zest or sprigs of fresh mint.

Serves 4

Per 1/2 cup (125 ml) blueberries and 2 tbsp (25 ml) candied almonds: 221 cal, 7 g pro, 14 g total fat (1 g saturated fat), 20 g carb, 5 g fibre, 0 mg chol, 25 mg sodium

Excellent source of: magnesium

Good source of: fibre

Flax Bean Brownies

Beans in brownies, you ask? A study published in the *Journal of the American Dietetic Association* found that when white kidney beans were used to replace part of the shortening in a brownie recipe, taste testers couldn't detect their presence. In fact, they rated the taste and texture of the brownies with beans the same as regular brownies.

My taste testers agreed: They couldn't tell that these brownies were made from legumes. I think you'll agree that these are some of the lightest and fluffiest brownies you've ever tasted.

1 cup	canned romano beans, drained and rinsed	250 ml
1/2 cup	canola oil	125 ml
1/2 tbsp	vanilla extract	7 ml
4	eggs, whole	4
3/4 cup	whole-wheat flour	175 ml
1 1/3 cups	granulated sugar	325 ml
1/2 cup	dark cocoa	125 ml
1 tbsp	whole flaxseed	15 ml
1 tsp	salt	5 ml
1 tsp	baking soda	5 ml
1 tsp	baking powder	5 ml

Preheat oven to 350°F (180°C).

Grease and flour an 8 x 8 inch (2 L) baking dish.

In a food processor, combine beans, oil, vanilla extract, and eggs. Blend to a smooth consistency.

In a mixing bowl, combine flour, sugar, cocoa, flaxseed, salt, baking soda, and baking powder.

Add bean mixture to dry ingredients, mixing well. Pour batter into baking dish.

Bake for 40 to 50 minutes or until brownies are cooked through (when a knife inserted in the centre comes out clean).

Serves 16

Per brownie: 184 cal, 4 g pro, 9 g total fat (1 g saturated fat), 25 g carb, 2 g fibre, 42 mg chol, 259 mg sodium

Excellent source of: vitamin K

Ginger-Flax Fruit Crisp

The ground flaxseed gives this dessert an infusion of fibre, while the gingerroot adds some bite. Feel free to use whatever locally grown fruit is available in place of the berries, apples, or peaches.

1/2 cup	whole-wheat flour	125 ml
1/2 cup	rolled oats	125 ml
2 tbsp	canola oil	25 ml
1 tbsp	ground flaxseed	15 ml
1 tbsp	whole flaxseed	15 ml
1 tbsp	brown sugar	15 ml
1 tsp	cinnamon	5 ml
1/4 tsp	nutmeg	1 ml
1/2 cup	mixed berries	125 ml
4	apples, peeled, cored, and sliced	4
2	peaches, peeled, cored, and sliced	2
1 tbsp	chopped gingerroot	15 ml

Preheat oven to 375°F (190°C).

In a large bowl, combine flour, oats, oil, ground and whole flaxseed, sugar, cinnamon, and nutmeg. Mix until crumbly.

In an 8 x 8 inch (2 L) glass baking dish, combine berries, apples, peaches, and gingerroot. Sprinkle flaxseed mixture over fruit.

Bake for 40 to 50 minutes or until fruit is soft and the topping begins to brown.

Serve warm.

Serves 6

Per 1 cup (250 ml) serving: 197 cal, 3 g pro, 7 g total fat (1 g saturated fat), 34 g carb, 5 g fibre, 0 mg chol, 3 mg sodium

Excellent source of: vitamin K

Good source of: fibre

Roasted Fruit Kebabs

This is a refreshing dessert to cap off a summer barbecue. The fruit needs only to be heated, so cooking time is short. For a variation on this recipe, soak the fruit in orange juice or brush with rum before grilling. Be sure the grill has been cleaned well before barbecuing the kebabs. I like to serve these kebabs with Lemon Ginger Fruit Dip (page 359).

12	bamboo skewers	12
2	apples, peeled, cored, and cut into 1 inch (2.5 cm) chunks	2
2	pears, peeled, cored, and cut into 1 inch (2.5 cm) chunks	2
2 cups	strawberries	500 ml
1	large orange, peeled and sectioned	1

Fill a shallow dish with water; soak skewers for 30 minutes.

Preheat clean grill to medium-low.

Thread 5 to 6 pieces of fruit onto each skewer, alternating types of fruit.

Lightly coat the grill with cooking spray. Grill kebabs, rotating every few minutes to prevent sticking, until lightly brown. Allow to cool before serving.

Serves 6

Per 2 undressed kebabs: 87 cal, 1 g pro, 1 g total fat (0 g saturated fat), 22 g carb, 4 g fibre, 0 mg chol, 1 mg sodium

Per 2 kebabs with Lemon Ginger Fruit Dip: 144 cal, 4 g pro, 1 g total fat (0 g saturated fat), 33 g carb, 4 g fibre, 1 mg chol, 45 mg sodium

Excellent source of: vitamin C

Good source of: fibre

Appendix 1

Leslie Beck's power foods checklist

Use this checklist to track which days of the week you eat the following power foods. The amount for 1 serving is listed in the corresponding chapter.

	Mon	Tues	Wed	Thurs	Fri	Sat	Sun
Power vegetables							
Leafy greens — 1 serving/day							
Cruciferous vegetables — 3 to 5 servings/week							
Bright orange vegetables — 1 serving/day							
Tomatoes — 5 servings/week							
Allium vegetables — 2 garlic cloves/week and multiple servings of onions							
Power fruit							
Berries — 1 to 2 servings/day							
Citrus fruit — 1 serving/day							
Pomegranate — 3 servings/week							

	Mon	Tues	Wed	Thurs	Fri	Sat	Sun
Power grains							
Whole grains — 3 to 4 servings/day (adults (20 years+); 2 to 3 servings/day (5–19 years)							
Power protein foods							
Fish and seafood — 2 servings/week							
Legumes and soy foods — 3 servings/week							
Nuts and seeds — 5 servings/week							
Power dairy							
Yogurt and kefir — 1 serving/day							
Power fats and oils							
Unsaturated fats — 2 to 3 servings/day							
Power beverages							
Tea (green, oolong, black) — 2 to 5 servings/day							
Coffee—up to 4 servings/day							

Appendix 2

Power herbs and spices

Believe it or not, herbs and spices are actually the first power foods, since they've been grown and cultivated for thousands of years. Herbs and spices not only add flavour to meals but also deliver potential health benefits. Today scientists are learning that many fresh herbs and spices pack the same—or greater—antioxidant punch as fresh fruits and vegetables. For instance, American researchers have found that gram for gram, oregano has 42 times as much antioxidant activity as apples, 30 times as much as potatoes, and 12 times as much as oranges. Studies carried out in test tubes and animals have also demonstrated the potential for phytochemical-rich herbs and spices to help fight cancer, heart disease, and type 2 diabetes.

The difference between herbs and spices is the part of the plant they come from. Herbs come from the leaf of the plant (e.g., parsley, oregano), whereas spices are from the buds (e.g., cloves), bark (e.g., cinnamon), roots (e.g., ginger), berries (e.g., peppercorns), and seeds (e.g., cumin).

In general, it's best to use fresh herbs in cooking, as they contain a higher level of antioxidant activity than their dried or processed counterparts. For instance, fresh garlic is much more powerful than dry garlic powder. (You'll learn how garlic helps fight disease on pages 96–99, Chapter 2.) To substitute fresh herbs for dried in a recipe, follow a ratio of 3 to 1. For example, 1 tablespoon (15 ml) of fresh thyme is equal to 1 teaspoon (5 ml) of dried.

Fresh herbs and spices not only boost your antioxidant intake but also flavour meals without adding sodium. Use the chart below to add a pinch of flavour and an antioxidant punch to your meals. (Potential health benefits are based on effects demonstrated in animal and lab studies.)

Herb or spice	Potential health benefits	Pair with/ suggested uses
Basil	Antioxidant, anti-bacterial, anti-inflammatory	Pasta sauces, pesto, pizza, grilled vegetables, salads, stews
Chili peppers	Anti-inflammatory, pain relief, decongestant, metabolism booster, prostate cancer prevention, blood sugar control	Asian and Mexican dishes, egg dishes, meat, poultry, seafood, curries, pasta sauces, soups, stews
Cilantro (coriander)	Blood sugar control, cholesterol lowering	Mexican dishes, salads, salsa, soups
Cinnamon	Anti–blood clotting, anti-microbial, blood sugar control, memory enhancer	Apples, fruit crisps, hot cereals, muffins, rice puddings, curries, Mexican dishes
Dill	Antioxidant, anti-bacterial	Eggs, fish, lamb, poultry, potatoes, salads
Ginger	Antioxidant, anti-inflammatory, anti-nausea (pregnancy), gastrointestinal relief, immune enhancer, colon cancer prevention	Asian stir-fries, meat, seafood, curries, marinades, dipping sauces, soups, fruit salads, fruit smoothies
Mint	Digestive relief (anti-spasmodic), anti-cancer, anti-bacterial	Lamb, marinades, pesto, salads, tomatoes, fruit salads

Herb or spice	Potential health benefits	Pair with/ suggested uses
Oregano	Anti-bacterial, antioxidant	Pasta sauces, pizza, salads, salad dressings, beef, lamb, grilled breads
Parsley	Antioxidant, anti-microbial	Eggs, meat, fish, shellfish, salads, soups, stews
Rosemary	Anti-inflammatory, immune enhancer, digestive relief	Beef, lamb, pork, poultry, fish, pastas, roasted root vegetables, salads, salad dressings, grilled breads
Sage	Antioxidant, anti-inflammatory, memory enhancer	Eggs, pork, poultry, poultry stuffing, pasta, rice dishes, soups
Thyme	Antioxidant, anti-microbial	Eggs, fish, poultry, poultry stuffing, marinades, rubs, pastas, soups, salads, salad dressings
Turmeric	Anti-inflammatory, antioxidant, anti-cancer, digestive health, improved liver function, cholesterol lowering	Eggs, fish, legumes, sautéed cauliflower, crudité dips

Appendix 3

A guide to reading nutrition labels

If you're like many health-conscious Canadians, chances are you've read a few nutrition labels on food packages. But knowing how to interpret serving sizes, fat grams, and percentage daily values—and then being able to apply this information to your own daily diet—is challenging for many people.

When shopping for the power foods I describe in the chapters of this book, you won't often need to read a nutrition label. That's because many of these powers foods don't carry a label—they're whole, unprocessed foods that are not sold in a package. Citrus fruits, fresh berries, avocado, leafy greens, cabbage, fresh fish, and dried legumes in bulk don't come with a label to tell you what's inside.

Of course, there are exceptions. Prepackaged greens, frozen vegetables and fruit, packaged whole-grain breads and ready-to-eat breakfast cereals, canned fish, canned legumes, bottled vegetable oils, nut butters, and packaged phytochemical-rich berry juices are required by law to carry a nutrition label and an ingredient list to help you make informed food purchases. Throughout my book I've provided tips on what to look for on a food label to enable you to select the most nutritious product.

Mandatory nutrition labelling is relatively new in Canada. As of December 12, 2005, most packaged foods were required by law to carry a Nutrition Facts box listing the calories, the amounts of total fat, saturated and trans fats, cholesterol, sodium, carbohydrate, fibre, sugars, protein, calcium, iron, and vitamins A and C for a specified serving. Small food companies were given until 2007 to add nutrition information to their packages.

As you may have noticed, there are exemptions to the labelling regulations. Fresh fruit and vegetables, raw meat and poultry (except ground), coffee beans, tea leaves, herbs and spices, alcoholic beverages, and foods prepared where they are sold (e.g., bakery goods) are not required to carry a nutrition label.

Nutrition labels are intended to make it easier for Canadians to compare brands of foods, assess the nutritional value of foods, and manage special diets, such as low sodium or high fibre. But labels are useful only if you know what the numbers mean, what to watch out for, and how to put the information into practice.

The following tips will help you sort through—and decipher—label information that's relevant to your diet.

The Nutrition Facts box

1. SERVING SIZE INFORMATION

The serving size is the first place to start and that's why it's listed first. The nutrient amounts that follow on the label are based on 1 serving of the food. This serving size is given in familiar household units—cups, tablespoons, or a portion of the food (e.g., a quarter of a pizza, one slice of bread)—and is followed by the metric equivalent.

Nutrition Facts Per 1 cup (264g)	
Amount	**% Daily Value**
Calories 260	
Fat 13g	20%
Saturated Fat 3g + Trans Fat 2g	25%
Cholesterol 30mg	
Sodium 660mg	28%
Carbohydrate 31g	10%
Fibre 0g	0%
Sugars 5g	
Protein 5g	
Vitamin A 4% • Vitamin C 2%	
Calcium 15% • Iron 4%	

For something that seems so simple, serving size information can be sometimes tricky. What you consider to be 1 serving—such as a bottle of fruit juice, sports drink, or soft drink—can actually be 2 or more. For example, the nutrition label on a 20 ounce (591 ml) bottle of Tropicana Twister Fruit Fusion provides 110 calories and 30 grams of sugars for a 1 cup (250 ml) serving. But most people won't measure out 1 cup (250 ml) and save the rest for later. Instead they'll guzzle all of what's in the bottle—260 calories and 70 grams of sugar (almost 18 teaspoons/90 ml worth).

Other items to watch out for include snack personal-sized pizzas, pita bread, flatbreads, and bagels. The nutrition information for many whole-grain bagels is given for half a bagel; if you eat the whole bagel, you'll need to double the numbers.

The bottom line: A serving size is not necessarily the whole package. Read the serving size and know how much you typically consume.

When comparing two brands of a similar food, make sure you're comparing nutrient numbers for identical serving sizes. For instance, most brands of salad dressing list numbers for 1 tablespoon (15 ml), but some specify 2 tablespoons (25 ml) as a serving.

2. CALORIES

The number of calories tells you how much energy you get from one serving of the food. The number of servings you consume determines how many calories you actually eat. How you prepare a food will also influence the calories you consume. Packaged rice and pasta dishes and muffin and cake mixes require you to add ingredients, such as oil, butter, milk, or eggs. To know how much you are consuming, always check calories and nutrient amounts under the "as prepared" heading.

By itself, the calorie count means little. Calorie requirements are different for everyone, depending on age, body size, sex, activity level, and whether you're pregnant or breastfeeding.

3. FAT, SATURATED AND TRANS FAT

The combined amount of saturated, polyunsaturated, monounsaturated, and trans fats is listed next on the nutrition label. If you're looking for lower fat cookies or crackers, you can compare brands on grams of total fat per serving. But a food product with a lot of fat grams isn't necessarily unhealthy. For instance, vinaigrette salad dressings, packages of nuts, and nut butters contain heart healthy fats. What's most important is to look at the number of grams of combined saturated and trans fats—two fats linked to a higher risk of heart disease because they raise LDL (bad) cholesterol.

The upper limit of saturated plus trans fat you should consume depends on your calorie intake. Current guidelines recommend consuming no more than 10% of daily calories from these unhealthy fats. For a 2000-calorie diet, that means no more than 22 grams of saturated plus trans fat per day. (The math: 2000 calories × 10% = 200 calories; 1 gram of fat = 9 calories; 200 ÷ 9 = 22 grams.)

4. CHOLESTEROL

You don't need to spend much time considering the cholesterol number. This wax-like substance found in animal foods has little or no effect on most people's blood cholesterol—it is far more important to limit saturated and trans fat to help lower elevated blood cholesterol. Your liver manufactures most of the cholesterol in your bloodstream. Nevertheless, consume 300 milligrams per day or less.

5. SODIUM

Most Canadians consume too much sodium, which can lead to high blood pressure, a strong risk factor for heart attack and stroke. Your upper daily sodium limit is 2300 milligrams. If all your meals aren't based on packaged foods (which they shouldn't be if you've adopted a power food diet), don't panic if one of your foods has a high number. A serving of lycopene-rich tomato juice with 700 milligrams of sodium is okay as long as you eat lower sodium foods for the rest of the day. However, you might want to pass on the instant soup or frozen dinner that delivers a whopping 1500 milligrams.

6. CARBOHYDRATE, FIBRE, AND SUGARS

Next on the label comes grams of total carbohydrate—all the starch, fibre, and sugar that's in one serving of the food. If you have diabetes and your diet requires you to count carbohydrates, this is useful information. Otherwise, the numbers that follow—fibre and sugars—are more important.

Most of us eat too little fibre. Women should strive for 25 grams per day; men, 38 grams. Look for foods with at least 2 grams of fibre per serving; breakfast cereals should deliver at least 5 grams per serving. Just because a package claims "made with whole grains" doesn't mean it has much fibre. General Mills Whole Grain Chocolate Lucky Charms have a measly 1 gram of fibre per serving. One serving (13 crackers) of Christie Vegetable Thins Multigrain has no fibre at all.

The sugar numbers include both naturally occurring sugars (e.g., fruit or milk sugars) and refined sugars added during food processing (e.g., sucrose, glucose-fructose, honey, corn syrup).

If you're limiting added sugars, you need to read the ingredient list. Sucrose, dextrose, glucose, fructose, honey, molasses, malt, corn syrup, rice syrup, cane juice, invert sugar, and fruit juice concentrate—you might be surprised to see how many types of sugar appear on the ingredient list of just one product.

7. PROTEIN

If you eat a mixed diet that contains meat, poultry, fish, eggs, legumes, and dairy, you're more than likely meeting your daily protein requirements. Since protein helps keep you feeling full longer after eating, choose snack foods that provide a little protein, such as granola bars and trail mix.

8. % DAILY VALUE

Fat, saturated plus trans fat, carbohydrate, fibre, sodium, vitamins A and C, calcium, and iron are also expressed as percentage of a daily value. Daily values are based on recommendations for a healthy diet and represent the contribution (from 0% to 100%) 1 serving of a food makes toward the particular nutrient's recommended intake.

Use the % daily value to see whether nutrients you are trying to consume more of (fibre, vitamins A and C, calcium, and iron) have high percentages in a food product. If you want to boost your fibre intake, when comparing two brands of a breakfast cereal, choose the one with the highest % daily value for fibre per similar serving size. If you want to buy a yogurt that provides the most calcium, choose the brand with the highest % daily value for calcium.

If 1 serving of food has a 15% daily value or more for fibre, vitamins A and C, calcium, or iron, it's considered a high source of these nutrients; a % daily value of 25% or more means it's an excellent source.

It's not always wise to strive for a higher % daily value. In the case of saturated plus trans fat and sodium, choose food products with a lower percentage. Foods with a 5% daily value or less for fat, cholesterol, and sodium are considered low in these nutrients. Foods with a 10% daily value or less for saturated plus trans fat is also low in these bad fats.

The ingredient list

All packaged foods must list ingredients in order, from greatest to least amount used. The first few ingredients usually make up the bulk of the food. Often, the fewer the ingredients the better, especially if there are a lot of unhealthy extras. If you're limiting added sugars, look for sucrose, dextrose, glucose, fructose, honey, molasses, malt, corn syrup, cane juice, and fruit juice concentrate listed on the ingredient list and avoid these products.

Ingredient lists are useful for people with food allergies or intolerances who must avoid certain ingredients. And scanning the ingredient list is often the only way you can tell if products are made from whole grains.

Nutrition claims

Manufacturers often make a nutrition claim on the packaging to help sell the product. Claims such as "low in fat," "light," "sodium free," and "zero trans fat" refer to 1 serving of the food. If you devour a box of low-fat cookies, your snack might not be low in fat after all. To make a claim, products must meet nutrient criteria set out by Health Canada. Here are a few common claims and what they mean (per serving):

- "Sodium free"—less than 5 milligrams of sodium
- "Low fat"—3 grams of fat or less
- "Low in saturated fat"—2 grams or less saturated and trans fat combined
- "Trans fat free"—less than 0.2 grams trans fat and low in saturated fat
- "Calorie-reduced"—at least 25% fewer calories than the regular version
- "High in fibre"—at least 4 grams of fibre
- "Light"—allowed only on foods that are either "reduced in fat" or "reduced in calories"; if it refers to taste, texture, or appearance, this must be explained on the label (e.g., "light in colour")

Don't judge a food solely on the basis of a nutrition claim. Read the Nutrition Facts box and ingredient list to get the whole picture. Just because a food is stamped "zero trans fat" doesn't mean it's low in fat, sodium, or calories. Potato chips deep-fried in non-hydrogenated corn oil may be better for your arteries, but they won't do your waistline any favours.

Diet and health claims

Food companies are also allowed to highlight a relationship between diet and disease on packages, providing they meet regulations about nutrient content. Claims involving the following five relationships have been permitted since 2003:

- A healthy diet low in sodium and high in potassium and reduced risk of high blood pressure
- A healthy diet with adequate calcium and vitamin D and reduced risk of osteoporosis
- A healthy diet low in saturated and trans fat and reduced risk of heart disease
- A healthy diet rich in vegetables and fruit and reduced risk of some types of cancers
- The non-carcinogenic benefits of non-fermentable carbohydrates in gums and hard candies

At the time of writing, Health Canada has reviewed the scientific data supporting additional health and diet claims that address the relationships between:

- Fruits, vegetables, and grain products that contain fibre, particularly soluble fibre, and coronary heart disease
- Fibre-containing grain products, fruits, and vegetables and cancer
- Dietary lipids (fats) and cancer
- Folate and neural tube defects

References

Chapter 1: What Your Body Needs

1. Zheng, W, DR Gustafson, R Sinha, et al. Well-done meat intake and the risk of breast cancer. *J Natl Cancer Inst* 1998, 90(22):1724–29.
2. Larsson, SC, and A Wolk. Meat consumption and risk of colorectal cancer: A meta-analysis of prospective studies. *Int J Cancer* 2006, 119(11):2657–64.
3. Albert, CM, K Oh, W Whang, et al. Dietary alpha-linolenic acid intake and risk of sudden cardiac death and coronary heart disease. *Circulation* 2005, 112(21):3232–38.

Chapter 2: Power Vegetables

1. Statistics Canada. The Canadian Community Health Survey. Overview of Canadians' Eating Habits 2004. Catalogue No. 82-620-XIE—No. 2. Ministry of Industry, 2006.
2. Ritter, L. Report of a panel on the relationship between public exposure to pesticides and cancer. Ad Hoc Panel on Pesticides and Cancer. National Cancer Institute of Canada. *Cancer* 1997, 80(10):2019–33.
3. Steinmetz, KA, JD Potter, and AR Folsom. Vegetables, fruit, and lung cancer in the Iowa Women's Health Study. *Cancer Res* 1993, 53(3):536–43.
4. Larsson, SC, L Bergkvist, and A Wolk. Fruit and vegetable consumption and incidence of gastric cancer: A prospective study. *Cancer Epidemiol Biomarkers Prev* 2006, 15(10):1998–2001.
5. Kushi, LH, PJ Mink, AR Folsom, KE Anderson, W Zheng, D Lazovich, and TA Sellers. Prospective study of diet and ovarian cancer. *Am J Epidemiol* 1999, 149(1):21–31.
6. Hung, HC, Joshipura KJ, Jiang R, et al. Fruit and vegetable intake and risk of major chronic disease. *J Natl Cancer Inst* 2004, 96(21):1577–84.
7. Joshipura, KJ, FB Hu, JE Mason, et al. The effect of fruit and vegetable intake on risk for coronary heart disease. *Ann Intern Med* 2001, 134(12):1106–14.
8. Joshipura, KJ, A Ascherio, JE Manson, et al. Fruit and vegetable intake in relation to risk of ischemic stroke. *JAMA* 1999, 282(13):1233–39.
9. Brown L, EB Rimm, JM Seddon, et al. A prospective study of carotenoid intake and risk of cataract extraction in U.S. men. *Am J Clin Nutr* 1999, 70(4):517–24.
10. Hammond, BR Jr, EJ Johnson, RM Russell, et al. *Invest Ophthalmol Vis Sci* 1997, 38(9):1795–1801.

11. Booth, SL, KE Broe, DR Gagnon, et al. Vitamin K intake and bone mineral density in women and men. *Am J Clin Nutr* 2003, 77(2):512–16.

12. Feskanich, D, P Weber, WC Willett, et al. Vitamin K intake and hip factures in women: A prospective study. *Am J Clin Nutr* 1999, 69(1):74–79.

13. Booth, SL, KL Tucker, H Chen, et al. Dietary vitamin K intakes are associated with hip fracture but not with bone mineral density in elderly men and women. *Am J Clin Nutr* 2000, 71(5):1201–08.

14. Morris, MC, DA Evans, CC Tangney, et al. Associations of vegetable and fruit consumption with age-related cognitive change. *Neurology* 2006, 67(8):1370–76.

15. Kang, JH, A Ascherio, and F Grodstein. Fruit and vegetable consumption and cognitive decline in aging women. *Ann Neurol* 2005, 57(5):713–20.

16. Steinmetz, KA, and JD Potter. Vegetables, fruit, and cancer prevention: A review. *J Am Diet Assoc* 1996, 96(10):1027–39.

17. Partos, Lindsey. Cauliflower "juice," a weapon against breast cancer. Jun 9, 2005. www.foodnavigator-usa.com/news/ng.asp?n=60546-cauliflower-cancer-weapon.

18. Patton, Dominique. Sauerkraut consumption may fight off breast cancer. Nov 4, 2005. www.foodnavigator-usa.com/news/ng.asp?id=63688.

19. Voorrips, LE, RA Goldbohm, DT Verhoeven, et al. Vegetable and fruit consumption and lung cancer risk in the Netherlands Cohort Study on diet and cancer. *Cancer Causes Control* 2000, 11(2):101–15. Neuhouser, ML, RE Patterson, MD Thornquist, et al. Fruits and vegetables are associated with lower lung cancer risk only in the placebo arm of the beta-carotene and retinol efficacy trial (CARET). *Cancer Epidemiol Biomarkers Prev* 2003, 12(4):350–58.

20. Zhao, B, A Seow, EJ Lee, et al. Dietary isothiocynates, glutathione S-transferase-M1, -T1 polymorphisms and lung cancer risk among Chinese women in Singapore. *Cancer Epidemiol Biomarkers Prev* 2001, 10(10):1063–67. Lewis, S, P Brennan, F Nyberg, et al. Re: Spitz, MR, Duphorne, CM, Detry, MA, Pillow, PC, Amos, CI, Lei, L, de Andrade, M, Gu, X, Hong, WK, and Wu, X. Dietary intake of isothiocynates: Evidence of a joint effect with glutathione S-transferase polymorphisms in lung cancer risk. *Cancer Epidemiol Biomark Prev,* 9:1017–20, 2000. *Cancer Epidemiol Biomarkers Prev* 2001, 10(10):1105–06. Spitz, MR, CM Duphorne, MA Detry, et al. Dietary intake of isothiocynates: Evidence of a joint effect with glutathione S-transferase polymorphisms in lung cancer risk. *Cancer Epidemiol Biomarkers Prev* 2000, 9(10):1017–20. London, SJ, JM Yuan, FL Chung, et al. Isothiocynates, glutathione S-transferase M1 and T1 polymorphisms, and lung-cancer risk: A prospective study of men in Shanghai, China. *Lancet* 2000, 356(9231):724–29.

21. Kolonel, LN, JH Hankin, AS Whittemore, et al. Vegetables, fruits, legumes, and prostate cancer: A multiethnic case-control study. *Cancer Epidemiol Biomarkers Prev* 2000, 9(8):795–804.

22. Michaud, DS, D Spiegelman, SK Clinton, et al. Fruit and vegetable intake and incidence of bladder cancer in a male prospective cohort. *J Natl Cancer Inst* 1999, 91(7):605–13.

23. Larsson, SC, N Hakansson, I Naslund, et al. Fruit and vegetable consumption in relation to pancreatic cancer risk: A prospective study. *Cancer Epidemiol Biomarkers Prev* 2006, 15(2):301–05.

24. Zhang, SM, DJ Hunter, BA Rosner, et al. Intakes of fruits, vegetables, and related nutrients and the risk of non-Hodgkin's lymphoma among women. *Cancer Epidemiol Biomarkers Prev* 2000, 9(5):477–85.

25. Joshipura, KJ, A Ascherio, JE Manson, et al. Fruit and vegetable intake in relation to risk of ischemic stroke. *JAMA* 1999, 282(13):1233–39.

26. Vallejo, F, FA Tomás-Barberán, and C García-Viguera. Phenolic compound contents in edible parts of broccoli inflorescences after domestic cooking. *J Sci Food Agric* 2003, 83(14):1511–16.

27. Holick, CN, DS Michaud, R Stolzenberg-Solomen, et al. Dietary carotenoids, serum beta-carotene, and retinol and risk of lung cancer in the alpha-tocopherol, beta-carotene cohort study. *Am J Epidemiol* 2002, 156(6):536–47.

28. Sahyoun, NR, PF Jacques, and RM Russell. Carotenoids, vitamins C and E, and mortality in an elderly population. *Am J Epidemiol* 1996, 144(5):501–11. Rimm, EB, MJ Stampfer, A Ascherio, et al. Vitamin E consumption and the risk of coronary heart disease in men. *N Engl J Med* 1993, 328(20):1450–56. Gaziano, JM, JE Manson, LG Branch, et al. A prospective study of consumption of carotenoids in fruits and vegetables and decreased cardiovascular mortality in the elderly. *Ann Epidemiol* 1995, 5(4):255–60. Osganian, SK, MJ Stampfer, E Rimm, et al. Dietary carotenoids and risk of coronary artery disease in women. *Am J Clin Nutr* 2003, 77(6):1390–99.

29. The Alpha-Tocopherol, Beta Carotene Cancer Prevention Study Group. The effect of vitamin E and beta carotene on the incidence of lung cancer and other cancers in male smokers. *N Engl J Med* 1994, 330(15):1029–35. Omenn, GS, GE Goodman, MD Thornquist, et al. Risk factors for lung cancer and for intervention effects in CARET, the Beta-Carotene and Retinol Efficacy Trial. *J Natl Cancer Inst* 1996, 88(21):1550–59.

30. Giovannucci, E, A Ascherio, EB Timm, et al. Intake of carotenoids and retinol in relation to risk of prostate cancer. *J Natl Cancer Inst* 1995, 87(23):1767–76.

31. Giovannucci, E, EB Rimm, Y Liu, et al. A prospective study of tomato products, lycopene, and prostate cancer risk. *J Natl Cancer Inst* 2002, 94(5):391–98.

32. Sesso, HD, S Liu, JM Gaziano, et al. Dietary lycopene, tomato-based food products and cardiovascular disease in women. *J Nutr* 2003, 133(7):2336–41.

33. Fleischauer, AT, C Poole, and L Arab. Garlic consumption and cancer prevention: Meta-analyses of colorectal and stomach cancers. *Am J Clin Nutr* 2000, 72(4):1047–52.

34. Gonzalez, CA, G Pera, A Agudo, et al. Fruit and vegetable intake and the risk of stomach and oesophagus adenocarcinoma in the European Prospective Investigation into Cancer and Nutrition (EPIC-EURGAST). *Int J Cancer* 2006, 118(10):2559–66.

35. Galeone, C, C Pelucchi, F Levi, et al. Onion and garlic use and human cancer. *Am J Clin Nutr* 2006, 84(5):1027–32.

36. Dorant, E, PA van den Brandt, and RA Goldbohm. A prospective cohort study on allium vegetable consumption, garlic supplement use, and the risk of lung carcinoma in the Netherlands. *Cancer Res* 1994, 54(23):6148–53.

37. Le Marchand, L, SP Murphy, JH Hankin, et al. Intake of flavonoids and lung cancer. *J Natl Cancer Inst* 2000, 92(2):154–60.

38. Gardner, CD, LD Lawson, E Block, et al. Effect of raw garlic vs commercial garlic supplements on plasma lipid concentrations in adults with moderate hypercholesterolemia: A randomized clinical trial. *Arch Intern Med* 2007, 167(4):346–53.

Chapter 3: Power Fruits

1. Halvorsen, BL, MH Carlsen, KM Phillips, et al. Content of redox-active compounds (ie, antioxidants) in foods consumed in the United States. *Am J Clin Nutr* 2006, 84(1):95–135.

2. Wu, X, GR Beecher, JM Holden, et al. Lipophilic and hydrophilic antioxidant capacities of common foods in the United States. *J Agric Food Chem* 2004, 52(12):4026–37.

3. Andres-Lacueva, C, B Shukitt-Hale, RL Galli, et al. Anthocyanins in aged blueberry-fed rats are found centrally and may enhance memory. *Nutr Neurosci* 2005, 8(2):111–20.

4. Duffy, KB, EL Spangler, DB Devan, et al. A blueberry-enriched diet provides cellular protection against oxidative stress and reduces a kainate-induced learning impairment in rats. *Neurobiol of Aging,* May 22, 2007 (published online ahead of print).

5. Joseph, JA, NA Denisova, G Arendash, et al. Blueberry supplementation enhances signaling and prevents behavioral deficits in an Alzheimer disease model. *Nutr Neurosci* 2003, 6(3):153–62.

6. Jepson, RG, L Mihaljevic, and J Craig. Cranberries for preventing urinary tract infections. *Cochrane Database Syst Rev* 2004, (2):CD001321. Stothers, L. A randomized trial to evaluate effectiveness and cost effectiveness of naturopathic cranberry products as prophylaxis against urinary tract infection in women. *Can J Urol* 2002, 9(3):1558–62. Kontiokari, T, K Sundqvist, M Nuutinen, et al. Randomised trial of cranberry-lingonberry juice and Lactobacillus GG drink for the prevention of urinary tract infections in women. *BMJ* 2001, 322(7302):1571. Avorn, J, M Monane, JH Gurwitz, et al. Reduction of bacteriuria and pyuria after ingestion of cranberry juice. *JAMA* 1994, 271(10):751–54.

7. Shmuely, H, J Yahav, Z Samra, et al. Effect of cranberry juice on eradication of Helicobacter pylori in patients treated with antibiotics and a proton pump inhibitor. *Mol Nutr Food Res* 2007, 51(6):746–51.

8. McHarg, T, A Rodgers, and K Charlton. Influence of cranberry juice on the urinary risk factors for calcium oxalate kidney stone formation. *BJU Int* 2003, 92(7):765–68.

9. Colditz, GA, LG Branch, RJ Lipnick, et al. Increased green and yellow vegetable intake and lowered cancer deaths in an elderly population. *Am J Clin Nutr* 1985, 41(1):32–36.

10. Gonzalez, CA, G Pera, A Agudo, HB Bueno-de-Mesquita, et al. Fruit and vegetable intake and the risk of stomach and oesophagus adenocarcinoma in the European Prospective Investigation into Cancer and Nutrition (EPIC-EUR-GAST). *Int J Cancer* 2006, 118(10):2559–66. McCullough, ML, AS Robertson, EJ Jacobs, A Chao, EE Calle, MJ Thun. A prospective study of diet and stomach cancer mortality in United States men and women. *Cancer Epidemiol Biomarkers Prev* 2001, 10(11):1201–05. Cipriani, F, E Buiatti, and D Palli. Gastric cancer in Italy. *Ital J Gastroenterol* 1991, 23(7):429–35.

11. Hakim, IA, RB Harris, and C Ritenbaugh. Citrus peel use is associated with reduced risk of squamous cell carcinoma of the skin. *Nutr Cancer* 2000, 37(2):161–68.

12. Gao, K, SM Henning, Y Niu, et al. The citrus flavonoid naringenin stimulates DNA repair in prostate cancer cells. *J Nutr Biochem* 2006, 17(2):89–95.

13. Hahn-Obercyger, M, AH Stark, and Z Madar. Grapefruit and oroblanco enhance hepatic detoxification enzymes in rats: Possible role in protection against chemical carcinogenesis. *J Agric Food Chem* 2005, 53(5):1828–32.

14. Joshipura, KJ, A Ascherio, JE Manson, et al. Fruit and vegetable intake in relation to risk of ischemic stroke. *JAMA* 1999, 282(13):1233–39.

15. Sumner, MD, M Elliott-Eller, G Weidner, et al. Effects of pomegranate juice consumption on myocardial perfusion in patients with coronary heart disease. *Am J Cardiol* 2005, 96(6):810–14.

16. Esmaillzadeh, A, F Tahbaz, I Gaieni, H Alavi-Majd, et al. Cholesterol-lowering effect of concentrated pomegranate juice consumption in type II diabetic patients with hyperlipidemia. *Int J Vitam Nutr Res* 2006, 76(3):147–51.

17. Pantuck, AJ, N Zomorodian, and AS Belldegrun. Phase-II Study of pomegranate juice for men with prostate cancer and increasing PSA. *Clin Cancer Res* 2006, 12(13):4018–26.

Chapter 4: Power Grains

1. Mellen, PB, TF Walsh, and DM Herrington. Whole grain intake and cardiovascular disease: A meta-analysis. *Nutr Metab Cardiovasc Dis,* Apr 19, 2007 (published online ahead of print).

2. Erkkila, AT, DM Herrington, D Mozaffarian, et al. Cereal fiber and whole-grain intake are associated with reduced progression of coronary-artery atherosclerosis in postmenopausal women with coronary artery disease. *Am Heart J* 2005, 150(1):94–101.

3. Mozaffarian, D, SK Kumanyika, RN Lemaitre, et al. Cereal, fruit, and vegetable fiber intake and the risk of cardiovascular disease in elderly individuals. *JAMA* 2003, 289(13):1659–66.

4. Mellen, PB, AD Liese, JA Tooze, et al. Whole-grain intake and carotid artery atherosclerosis in a multiethnic cohort: The Insulin Resistance Atherosclerosis Study. *Am J Clin Nutr* 2007, 85(6):1495–1502.

5. Weickert, MO, M Mohlig, CF Schofl, et al. Cereal fiber improves whole-body insulin sensitivity in overweight and obese women. *Diabetes Care* 2006, 29(4):775–80. Sahyoun, NR, PF Jacques, XL Zhang, et al. Whole-grain intake is inversely associated with the metabolic syndrome and mortality in older adults. *Am J Clin Nutr* 2006, 83(1):124–31. McKeown, NM, JB Meigs, S Liu, et al. Carbohydrate nutrition, insulin resistance, and the prevalence of the metabolic syndrome in the Framingham Offspring Cohort. *Diabetes Care* 2004, 27(2):538–46. Liese, AD, AK Roach, KC Sparks, et al. Whole-grain intake and insulin sensitivity: The Insulin Resistance Atherosclerosis Study. *Am J Clin Nutr* 2003, 78(5):965–71.

6. Montonen, J, P Knekt, R Jarvinen, et al. Whole-grain and fiber intake and the incidence of type 2 diabetes. *Am J Clin Nutr* 2003, 77(3):622–29.

7. Schulze, MB, M Schulz, C Heidemann, et al. Fiber and magnesium intake and incidence of type 2 diabetes: A prospective study and meta-analysis. *Arch Intern Med* 2007, 167(9):956–65.

8. Jacobs Jr., DR, L Marquart, J Slavin, and LH Kushi. Whole-grain intake and cancer: An expanded review and meta-analysis. *Nutr Cancer* 1998, 30(2):85–96.

9. Larsson, SC, E Giovannucci, L Bergkvist, and A Wolk. Whole grain consumption and risk of colorectal cancer: A population-based cohort of 60,000 women. *Br J Cancer* 2005, 92(9):1803–07.

10. Schatzkin, A, T Mouw, Y Park, et al. Dietary fiber and whole-grain consumption in relation to colorectal cancer in the NIH-AARP Diet and Health Study. *Am J Clin Nutr* 2007, 85(5):1353–60.

11. Decision News Media SAS. Flaxseed's role in breast cancer prevention suggested. Aug 31, 2001. www.nutraingredients-usa.com/news/ng.asp?n=20958-flaxseed-s-role.

12. Liu, S, WC Willett, JE Manson, and FB Hu. Relation between changes in intakes of dietary fiber and grain products and changes in weight and development of obesity among middle-aged women. *Am J Clin Nutr* 2003, 78(5):920–27.

13. Jacobs, DR, LF Andersen, and R Blomhoff. Whole-grain consumption is associated with a reduced risk of noncardiovascular, noncancer death attributed to inflammatory diseases in the Iowa Women's Health Study. *Am J Clin Nutr* 2007, 85(6):1606–14.

Chapter 5: Power Protein Foods

1. Mozaffarian, D, and EB Rimm. Fish intake, contaminants, and human health: Evaluating the risks and the benefits. *JAMA* 2006, 296(15):1885–99.

2. Marchioli, R, F Barzi, E Bomba, et al. Early protection against sudden death by n-3 polyunsaturated fatty acids after myocardial infarction. *Circulation* 2002, 16(105):1897–1903.

3. Farmer, A, V Montori, S Dinneen, and C Clar. Fish oil in people with type 2 diabetes mellitus. *Cochrane Database Syst Rev* 2001, 3:CD003205.

4. Auestad, N, DT Scott, JS Janowsky, et al. Visual, cognitive, and language assessments at 39 months: A follow-up study of children fed formulas containing long-chain polyunsaturated fatty acids to 1 year of age. *Pediatrics* 2003, 112(3 Pt 1):e177–83.

5. Morris, MC, DA Evans, JL Bienias, et al. Consumption of fish and n-3 fatty acids and risk of incident Alzheimer disease. *Arch Neurol* 2003, 60(7):940–46.

6. Kalmijn, S, LJ Launer, A Ott, et al. Dietary fat intake and the risk of incident dementia in the Rotterdam Study. *Ann Neurol* 1997, 42(5):776–82.

7. Seddon, JM, S George, and B Rosner. Cigarette smoking, fish consumption, omega-3 fatty acid intake, and associations with age-related macular degeneration: The US Twin Study of Age-Related Macular Degeneration. *Arch Ophthalmol* 2006, 124(7):995–1001. Chua B, V Flood, E Rochtchina, et al. Dietary fatty acids and the 5-year incidence of age-related maculopathy. *Arch Ophthalmol* 2006, 124(7):981–86. Seddon, JM, J Cote, and B Rosner. Progression of age-related macular degeneration: Association with dietary fat, transunsaturated fat, nuts, and fish intake. *Arch Ophthalmol* 2003, 121(12):1728–37. Seddon, JM, B Rosner, RD Sperduto, et al. Dietary fat and risk for advanced age-related macular degeneration. *Arch Ophthalmol* 2001, 119(8):1191–99. Cho E, S Hung, WC Willett, et al. Prospective study of dietary fat and the risk of age-related macular degeneration. *Am J Clin Nutr* 2001, 73(2):209–18.

8. Augustsson, K, DS Michaud, EB Rimm, et al. A prospective study of intake of fish and marine fatty acids and prostate cancer. *Cancer Epidemiol Biomarkers Prev* 2003, 12(1):64–67.

9. Chavarro, JE, MJ Stampfer, H Li, et al. A prospective study of polyunsaturated fatty acid levels in blood and prostate cancer risk. *Cancer Epidemiol Biomarkers Prev* 2007 (published online ahead of print), doi: 10.1158/1055-9965. EPI-06-1033.

10. Hites, RA, et al. Global assessment of polybrominated diphenyl ethers in farmed and wild salmon. *Environ Sci Technol* 2004, 38(19):4945–49.

11. Hites, RA, et al. Global assessment of organic contaminants in farmed salmon. *Science* 2004, 303(5655):226–29.

12. Mozaffarian, D, and EB Rimm. Fish intake, contaminants, and human health: Evaluating the risks and the benefits. *JAMA* 2006, 296(15):1885–99.

13. Ibid.

14. Bazzano, LA, J He, LG Ogden, et al. Legume consumption and risk of coronary heart disease in US men and women: NHANES I Epidemiologic Follow-up Study. *Arch Intern Med* 2001, 161(21):2573–78.

15. Hu FB, EB Rimm, MJ Stampfer, et al. Prospective study of major dietary patterns and risk of coronary heart disease in men. *Am J Clin Nutr* 2000, 72(4):912–21.

16. Anderson, JW, and AW Major. Pulses and lipaemia, short- and long-term effect: Potential in the prevention of cardiovascular disease. *Br J Nutr* 2002, 88(Suppl 3):S263–71.

17. Sacks, FM, LP Svetkey, WM Vollmer, LJ Appel, GA Bray, D Harsha, E Obarzanek, PR Conlin, ER Miller 3rd, DG Simons-Morton, N Karanja, and PH Lin; DASH-Sodium Collaborative Research Group. Effects on blood pressure of reduced dietary sodium and the Dietary Approaches to Stop Hypertension (DASH) diet. DASH-Sodium Collaborative Research Group. N Engl J Med 2001, 344(1):3–10; Conlin, PR, D Chow, ER Miller 3rd, LP Svetkey, et al. The effect of dietary patterns on blood pressure control in hypertensive patients: Results from the Dietary Approaches to Stop Hypertension (DASH) trial. Am J Hypertens 2000, 13(9):949–55.

18. Jacobsen, BK, SF Knutsen, and GE Fraser. Does high soy milk intake reduce prostate cancer incidence? The Adventist Health Study (United States). Cancer Causes Control 1998, 9(6):553–57.

19. Kolonel, LN, JH Hankin, AS Whittemore, et al. Vegetables, fruits, legumes and prostate cancer: A multiethnic case-control study. Cancer Epidemiol Biomarkers Prev 2000, 9(8):795–804.

20. Schuurman, AG, RA Goldbohm, E Dorant, and PA van den Brandt. Vegetable and fruit consumption and prostate cancer risk: A cohort study in the Netherlands. Cancer Epidemiol Biomarkers Prev 1998, 7(8):673–80.

21. Trock, BJ, L Hilakivi-Clarke, and R Clarke. Meta-analysis of soy intake and breast cancer risk. J Natl Cancer Inst 2006, 98(7):459–71.

22. Shu, XO, F Jin, Q Dai, W Wen, et al. Soyfood intake during adolescence and subsequent risk of breast cancer among Chinese women. Cancer Epidemiol Biomarkers Prev 2001, 10(5):483–88.

23. Strom, BL, R Schinnar, EE Ziegler, et al. Exposure to soy-based formula in infancy and endocrinological and reproductive outcomes in young adulthood. JAMA 2001, 286(7):807–14; Giampietro, PG, G Bruno, G Furcolo, et al. Soy protein formulas in children: No hormonal effects in long-term feeding. J Pediatr Endocrinol Metab 2004, 17(2):191–96.

24. Salmeron, J, A Ascherio, EB Rimm, et al. Dietary fiber, glycemic load, and risk of NIDDM in men. Diabetes Care 1997, 20(4):545–50; Salmeron, J, JE Manson, MJ Stampfer, et al. Dietary fiber, glycemic load, and risk of non-insulin-dependent diabetes mellitus in women. JAMA 1997, 277(6):472–77. Willett, W, J Manson, and S Liu. Glycemic index, glycemic load, and risk of type 2 diabetes. Am J Clin Nutr 2002, 76(1):S274–80.

25. Thomas, D, E Elliott, and L Baur. Low glycaemic index or low glycaemic load diets for overweight and obesity. Cochrane Database Syst Rev 2007 Jul 18; 3:CD005105.

26. Albert, CM, JM Gaziano, WC Willett, and JE Manson. Nut consumption and decreased risk of sudden cardiac death in the Physicians' Health Study. Nutr Metab Cardiovasc Dis 2001, 11(6):372–77.

27. Hu, FB, MJ Stampfer, JE Manson, et al. Frequent nut consumption and risk of coronary heart disease in women: Prospective cohort study. BMJ 1998, 317(7169):1341–45.

28. Kelly Jr, JH, and J Sabate. Nuts and coronary heart disease: An epidemiological perspective. *Br J Nutr* 2006, 96(Suppl 2):S61–67. PMID:17125535. Published online by Cambridge University Press, April 19, 2007.

29. Spiller, GA, DA Jenkins, O Bosello, et al. Nuts and plasma lipids: An almond-based diet lowers LDL-C while preserving HDL-C. *J Am Coll Nutr* 1998, 17(3):285–90.

30. Jiang, R, JE Manson, MJ Stampfer, et al. Nut and peanut butter consumption and risk of type 2 diabetes in women. *JAMA* 2002, 288(20):2554–60.

Chapter 6: Power Dairy Foods

1. Sazawal, S, G Hiremath, U Dhingra, et al. Efficacy of probiotics in prevention of acute diarrhoea: A meta-analysis of masked, randomised, placebo-controlled trials. *Lancet Infect Dis* 2006, 6(6):374–82.

2. Johnston, BC, AL Supina, and S Vohra. Probiotics for pediatric antibiotic-associated diarrhea: A meta-analysis of randomized placebo-controlled trials. *CMAJ* 2006, 175(4):377–83.

3. Adolfsson, O, SN Meydani, and RM Russell. Yogurt and gut function. *Am J Clin Nutr* 2004, 80(2):245–56.

4. Hertzler, SR, and SM Clancy. Kefir improves lactose digestion and tolerance in adults with lactose maldigestion. *J Am Diet Assoc* 2003, 103(5):582–87.

5. Labayen, I, L Forga, A Gonzalez, et al. Relationship between lactose digestion, gastrointestinal transit time and symptoms in lactose malabsorbers after dairy consumption. *Aliment Pharmacol Ther* 2001, 15(4):543–49.

6. Xiao, JZ, S Kondo, N Takahashi, et al. Effects of milk products fermented by Bifidobacterium longum on blood lipids in rats and healthy adult male volunteers. *J Dairy Sci* 2003, 86(7):2452–61.

7. Agerholm-Larsen, L, A Raben, N Haulrik, et al. Effect of 8 week intake of probiotic milk products on risk factors for cardiovascular diseases. *Eur J Clin Nutr* 2000, 54(4):288–97.

8. Hilton, E, HD Isenberg, P Alperstein, et al. Ingestion of yogurt containing Lactobacillus acidophilus as prophylaxis for candidal vaginitis. *Ann Intern Med* 1992, 116(5):353–57.

9. Shalev, E, S Battino, E Weiner, et al. Ingestion of yogurt containing Lactobacillus acidophilus compared with pasteurized yogurt as prophylaxis for recurrent candidal vaginitis and bacterial vaginosis. *Arch Fam Med* 1996, 5(10):593–96.

10. Bibiloni, R, RN Fedorak, GW Tannock, et al. VSL#3 probiotic-mixture induces remission in patients with active ulcerative colitis. *Am J Gastroenterol* 2005, 100(7):1539–46.

11. Rafter, J, M Bennett, G Caderni, et al. Dietary synbiotics reduce cancer risk factors in polypectomized and colon cancer patients. *Am J Clin Nutr* 2007, 85(2):488–96.

Chapter 7: Power Fats and Oils

1. Mensink, RP, PL Zock, AD Kester, and MB Katan. Effects of dietary fatty acids and carbohydrates on the ratio of serum total to HDL cholesterol and on serum lipids and apolipoproteins: A meta-analysis of 60 controlled trials. *Am J Clin Nutr* 2003, 77(5):1146–55.

2. Albert, CM, K Oh, W Whang, et al. Dietary alpha-linolenic acid intake and risk of sudden cardiac death and coronary heart disease. *Circulation* 2005, 112(21):3232–38.

3. Mozaffarian, D, A Ascherio, FB Hu, et al. Interplay between different polyunsaturated fatty acids and risk of coronary heart disease in men. *Circulation* 2005, 111(2):157–64.

4. Masala, G, M Ceroti, V Pala, et al. A dietary pattern rich in olive oil and raw vegetables is associated with lower mortality in Italian elderly subjects. *Br J Nutr* 2007, 98(2):406–15.

5. Trichopoulou, A, T Costacou, C Bamia, and D Trichopoulos. Adherence to a Mediterranean diet and survival in a Greek population. *N Eng J Med* 2003, 348(26):2599–608.

6. Haban P, J Klvanova, E Zidekova, and A Nagyova. Dietary supplementation with olive oil leads to improved lipoprotein spectrum and lower n-6 PUFAs in elderly subjects. *Med Sci Monit* 2004, 10(4):PI49–54.

7. Lopez Ledesma, R, AC Frati Munari, BC Hernandez Dominguez, et al. Monounsaturated fatty acid (avocado) rich diet for mild hypercholesterolemia. *Arch Med Res* 1996, 27(4):519–23.

Chapter 8: Power Beverages

1. Michael Kahn. Three drinks a day ups breast cancer risk: Study. September 27, 2007, www.reutershealth.com/en/index.html.

2. Paganga, G, N Miller, and CA Rice-Evans. The polyphenolic content of fruit and vegetables and their antioxidant activities. What does a serving constitute? *Free Radic Res* 1999, 30(2):153–62.

3. Sun, CL, JM Yuan, WP Koh, and MC Yu. Green tea, black tea and breast cancer risk: A meta-analysis of epidemiological studies. *Carcinogenesis* 2006, 27(7):1310–15.

4. Nakachi, K, K Suemasu, K Suga, et al. Influence of drinking green tea on breast cancer malignancy among Japanese patients. *Jpn J Cancer Res* 1998, 89(3):254–61.

5. Larsson, SC, and A Wolk. Tea consumption and ovarian cancer risk in a population-based cohort. *Arch Intern Med* 2005, 165(22):2683–86.

6. Zhang, M, AH Lee, CW Binns, and X Xie. Green tea consumption enhances survival of epithelial ovarian cancer. *Int J Cancer* 2004, 112(3):465–69.

7. Sano, J, S Inami, K Seimiya, et al. Effects of green tea intake on the development of coronary artery disease. *Circ J* 2004, 68(7):665–70.

8. Shimazu, T, S Kuriyama, A Hozawa, et al. Dietary patterns and cardiovascular disease mortality in Japan: A prospective cohort study. *Int J Epidemiol*, April 11, 2007 (published online ahead of print), PMID: 17317693.

9. Yang, YC, FH Lu, JS Wu, et al. The protective effect of habitual tea consumption on hypertension. *Arch Intern Med* 2004, 164(14):1534–40.

10. Haqqi, TM, DD Anthony, S Gupta, et al. Prevention of collagen-induced arthritis in mice by a polyphenolic fraction from green tea. *Proc Natl Acad Sci USA* 1999, 96(8):4524–29.

11. Gardner, EJ, CH Ruxton, and AR Leeds. Black tea—helpful or harmful? A review of the evidence. *Eur J Clin Nutr* 2007, 61(1):3–18.

12. Geleijnse, JM, LJ Launer, DA van der Kuip, et al. Inverse association of tea and flavonoid intakes with incident myocardial infarction: The Rotterdam Study. *Am J Clin Nutr* 2002, 75(5):880–86.

13. Mukamal, KJ, M Maclure, JE Muller, et al. Tea consumption and mortality after acute myocardial infarction. *Circulation* 2002, 105(21):2476–81.

14. Salazar-Martinez, E, WC Willett, A Ascherio, et al. Coffee consumption and risk for type 2 diabetes mellitus. *Ann Intern Med* 2004, 140(1):1–8.

15. Pereira, MA, ED Parker, and AR Folsom. Coffee consumption and risk of type 2 diabetes mellitus: An 11-year prospective study of 28,812 postmenopausal women. *Arch Intern Med* 2006, 166(12):1311–16.

16. van Dam, RM, and FB Hu. Coffee consumption and risk of type 2 diabetes: A systematic review. *JAMA* 2005, 294(1):97–104.

17. Andersen, LF, DR Jacobs Jr, MH Carlsen, and R Blomhoff. Consumption of coffee is associated with reduced risk of death attributed to inflammatory and cardiovascular diseases in the Iowa Women's Health Study. *Am J Clin Nutr* 2006, 83(5):1039–46.

18. Lopez-Garcia, E, RM van Dam, WC Willett, et al. Coffee consumption and coronary heart disease in men and women: A prospective cohort study. *Circulation* 2006, 113(17):2045–53.

19. Sofi, F, AA Conti, AM Gori, et al. Coffee consumption and risk of coronary heart disease: A meta-analysis. *Nutr Metab Cardiovasc Dis* 2007, 17(3):209–23.

20. Ascherio, A, SM Zhang, MA Hernan, et al. Prospective study of caffeine consumption and risk of Parkinson's disease in men and women. *Ann Neurol* 2001, 50(1):56–63.

21. Ross, GW, RD Abbott, H Petrovitch, et al. Association of coffee and caffeine intake with the risk of Parkinson disease. *JAMA* 2000, 283(20):2674–79.

22. Larsson, SC, and A Wolk. Coffee consumption and risk of liver cancer: A meta-analysis. *Gastroenterology* 2007, 132(5):1740–45.

23. American Chemical Society Meeting and Exposition, Washington, DC, Aug 27–Sept 1, 2005. News release, American Chemical Society.

General index

Recipe index